AF411639

M. Zehender
G. Breithardt · H. Just

Editors

From Molecule to Men

Molecular Basis
of Congenital
Cardiovascular
Disorders

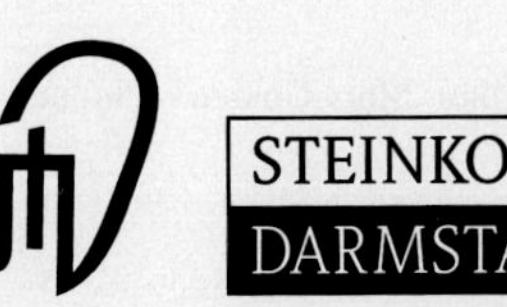

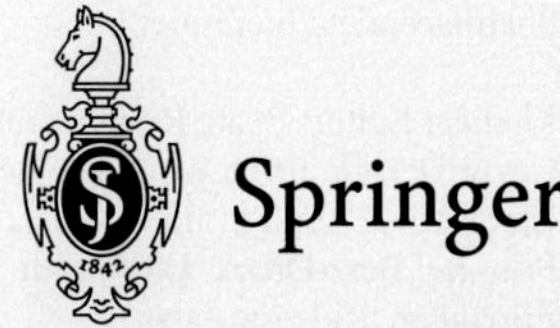

STEINKOPFF
DARMSTADT

Springer

Editors' addresses:

PD Dr. M. Zehender · Prof. Dr. H. Just
Universität Freiburg – Med. Klinik III
Abt. Kardiologie und Angiologie
Hugstetter Straße 55
79106 Freiburg

Prof. Dr. G. Breithardt
Medizinische Klinik und Poliklinik
Innere Medizin C
Albert-Schweitzer-Straße 33
48149 Münster

Die Deutsche Bibliothek – CIP-Einheitsaufnahme

From molecule to men : molecular basis of congenital cardiovascular
disorders / M. Zehender ... ed. – Darmstadt : Steinkopff ; New York :
Springer, 2000
  ISBN 3-7985-1168-3

Medical Editor: Beate Rühlemann – English Editor: Mary Gossen – Production: Heinz J. Schäfer
Cover Design: Erich Kirchner, Heidelberg
Typesetting: Typoservice, Griesheim
Printing: Betz-Druck, Darmstadt
Printed on acid-free paper

Foreword

From molecule to men: Medical research has indeed taken this direction, and major improvements of our understanding of the pathophysiology and epidemiology of disease have been achieved. The molecular basis of the congenital cardiovascular disorders has been extended from relatively few congenital malformations into everyday illnesses such as diabetes mellitus, hyperlipoproteinaemea, and arterial hypertension. The monogenic and, more difficult, polygenic basis for a vast majority of cardiovascular disorders are being defined more precisely from year to year. Clinically important consequences for diagnosis, prognosis, and treatment have been acomplished, for example, in the case of the cardiomyopathies and/or the long QT syndrome.

Although we realize that the expansion of our knowledge is likely to continue at a rapid pace, it was deemed necessary to summarize what has been achieved so far and to define our current position. Three reasons are evident:

1. The practising physician needs updated state-of-the-art messages from time to time. He faces the need of decision-making every day, and he deserves expert help in a situation where the ever-expanding subspecialities have to concentrate and focus the new information and to combine the message from the different fields into packages that can be handled clinically.
2. Both basic science and clinical research face the need to coordinate their efforts. This is not only so for reasons of limited financial resources, but also for the need of mutual understanding. Clinical research at its frontiers relies in large part on basic science. In some fields, especially in molecular genetics, basic scientists dominate the field. Here remains the clinician's role in the definition of the right questions to be asked. In other fields where the clinician leads the pace, for example in direct patient-oriented research at the bedside or in the large field of multi-center studies, advice from basic scientists is indispensable for the definition of questions that can be answered.
3. Where do we go from here? The very nature of science is its ever-expanding structure: Each question answered generates more new questions. It is not only for the limited financial resources, but also in the interest of directed, focused research that the right questions must be selected, the methodologies available be examined, and a research plan be defined. The experience has been that asking questions and outlining the direction how to find answers can best be achieved, when scientists from different fields get together.

The Society for Cooperation in Medical Sciences has recognized this need and has conducted the Gargellen conferences since 1986. The conferences organized were

Cardiac Energetics 1987
Inotropic Stimulation and Myocardial Energetics 1989
Endothelial Mechanisms of Vasomotor Control 1991
Cellular and Molecular Alterations in the Failing Human Heart 1992
Cardiac Adaptation in Heart Failure. Risks Due to Myocardial Phenotype Changes 1992
Arteriosclerosis. New Insights into Pathogenetic Mechanisms and Prevention 1993
Myocardial Ischemia and Arrhythmia 1994
Endothelial Dysfunction and Cell Adhesion 1994
Nitrates in Cardiovascular Disease. Basic Mechanisms of Action, Tolerance Phenomena, Clinical Application, 1995

Regulation of Myocardial Contractility and Cardiac Growth 1995

Heart Rate as a Determinant of Cardiac Function. Basic Mechanisms and Clinical Significance 1996

Positive Inotropes in Cardiovascular Medicine. Perspectives and Limitations in Theory and Practice 1996

Alterations of Exitation Contraction Coupling in the Failing Human Heart 1996

Recent Advances in Hemostasiology with Particular Reference to Pulmonary Embolism 1997

From Molecule to Man. Molecular Basis of Congenital Cardiovascular Disorders 1998.

The symposium mentioned last was held as the tenth Gargellen conference. These conferences have been very successful in the translation of basic science achievements into clinical research and clinical application. The series of symposia reflects not only the advancements of the frontiers in clinical science during the last decade, but it also signals a major paradigm change in cardiovascular medicine:

Cardiology and angiology have traditionally been oriented and based upon methods of physics and applied engineering. Measurements of pressure, flow, voltage, and the like together with the analysis of form, structure, and function of the heart and the blood vessels with imaging techniques such as X-ray, angiocardiography, echocardiography, electron beam tomography, and nuclear magnetic resonance techniques have been the basis for major achievements in medicine altogether. I name the pacemaker, the intensive-care unit, the respirator, coronary angiography, coronary bypass surgery, interventional catheter techniques, applied electrophysiology. The development of pharmacotherapeutic principles and new drugs, such as vasodilators, antiarrhythmics, antihypertensives, betablockers, inotropes, and the like has been achieved with these techniques.

Biochemistry and more recently molecular biology have to some extent been neglected or even ignored. It has been only with the development of fibrinolytic agents and more recently insights into hemostasiology, and, even more so, with the understanding of the hyperlipoproteinaemias and the development of lipid-lowering drugs that a major change of paradigm in cardiovascular medicine has occurred. Now biochemistry and molecular biology, respectively molecular genetics, have taken the lead in cardiovascular medicine.

The Gargellen conferences signal this recent development. Nevertheless, cardiologists will have to learn to expertly use their physical and technical methodology and to develop them further as well. In addition, however, the lead into the future will be given to biochemistry and molecular biology. They will be the sciences of the foreseeable future. Major achievements in understanding of disease and major new diagnostic and therapeutic techniques will be developed. The tenth Gargellen conference was intended as a step on the way into the future.

My thanks go to PD Dr. Manfred Zehender and his group who have expertly organized and conducted the conference. My thanks go to my residents and fellows of the Medizinische Universitätsklinik in Freiburg, who have understood the signs of the future and have followed me on this way over the years.

Last but not least I would like to thank the sponsors who have made the conference possible and who have contributed to its very substance in a remarkable and objective way. Ms. Sabine Ibkendanz from the Dr. D. Steinkopff Verlag deserves our thanks for expert help in the publication.

It is with great respect and the fondest appreciation that we thank Prof. Stanley H. Taylor, MD, PhD, Leeds. As a founding member of the Society for Cooperation in Medical Sciences he has immensely contributed to our conferences. He has foreseen and supported the paradigm change in cardiovascular medicine as documented in his concluding article of this book. He passed away not long after completion of his article full of plans for future activities. A great physician researcher and friend has left us for ever. Be this book dedicated to him! He continues to live in our memory.

Professor Dr. med. Dr. hc F. J. G. H. Hanjörg Just, FESC, FRCP
President of the Society for Cooperation in Medical Sciences
Em. Director of the Medizinische Universitätsklinik, Abteilung Innere Medizin III, Kardiologie, Angiologie, Freiburg im Breisgau

Contents

Genetics of dilated cardiomyopathy

L. Thierfelder

Max-Delbrück-Centrum für Molekulare Medizin (MDC) und
Franz-Volhard Klinik am Virchow Klinikum der Humboldt-Universität zu Berlin, Germany

Abstract

Dilated cardiomyopathy (DCM) is a primary heart muscle disorder characterized by cardiac dilatation and impaired systolic function. In approximately half of all DCM patients a specific etiology can be identified and in the remaining cases DCM is termed idiopathic. There is wide variation of the clinical presentation in DCM. The majority of patients manifest classical disease, i.e., heart failure due to left (and right) ventricular systolic dysfunction. However, some cases may first come to clinical attention because of supraventricular arrhythmias such as sinus node dysfunction, AV-block or atrial fibrillation. Although a multitude of etiologies may be responsible for DCM (e.g., viral, immunological, toxic), the disease is inherited in at least 30–40 % of cases. Most genetic forms of DCM are caused by autosomal dominant gene defects. Six dominant disease loci on chromosomes 1p1-q1, 1q32, 3p22-p25, 6q23, 9q13, and 10q21-q23 have been mapped by linkage analyses. Cardiac actin chromosome 15q14-22 was recently suspected as a DCM disease gene, and two point mutations were identified. Presumably these mutations cause perturbations in anchoring the thin filament to the Z-band of the sarcomere. The effect may be destabilization of the force generating apparatus. The prevalence of actin mutations in DCM is, however, unknown and it remains unclear whether mutations in other cytoskeletal proteins account for the remaining cases of autosomal dominant DCM. Mutations in another gene, dystrophin, can cause X-linked forms of DCM. In contrast to Duschenne or Becker muscular dystrophy, skeletal muscles are clinically unaffected in X-linked DCM. However, X-linked DCM as well as autosomal recessive mutations and mutations in mitochondrial DNA are rare causes for genetic forms of DCM.

Clinical genetics

Dilated cardiomyopathy (DCM) is a primary disorder of the cardiac muscle morphgologically and functionally characterized by (often global) cardiac dilatation and, respectively, by a reduced systolic function (5). According to WHO criteria, the left ventricular end-diastolic diameter in DCM patients exceeds 2.6 cm/m^2 BSA and fractional shortening is less than 25 % (27). DCM has an estimated prevalence of 36.5/100,000 (16). This figure which is based on a study conducted between 1975 and 1985 probably underestimates the true prevalance as only symptomatic cases were included in this epidemiologic survey. However, cases with little or no symptoms may represent a significant portion of the DCM population. Symptomatic DCM patients may suffer from chronic heart failure, cardiac arrhythmias, and sudden cardiac death. Approximately 20 % of DCM patients die within 5 years of disease onset (9). DCM is the most frequent indication for heart transplantation (16).

A long list of different etiologies can cause cardiac dilatation with impairment of systolic function but only for approximately half of all cases a definitve causative agent can be identified. Multiple myocardial infarcts account for ischemic cardiomyopathy, chronic arterial hypertension for hypertensive heart disease with cardiac dilatation, endocrinologic disorders, such as hypothyroidism for the myxedema heart, etc. For the remaining cases (approximately 50 %), no etiologic factor is known. These cases are termed idiopathic DCM reflecting our lack of insight into the pathophysiology in this condition. There are four major groups of potential etiologic factors for idiopathic DCM: DCM may be a late consequence of viral (12) or non-viral infections; the disease may develop as an autoimmunologic process triggered, e.g., by infections (4, 28, 29); DCM may develop after ingestion of toxins, such as with chronic alkohol abuse (26) or due to intake of alkylating agents (8). Finally, genetic factors may account for up to 30–50 % of all DCM cases (19).

It has long been suspected that DCM can be inherited in a Mendelian fashion. When a careful family history is taken, 5–10 % of patients are identified who report of other DCM cases in their families (18). This strategy will only identify relatives with symptomatic disease. However, if not only a family history is taken but instead clinical, electrocardiographic, and echocardiographic tests are performed in relatives of DCM patients, it was shown that DCM may be a genetic condition in 20–30 % of cases (19). This assumption has recently been confirmed by two independent research teams (1, 10). The proportion of genetic forms in DCM ranged in all three studies from 30–50 % (if borderline cases are included). Formal segregation anlyses have suggested that most genetic cases of DCM are due to autosomal dominant single gene defects (19). Rarely, DCM in a family shows X-linked transmission. If not associated with a skeletal muscle phenotype (such as in Duchenne or Becker muscular dystrophy) DCM is considered X-linked (7, 21, 31)). Autosomal recessive cases (13) or DCM caused by mutations in the mitochondrial genome (30) are only rarely seen in clinical practice.

Molecular genetics

DCM with autosomal dominant inheritance

Segregation analyses have shown that familial DCM is in most cases due to single gene defects. An autosomal dominant inheritance pattern with incomplete penetrance is 10^{10} more likely compared to autosomal recessive transmission or sporadic genetic defects (19). Linkage analyses in large pedigrees with autosomal dominant DCM indicated extensive genetic heterogeneity in DCM. Analysis of highly informative polymorphic DNA microsatellites revealed six different genomic loci carrying DCM disease genes. Kass et al.

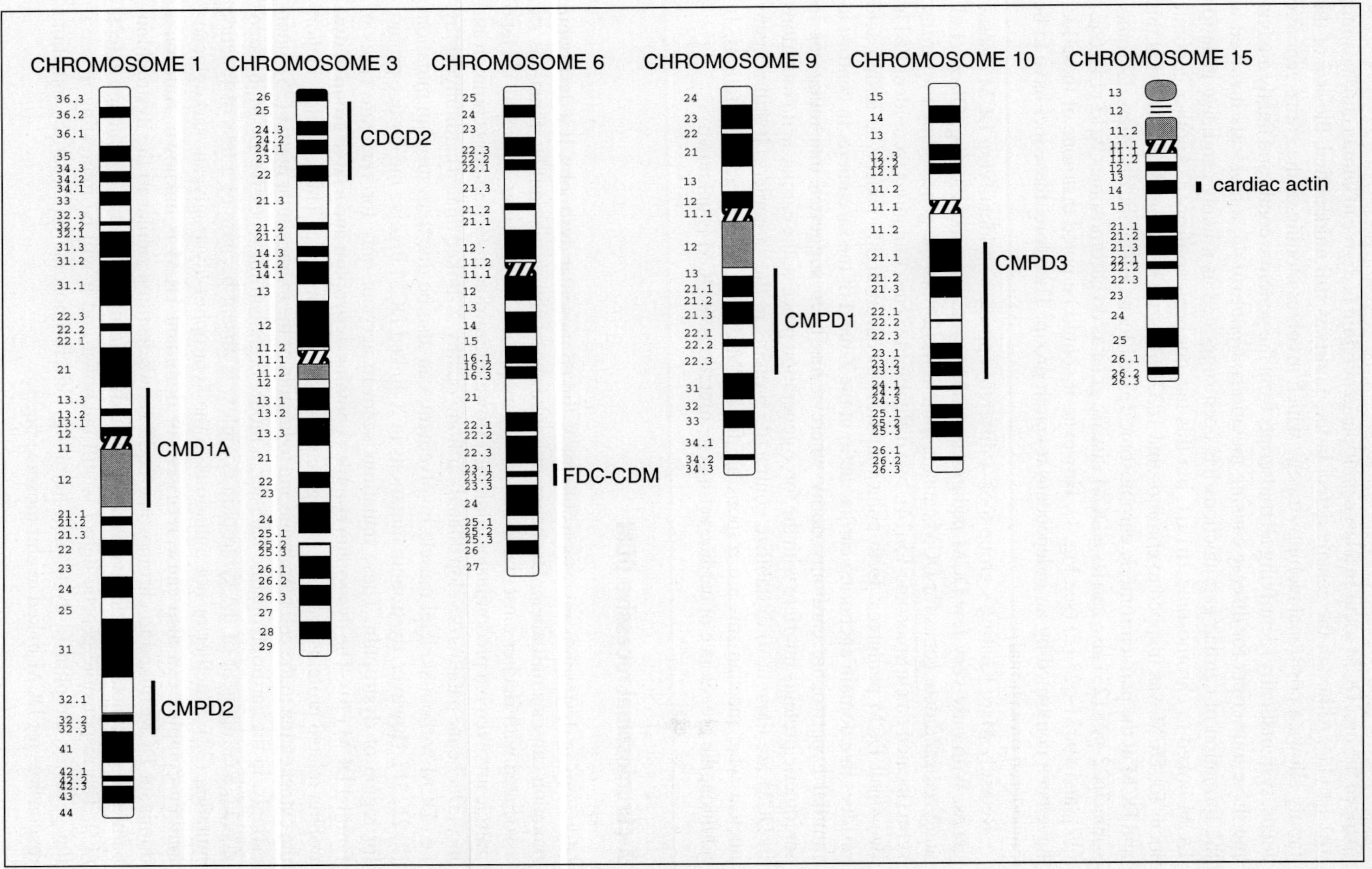

Fig. 1. Schematic representation of human autosomes carrying DCM disease genes

mapped the first DCM locus in a large multiple generation pedigree to human chromosome 1p1-q1 (11). Although the genetic defect in this family is still unidentified, the size of the family allows a positional cloning strategy which involves cloning of the entire genomic locus, systematically identifying all transcripts from the genomic contig and finally analyzing these transcripts for disease causing mutations. *Connexin 45*, a molecule involved in the formation of cardiac gap junctions has been suggested as a likely candidate gene for DCM linked to chromosome 1p1-q1, but this has not been confirmed. Another genomic locus for DCM was mapped to chromosome 1q32 (6), but it is still unclear if DCM at this and DCM at the pericentromeric chromosome 1p1-q1 locus are allelic disorders. Chromosome 3p22-p25 (23) also carries a DCM disease gene as do chromosomes 9q13 (14), 6q23 (17), and 10q21-q23 (2) (see Fig. 1). However, it should be noted that none of these loci have been confirmed by an independent research group. Therefore, these loci have to be considered provisional.

Recently Marc Keating's group took a different approach in identifying DCM disease genes. With only very few DCM pedigrees available for positional cloning, Olson et al. analyzed candidate genes for DCM causing mutations (24). In the gene coding for cardiac actin (located on chromosome 15q14), two different missense mutations were identified in two small DCM pedigrees. Both point mutations occur at highly conserved amino acid residues in a domain anchoring cardiac actin in the Z band of the sarcomere. In contrast to familial hypertrophic cardiomyoapthy where it has been suggested that mutations in sarcomeric proteins interfere with the force generation process, the cardiac actin mutations in DCM are thought to destabilize contractile proteins in the sarcomere. It still remains unclear what mechanisms are responsible for DCM due to cardiac actin mutations. In addition, the prevalence of cardiac actin gene mutations in DCM is unknown.

X-chromosomal recessive DCM

Mutations in dystrophin are responsible for X-linked muscular dystrophy. If a dystrophin mutation causes a null allele, Duchenne muscular dystrophy results; milder mutations are associated with Becker muscular dystrophy. In most cases of muscular dystrophy skeletal muscle involvement predominates clinically. However, cardiac involvement is common and most Duchenne patients develop dilated cardiomyopathy. X-linked dilated cardiomyoapthy, i.e., DCM without skeletal muscle involvement, can also be due to dystrophin mutations (7, 21, 31). However, dystrophin mutations in X-linked DCM involve the cardiac promotor region of dystrophin. These mutations seem to account only for very rare cases of familial DCM (20). The dystrophin complex contains dystrophin and a large group of dystrophin related proteins (various sarcoglycans, dystroglycans, etc.). This complex anchors the cytoskeleton to the cell membrane and to laminin of the extracellular matrix (25). Interestingly, in the cardiomyopathic hamster, a model organism for recessive DCM, δ-sarcoglycan, a component of the syntrophin complex, is absent because of a loss of function mutation (22). Whether or not mutations in the syntrophin-/dystroglycan-/sarkoglycan-/laminin complex can also cause recessive or dominant DCM is unknown. Autosomal dominant DCM linked to chromosome 6q23 shows features similar to the dystrophinopathies, e.g., skeletal muscle involvement, dilated cardiomyopathy, and conduction defects (17). The responsible genetic defect is still unknown and it will be interesting to see if the gene for utrophin (a dystrophin homolog) on chromosome 6q23 carries mutations responsible for DCM linked to chromosome 6q23.

Autosomal recessive DCM

In autosomal recessive diseases both alleles of a gene are mutated and usually no functinal gene product is present (loss of function mutations). Various genes of the fatty acid oxidation pathway can carry mutations in autosomal recessive forms of DCM (13). The most prominent of these defects is carnitine deficiency. This disorder usually manifests in childhood and can be corrected by carnitine substitution.

DCM and mutations of the mitochondrial genome

Mitochondria contain genetic information of about 16 kb circular DNA. This non-nuclear DNA originates from maternal egg cells and is transmitted independently from chromosomal DNA. Thirteen different genes coding for proteins of the oxidative phosphorylation pathway, ribosomal, and transfer RNA are encoded through mitochondrial DNA. Mitochondrial DNA can contain deletions or point mutations associated with cardiomyopathies (13). However, proof that a mutation in mitochondrial DNA is responsible for DCM in a given patient is often difficult because mitochondria are genetically heterogenous (heteroplasmy) and the spontaneous rate of mutations in mitochondria is high. A prerequisite for the assumption that a mitochondrial mutation is disease causing is inheritance of the mutation and the disease from the mother.

Genotype/phenotype correlations in autosomal dominant DCM

From linkage studies, it became evident that autosomal dominant DCM is genetically heterogenous and this heterogeneity also translates into clinical subclasses. Three clinical characteristics distinguish the various genetic forms of DCM: age of onset, conduction defects preceding mechanical impairment, and skeletal muscle involvement. DCM linked to chromosome 1p1-q1 (CMD1A (11)), 3p22-p25 (CDCD2 (23)), and 6q23 (FDC-CDM (17)) typically shows preceding conduction defects in the second to third decade of life, frequently requiring interventions such as pace maker implantation before systolic dysfunction is apparent in the forties or fifties.

In contrast, DCM usually manifests early in life with heart failure because of systolic dysfunction when the disease is linked to chromosome 1q32 (6), 9q13 (14), 10q21-q23 (2) or 15q14 (24). Skeletal muscle involvement is usually absent.

Autosomal dominant atrial fibrillation has recently been linked to the long arm of chromosome 10 (3) and, according to published data, this locus overlaps genetically with the DCM locus chromosome 10q21-q23 (2). Furthermore, two of 12 affected family members with atrial fibrillation demonstrated increased left ventricular diameters and a reduced left ventricular ejection fraction. Therefore, familial DCM and familial atrial fibrillation at chromosome 10q may be allelic disorders, i.e., specific mutations in one (or different) isoforms may cause a "ventricular" phenotype in one case and an "atrial" disease in the other (15).

References

1. Baig K, Goldman J, Caforio A et al. (1998) Familial dilated cardiomyopathy: Cardiac abnormalities are common in asymptomatic relatives and may represent early disease. J Am Coll Cardiol 31: 195–201
2. Bowles KR, Gajarski R, Porter P et al. (1996) Gene mapping of familial autosomal dominant dilated cardiomyopathy to chromosome 10q21-23. J Clin Invest 98: 1355–60

3. Brugada R, Tapscott T, Czernuszewicz GZ et al. (1997) Identification of a genetic locus for familial atrial fibrillation [see comments]. N Engl J Med 336: 905–11
4. Caforio AL (1994) Role of autoimmunity in dilated cardiomyopathy. Br Heart J 72: S30–4
5. Dec GW, Fuster V (1994) Idiopathic dilated cardiomyopathy [see comments]. N Engl J Med 331: 1564–75
6. Durand JB, Bachinski LL, Bieling LC et al. (1995) Localization of a gene responsible for familial dilated cardiomyopathy to chromosome 1q32. Circulation 92: 3387–9
7. Franz WM, Cremer M, Herrmann R et al. (1995) X-linked dilated cardiomyopathy. Novel mutation of the dystrophin gene. Ann N Y Acad Sci 752: 470–91
8. Freter CE, Lee TC, Billingham ME et al. (1986) Doxorubicin cardiac toxicity manifesting seven years after treatment. Case report and review. Am J Med 80: 483–5
9. Gillum RF (1986) Idiopathic cardiomyopathy in the United States, 1970–1982. Am Heart J 111: 752–5
10. Grünig E, Tasman J, Kücherer H et al. (1998) Frequency and phenotypes of familial dilated cardiomyopathy. J Am Coll Cardiol 31: 186–194
11. Kass S, MacRae C, Graber HL et al. (1994) A gene defect that causes conduction system disease and dilated cardiomyopathy maps to chromosome 1p1-1q1. Nat Genet 7: 546–51
12. Keeling PJ, Tracy S (1994) Link between enteroviruses and dilated cardiomyopathy: Serological and molecular data. Br Heart J 72: S25–9
13. Kelly DP, Strauss AW (1994) Inherited cardiomyopathies [see comments]. N Engl J Med 330: 913–9
14. Krajinovic M, Pinamonti B, Sinagra G et al. (1995) Linkage of familial dilated cardiomyopathy to chromosome 9. Heart Muscle Disease Study Group. Am J Hum Genet 57: 846–52
15. MacRae CA (1997) Familial atrial fibrillation [letter]. N Engl J Med 337: 350
16. Manolio TA, Baughman KL, Rodeheffer R et al. (1992) Prevalence and etiology of idiopathic dilated cardiomyopathy (summary of a National Heart, Lung, and Blood Institute workshop [see comments]. Am J Cardiol 69: 1458–66
17. Messina DN, Speer MC, Pericak Vance MA et al. (1997) Linkage of familial dilated cardiomyopathy with conduction defect and muscular dystrophy to chromosome 6q23. Am J Hum Genet 61: 909–17
18. Mestroni L, Miani D, Di Lenarda A et al. (1990) Clinical and pathologic study of familial dilated cardiomyopathy. Am J Cardiol 65: 1449–53
19. Michels VV, Moll PP, Miller FA et al. (1992) The frequency of familial dilated cardiomyopathy in a series of patients with idiopathic dilated cardiomyopathy. N Engl J Med 326: 77–82
20. Michels VV, Pastores GM, Moll PP et al. (1993) Dystrophin analysis in idiopathic dilated cardiomyopathy. J Med Genet 30: 955–7
21. Muntoni F, Cau M, Ganau A et al. (1993) Brief report: Deletion of the dystrophin muscle-promoter region associated with X-linked dilated cardiomyopathy [see comments]. N Engl J Med 329: 921–5
22. Nigro V, Okazaki Y, Belsito A et al. (1997) Identification of the Syrian hamster cardiomyopathy gene. Hum Mol Genet 6: 601–7
23. Olson TM, Keating MT (1996) Mapping a cardiomyopathy locus to chromosome 3p22-p25. J Clin Invest 97: 528–32
24. Olson TM, Michels VV, Thibodeau SN et al. (1998) Actin mutations in dilated cardiomyopathy, a heritable form of heart failure. Science 280: 750–2
25. Ozawa E, Yoshida M, Suzuki A et al. (1995) Dystrophin-associated proteins in muscular dystrophy. Hum Mol Genet: 1711–6
26. Regan TJ (1984) Alcoholic cardiomyopathy. Prog Cardiovasc Dis 27: 141–52
27. Richardson P, McKenna W, Bristow M et al. (1996) Report of the 1995 World Health Organization/International Society and Federation of Cardiology Task Force on the Definition and Classification of cardiomyopathies. Circulation 93: 841–2
28. Schultheiss HP (1993) Disturbance of the myocardial energy metabolism in dilated cardiomyopathy due to autoimmunological mechanisms. Circulation 87: Iv43–8
29. Schultheiss HP, Schulze K, Schauer R et al. (1995) Antibody-mediated imbalance of myocardial energy metabolism. A causal factor of cardiac failure? Circ Res 76: 64–72
30. Suomalainen A, Paetau A, Leinonen H et al. (1992) Inherited idiopathic dilated cardiomyopathy with multiple deletions of mitochondrial DNA. Lancet 340: 1319–20
31. Towbin JA, Hejtmancik JF, Brink P et al. (1993) X-linked dilated cardiomyopathy. Molecular genetic evidence of linkage to the Duchenne muscular dystrophy (dystrophin) gene at the Xp21 locus. Circulation 87: 1854–65

Author's address:
Prof. Dr. L. Thierfelder
Robert-Rössle Str. 10
13122 Berlin
e-mail: lthier@mdc-berlin.de

Registry of families with inherited dilated cardiomyopathy for molecular analyses

W.-M. Franz[1], O. J. Müller[1], E. Grünig[2], M. Cremer[3], H. A. Katus[1]

[1] Medizinische Klinik II, Medizinische Universität zu Lübeck, Germany
[2] Innere Medizin III, Universität Heidelberg, Germany
[3] Inst. f. Anthropologie und Humangenetik, Universität München, Germany

Abstract

Despite several reports on the genetic cause of dilated cardiomyopathy (DCM), most cases are believed to be sporadic and specific clinical findings are not well defined. Therefore, we initiated a registry of patients with idiopathic DCM to analyze the frequency and clinical characteristics of this inherited disorder. In a first evaluation, 445 consecutive patients with angiographically proven DCM were included. Pedigrees were constructed, and 970 first and second-degree family members were examined. Familial DCM was confirmed in 48 (10.8 %) of the 445 index patients and was suspected in 108 (24.2 %) patients. Among the families of the 48 index patients with confirmed familial disease, five phenotypes (A–E) of familial DCM could be identified in 19 independent families: (A) 2 families with juvenile DCM with subclinical muscular dystrophy and elevated CK-MM levels, (B) 5 families with juvenile DCM without an increase of CK-MM, (C) 5 families with DCM and segmental hypokinesia of the left ventricle, (D) 6 families with DCM and early conduction defects, and (E) only 1 DCM family with sensorineural hearing loss. Genetic analyses of a DCM family with phenotype A revealed an X-linked inheritance. DNA and protein analyses identified a mutated rod region of the dystrophin gene to be associated with this rapidly progressive disorder in young males. The present results indicate that DCM may be a genetic disorder in approximately 35 % of all cases. The common phenotypes of DCM may facilitate screening for genetic defects and help in risk stratification. In particular, young men with suspected DCM (phenotype A and B) show a rapid progression of the disease and should, therefore, be closely evaluated for heart transplantation.

Introduction

Dilated cardiomyopathy (DCM) constitutes a group of heart muscle diseases characterized by "dilatation and impaired contraction of the left or both ventricles. It may be idiopathic, familial/genetic, viral and/or immune, alcoholic/toxic or associated with recognized cardiovascular disease in which the degree of myocardial dysfunction is not explained by the abnormal loading conditions or the extent of ischemic damage" (30). DCM represents a

Table 1. Chromosomal localization of genes with inherited DCM

locus	gene
1 (1p1-q1)	– – –
1 (1q32)	– – –
3 (3p22-p25)	– – –
6 (6q23)	– – –
9 (9q13-q22)	– – –
10 (10q21-q23)	– – –
15 (15q14)	cardiac actin
X (Xp21)	dystrophin
X (Xq28)	– – –

significant health problem leading to progressive refractory heart failure, the most frequent indication for heart transplantation. This condition is associated with a high rate of sudden death due to ventricular arrhythmias with a rate of mortality from 15 – 50 % at 5 years (18). The prevalence of DCM in the US population was estimated to be 36.5 per 100,000 persons (6). Etiology and the pathogenic mechanisms of most cases are unknown, and therefore the most frequent diagnosis is „idiopathic cardiomyopathy". The importance of genetic factors has been underestimated for a long time. In 1981, the percentage of familial cases was estimated to be only 2 % (12). However, in recently published prospective studies on patients with DCM and their family members 20 – 25 % of index patients were classified as inherited disorders (15, 16). Because the diagnosis of familial DCM depends on both the completeness of the pedigree analysis and the diagnostic criteria used, the true frequency of familial DCM may be still underestimated. A careful analysis of the family members of patients with DCM may reveal a typical phenotype within a single family. Based on these phenotypic characteristics of familial DCM, molecular causes of the disease were identified. Genetic analyses have linked chromosome 1 (p1-q1) (8, 15), 3 (p22-p25) (26), 6 (6g23) (23), and 9 (q13-q22) (19) to DCM families with characteristic conduction defects. Linkage to chromosome 10 (q21-q23) was identified in a DCM family with mitral valve prolapse (2). DNA and protein analyses identified dystrophin (Xp21), cardiac actin (15q14) and mutations of the mitochondrial DNA to be associated with familial DCM (Table 1) (11, 25, 27, 33, 36, 40). While mutations of mitochondrial DNA lead to alterations of the energy production, mutations of dystrophin or actin may lead to a destabilization of the plasma membrane or destruction of the Z-band respectively, thus, deteriorating the cytoskeletal architecture.

Here, we describe our registry of families with invasively proven DCM and introduce a family with X-linked dilated cardiomyopathy based on a mutated rod region of the dystrophin gene.

Methods

Index Patients

In this study, 481 consecutive patients with DCM were analyzed (14). DCM was confirmed by left ventricular and coronary angiography performed at the University Hospital of

Heidelberg. The diagnosis of DCM was based on the WHO criteria (30). Only patients with an angiographic left ventricular ejection fraction < 50 % were included. Exclusion criteria were coronary artery disease (> 50 % diameter stenosis of at least one major coronary artery), valvular or congenital heart disease, long-standing hypertension with diastolic blood pressure > 95 mmHg, active myocarditis, type I insulin-dependent diabetes mellitus, hypothyroidism, amyloid disease, thalassemia, sarcoidosis, hypertrophic cardiomyopathy with dilative course, alcohol ingestion > 100 g/d, and a history of exposure to cardiotoxic drugs.

Definition of familial disease

Familial DCM was defined as confirmed when, in addition to the index patient, at least one first- or second-degree relative had DCM documented either by left heart catheterization or by autopsy. Familial DCM was defined as suspected when at least one additional first-degree family member had either died suddenly or died of chronic heart failure before the age of 65 years, or when impaired left ventricular function was documented by echocardiography.

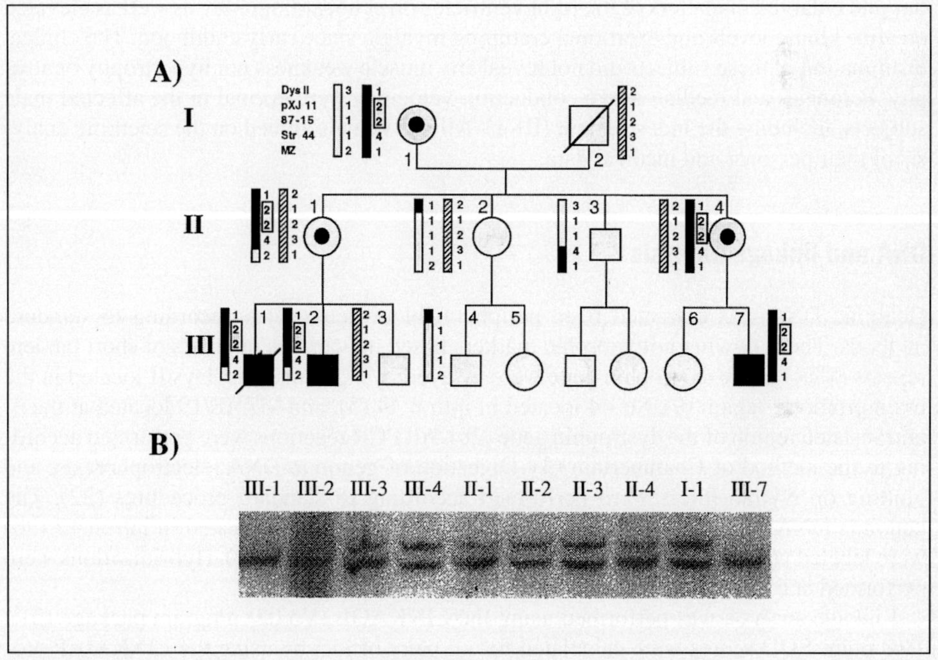

Fig. 1. (A) Pedigree of family X with X-linked DCM. Each individual is specified by the generation (I, II, III) and number (1-7). Phenotypically affected male DCM patients are represented by a filled square. Heterozygous female carriers are marked with a filled dot within the circle. Crossed symbols represent death. Bars with numbers represent the allelic configuration for the 5 genomic markers (Dys II, XJ 1.1, 87-15, Str 44, and MZ 18/19) investigated. Open bars represent the disease unrelated Xp21 region; filled bars represent the disease related Xp21 region. Hatched bars represent the male non-carrier Xp21 region. Boxes mark the cosegregation of the alleles (XJ 1.1, 87-15) with the DCM. (B) SSCP-analysis of the PCR amplified exon 29 of the indicated members of family X. Lymphocyte derived genomic DNA was used as a template for amplification with the primers e29F and e29R.

Familial DCM of phenotype A

The index patient (III-1) of family X (Fig. 1A) was a 21-year-old man of normal intelligence, who presented with elevated serum CK-MM levels and dyspnoe due to pulmonary edema. On echocardiography left ventricular shortening fraction was 16 % and the end-diastolic diameters of the right and left ventricles were markedly enlarged to 3.5 and 7.9 cm respectively. Impaired left and right heart function was confirmed by heart catheterization (left ventricular ejection fraction = 20%, cardiac index = 1.5 l/min, mean pulmonary artery pressure = 35 mmHg). Coronary angiography was normal. Mild mitral and moderate tricuspidal regurgitation were observed. Endomyocardial biopsies taken from left ventricular myocardium revealed histological changes compatible with DCM. There was no evidence of inflammatory heart disease. On neurological examination, he had normal muscle strength in all muscle groups, normal muscle tone, no muscle atrophies, normal bilateral reflexes and no sensory deficits. Diagnostic muscle biopsies from the vastus lateralis muscle showed a mildly myopathic picture with increased variation of fiber size and some endo- and perimyseal fibrosis. During the course in the hospital, his cardiac function deteriorated rapidly requiring emergency transplantation. The patient died of a septic shock after heart transplantation.

The family history disclosed that a brother of his maternal grandmother (I-1) had died of clinically diagnosed cardiomyopathy at the age of 29 years. The youngest brother (III-2) and a maternal cousin (III-7) of the index patient had electrocardiographic abnormalities and enlarged diameters of the right ventricles on echocardiography as well as elevated creatine kinase levels and exertional cramping myalgia since early childhood. The clinical examination of these subjects did not reveal any muscle weakness nor hypertrophy or atrophy. Peroneal- and median-nerve conduction velocities were normal in the affected male subjects, including the index patient (III-1). All individuals agreed on the scientific analysis of their personal and medical data.

DNA and linkage analysis

Genomic DNA was extracted from peripheral blood leukocytes according to standard methods. The following polymorphic markers based on variable numbers of short tandem repeats (STR) in the dystrophin gene were assayed by PCR analysis: Dys II located in the brain promoter region (9), Str 44 located in intron 44 (5), and MZ 18/19 located at the 3' untranslated region of the dystrophin gene (28). All PCR reactions were performed according to the method of Chamberlain (3). Digestion of genomic DNA, electrophoresis, and blotting on Nytran filters were performed according to standard procedures (22). The genomic DNA probes XJ1.1 located in intron 7 (37) and 87-15 located in intron 17 (20) were labeled with ^{32}P using the random primed labeling method (10). Hybridizations were performed at 65 °C using the buffer of Church et al. (4).

Linkage analysis was performed using the LINKAGE (V5.03) program package (21). Two point LOD scores were calculated for all pairs of loci by using the LINKMAP program (21). The mode of inheritance was assumed to be X-linked. Penetrance was considered to be 100 %. The disease prevalence was assumed to be 1:10,000. Allele frequency was used according to Towbin (36).

For detection of single-strand conformation polymorphisms (SSCP), DNA was extracted from peripheral leukocytes and amplified by PCR using the following external primers, which bind in the flanking intronic regions of exon 28, 29, and 30: e28F (5'-TTCACATTTACTTTTCTACC-3') and e28R (5'-ATTTACAACTTACATC-3'); e29F (5'-

CATTTGCTGATAATCCAATG-3´) and e29R (5´-TCTGAGAGCTCTATCTGC-3´); e30F (5´-ATCGTTTTACCTGATACAG-3´) and e30R (5´-GATTCCCAGATGTACTTG-3´).

Sources of tissues

After informed consent had been obtained, a biopsy of the vastus lateralis muscle was performed in six patients (II-1, II-4, III-1, III-2, III-4, III-7) of family X. Normal skeletal muscle tissue obtained from the department of orthopedic surgery served as control. Myocardial tissue was obtained from the explanted heart of our index patient (III-1). Control heart tissue deriving from papillary muscles of a patient with mitral valve replacement was obtained from the department of cardiac surgery.

Immunofluorescence and westernblot

Immunofluorescence was carried out as previously described (11). Monoclonal antibodies (Medac Molecular Biology, Hamburg) directed against the rod region (dys-1), the C-terminus (dys-2), and the N-terminus (dys-3) of dystrophin (dys) were used in the following dilutions: dys-1 (1:10), dys-2 (1:100), dys-3 (1:200). Electrophoresis was carried out as previously described (11) applying 200 μg of protein per lane. Westernblots were probed with the same anti-dystrophin and -spectrin antibodies.

Results

Frequency of familial DCM

In 445 (92.5 %) out of 481 index patients with DCM a detailed family history was obtained and pedigrees were constructed. Evidence for a familial disease was gained in 156 patients. Based on invasive investigations or autopsy, DCM was proven in relatives of 48 index patients (10.8 %) (confirmed familial DCM). Out of these 48 families, 65 additional members had confirmed DCM. Remarkably, 38 of the 65 were newly identified DCM cases. In 108 (24.2 %) of the 445 index patients, familial DCM was assumed to be present based on a history of unexplained heart failure (n = 23), sudden cardiac death (n = 75), or unexplained depressed left ventricular function on echocardiography (n = 10) (suspected familial DCM). In the remaining 289 (65 %) of the 445 index patients, family history did not reveal evidence for additional family members with DCM (nonfamilial DCM). However, concomitant cardiac abnormalities, such as unspecific ECG changes (n = 69), mitral valve prolapse (n = 22), Wolff-Parkinson-White (WPW) syndrome (n = 12), atrial septal aneurysm (n = 4), atrial septal defect (n = 2), ventricular septal defect (n = 1) or pulmonary stenosis (n = 1) were found in 120 of the 970 family members with normal left and right ventricular function. In five index patients with familial and four with sporadic disease, DCM was associated with WPW syndrome.

Table 2. Phenotypes of familial DCM.

Phenotype A (DCM with subclinical muscular dystrophy)	Cardiac symptoms predominant with elevated CK-MM	X-chromosomal	Xp21 dystrophin
Phenotype B (DCM with rapid progressive course in young males)	Early onset and rapid progression with normal CK-MM	X-chromosomal?	unknown Xq28?
Phenotype C (DCM with segmental hypokinesia of LV)	Regionally impaired LV function, stable course	autosomal-dominant	unknown
Phenotype D (DCM with early conduction system disease)	AV block, Atrial fibrillation	autosomal-dominant	1p1-1q1 3p22-3p25 9q13-9q23
Phenotype E (DCM with sensorineural hearing loss)	Severely impaired LV and RV function, Bilateral pantonal hearing loss	maternal or autosomal-dominant	Mitochondrial DNA- mutations?

Phenotypes in patients with confirmed familial DCM

In 28 of the 48 families with confirmed familial DCM, at least two members with confirmed DCM and two with suspected DCM were identified in at least two generations. Five distinct phenotypic presentations varying in mode of inheritance, clinical symptoms, disease progression, and prognosis could be identified in 19 of these 28 families (Table 2). Nine families could not be classified because of their heterogenous clinical picture.

Phenotype A: Juvenile DCM with subclinical muscular dystrophy and elevated CK-MM levels

Two families were found in which six juvenile patients with a mean age of 28.4 years showed a rapidly progressive course of DCM, with elevated serum activity of creatine kinase (CK-MM) but normal CK-MB or cardiac troponin T. During a mean follow-up period of 4 years, two male patients died, and one underwent heart transplantation. All patients revealed impaired biventricular function. Depressed left ventricular function was only observed in two females at the age of 46 and 68 years. The pedigree of one family with phenotype A is presented in Fig. 1A. In this representative family, a novel mutation within the rod region of the dystrophin gene was detected by genetic linkage, protein and SSCP analyses (see below).

Phenotype B: Juvenile DCM without an increase of CK-MM

This phenotype was observed in five families in which 14 members were classified as confirmed and 10 as suspected DCM. Similar to group A, the clinical course of DCM was rapidly progressive in all nine male patients (mean age at diagnosis 23.6 years). During a mean follow-up period of 5.2 years, two patients deteriorated, 6 underwent heart transplantation, and one died. Serum CK-MM levels were normal and in one family dystrophinopathy was ruled out by histopathologic and molecular genetic analyses. Mean age at diagnosis and functional status after a 6- to 12-month follow-up in the male patients was clearly different from DCM patients in the following groups C to F.

Phenotype C: Familial DCM with segmental hypokinesia

In five families comprising 14 patients, DCM was characterized by an autosomal dominant trait and by abnormalities of the regional wall motion. Due to the presence of impaired left ventricular function in a defined area, coronary artery disease was suspected in 10 out of 14 patients. However, subsequent coronary angiographies did not change significantly over a follow-up period of 4–10 years. An autosomal dominant mode of inheritance was likely in these families.

Phenotype D: Familial DCM with early conduction defects

This group comprises six families. Of the 76 members examined, 20 developed DCM. In all 20 patients, either atrial fibrillation (n=14) or atrioventricular (AV) block (n=7) was documented before impaired left ventricular function could be documented. In this group, the incidence of atrial fibrillation and AV block was significantly higher compared to groups A, C, and F. The pattern of inheritance was compatible with an autosomal dominant trait.

Phenotype E: Familial DCM with sensorineural hearing loss

In only one family DCM was associated with bilateral sensorineural hearing loss in 3 of 27 family members examined. The mode of inheritance in this family is most likely autosomal dominant or maternal.

Genetic linkage analysis

In order to show that the dystrophin gene is associated with DCM of phenotype A, genetic linkage analysis of family X was performed (Fig. 1A). Family members presenting the following criteria were considered as diseased: (1) increased CK-MM levels, (2) exertional cramping myalgia, (3) echocardiographic right or left ventricular dilatation, and (4) unspecific ECG changes. Allelic configurations of five different DNA loci were investigated using the polymorphic DNA probes, Dys II, XJ1.1, 87-15, Str 44, and MZ 18/19. All DNA probes used have previously been mapped within the dystrophin gene on Xp21 (Fig. 2). Using two-point linkage analysis, evidence of linkage was found for the genomic probe XJ1.1 with a pairwise LOD score of +1.93 at ϕ=0 (Fig. 2). The intronic probe XJ1.1 (DXS206) is known to be located in the Xp21.2 region (29, 35) within the proximal (5') portion of the dystrophin gene between exon 7 and exon 8. Autoradiographs of the XJ1.1 polymorphism demonstrated that the 3.1 kb band (allele 2) was observed in all affected males and female carriers and was absent in all unaffected males. With respect to the adjacent polymorphic marker 87-15 located in intron 17 (20), a pairwise LOD score of +0.73 was calculated, which does

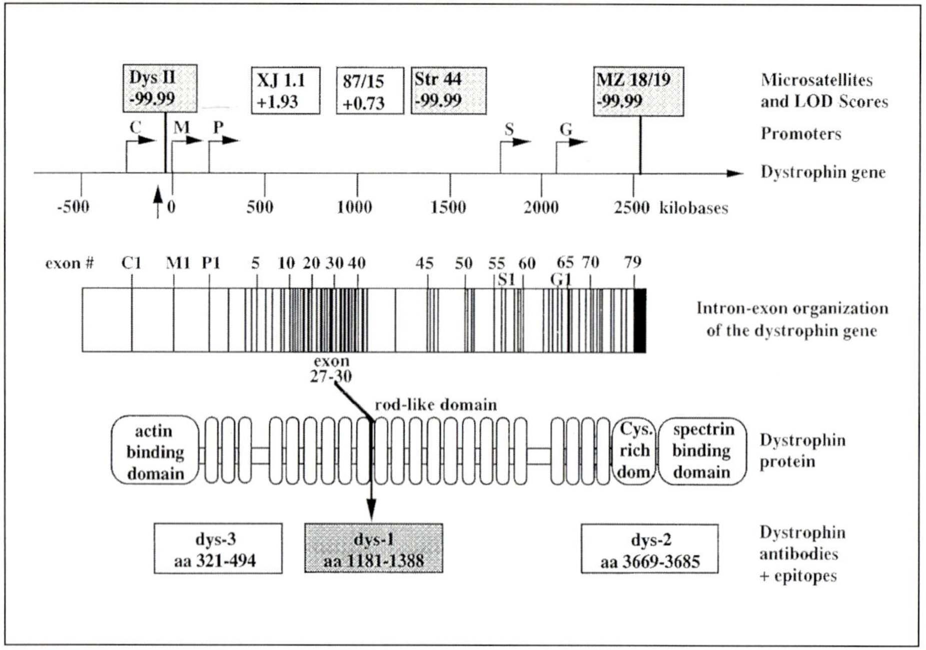

Fig. 2. The dystrophin gene (1). Top line: genomic map of the dystrophin gene spanning approximately 2.4 million bases of the short arm of X-chromosome. Above, polymorphic DNA markers and pairwise LOD scores for f=0. At least five distinct promoters drive independent cell-type specific expression of dystrophin. The C (cortical)-, M (muscle)-, and P (Purkinje cell)-dystrophins, the "full-length" forms, each use their own first exon. The S (Schwann cell)- and G (general or glial)-dystrophin promoters encode C-terminal proteins Dp 116 and Dp 71, respectively. Middle line: a map of the complex exon-intron organization, in which at least 79 (plus 4 additional first) exons encode its 14 kilobase mRNA. Bars represent approximate relative exon positions. Bottom line: schematic map of the four domains, actin binding, rod-like, cystein-rich, and spectrin-associated domain, forming the dystrophin polypeptide. Below, local distribution of the antigenic sites (aa= aminoacids) reacting with the domain-specific, monoclonal anti-dystrophin antibodies (dys-1, dys-2, dys-3).

not exclude linkage with the phenotype (Fig. 2). The other markers 5' (Dys II) and 3' (Str 44 and MZ 18/19) revealed a negative LOD score of –99.99 at ϕ=0 excluding cosegregation with the disease locus. Recombinations noted with markers in the dystrophin region were within Dys II (subject II-2, III-4), Str 44 (subject II-3), and MZ 18/19 (subject II-1, III-1, III-3), suggesting that the mutation causing X-linked DCM lies centromeric to Str 44 and telomeric to Dys II as indicated in Fig. 2. Thus, genetic linkage analysis has marked the DNA region relevant for this disease 3' of the brain promoter (Dys II) within the polymorphic markers XJ1.1 and 87-15 and 5' of intron 44 (Str 44). This region includes the epitope of the monoclonal dys-1 antibody, which is located between exon 27 and 30.

Dystrophin protein analyses

Immunofluorescence staining of heart (III-1) and skeletal muscle of the index patient (III-1), his brother (III-2) as well as his maternal cousin (III-7) revealed a pathological dystrophin pattern: there was a complete lack of staining with the monoclonal antibody dys-1 directed against the amino acids 1181-1388 within the rod portion of the dystrophin molecule. In contrast, the antibodies directed against epitopes on both N-terminal (dys-3) and C-terminal (dys-2) sequences of the dystrophin protein showed patchy dystrophin staining of reduced intensity on the sarcolemma of skeletal and cardiac myofibers. Control stains using anti-spectrin were normal in both cardiac and skeletal muscle tissues indicating good preservation of the sarcolemma in these specimen. There was no apparent change of molecular weight of the 427 kd dystrophin protein on Western Blot. In contrast to dys-2 and dys-3 antibodies, no reactivity was detected with dys-1 in heart (III-1) nor skeletal muscle (III-1, III-2, III-7) homogenates (data not shown).

DNA analyses of the dys-1 epitope

Based on the observation that the monoclonal antibody dys-1 directed against the midrod region of dystrophin gave no positive signal in heart or skeletal muscle of our family with X-linked DCM (11), we analyzed this epitope encoded by the nucleotides 3751 to 4372. SSCP analyses of the related exons 27-30 revealed a polymorphic banding pattern only for exon 29 in all affected males (Fig. 1B).

Discussion

We have initiated a registry of families with idiopathic DCM. The patient history as well as blood samples for genetic linkage analyses have been collected. According to the analysis of 451 patients with invasively documented DCM, 35 % have most likely inherited this genetic defect. The frequency of familial aggregation of DCM documented in our study is slightly higher than previously reported by others (16, 24). The importance of familial screening may be underlined by the fact that 38 new DCM cases were detected in this trial.

In our registry, five different clinical phenotypes could be discerned. Phenotype A and B are characterized by a rapid progressive cardiomyopathy in teenage males presenting with congestive heart failure without clinical signs of skeletal myopathy. Typically, patients die of biventricular heart failure within a year after the first symptoms. Affected women may present with atypical chest pain in their 50s or 60s, when the heart size and left ventricular function are often considered normal. At this age, some female patients may also show impaired left ventricular function which is stable at follow-up. Families have been divided in phenotype A or B according to their serum CK-MM levels. Patients with phenotype A revealed elevated CK-MM activities with subclinical myopathy. Molecular genetic analyses detected a linkage to the X-chromosomal dystrophin gene at Xp21. Phenotype B is associated with normal CK-MM levels. The defect follows most probably an X-linked trait but does not appear to be associated with a dystrophinopathy. The molecular cause of phenotype B still remains to be elucidated. Candidates could be genes on Xq28 as this locus was linked to a severe form of X-chromosomal DCM (7).

Familial DCM may also manifest as a segmental disease of the left ventricular myocardium (phenotype C). Segmental hypokinesia was described earlier in patients with sporadic disease (34, 38); however, familial aggregation of this type of DCM has not been previously reported. The five families of phenotype D are characterized by an autosomal inheritance and the association of DCM with AV block or atrial fibrillation early in the disease process. This phenotype resembles that of families described previously in which linkage of DCM with polymorphic markers located on the centromeric region of chromosome 1 (8, 15), chromosome 3p (26), and chromosome 9 (19) has been reported. In phenotype E, DCM was associated with sensorineural hearing loss. Because maternal inheritance is most likely in this family, this phenotype might be caused by mutations of mitochondrial DNA, which has been reported previously in patients with DCM and neurologic symptoms (17, 31, 32, 33). Other candidate genes that might be responsible for DCM of this phenotype may include Shaker 1 and USH1b genes encoding nonsarcomeric myosins. Mutations in these genes have recently been identified as causing deafness or severe bilateral hearing loss (13, 39).

Genotypic characterization of the X-linked DCM family of phenotype A

Using five different polymorphic markers for linkage analysis the region most likely corresponding to this disease was narrowed down to the genomic segment 3' of the brain dystrophin promoter (Dys II marker) and 5' of intron 44 (Str 44 marker). The LOD score of 1.93 (ϕ=0) was highest for the polymorphic marker XJ 1.1, the same which was described in two other families (36).

In our DCM family, a major deletion of exons or of a promoter element was excluded by Southernblot, multiplex PCR analysis, and additional amplifications of the first 850 bp of the muscular promoter region (11). Protein data using a panel of three different antibodies (Ab) showed a constant lack of binding to dys-1 Ab in all of our affected male individuals. The lack of reaction with the dys-1 Ab cannot be explained by a disruption of the reading frame, since both the N- and C-terminal Ab (dys-2 and dys-3) did bind as expected. We conclude that there could be a distinct sequence change of the antigenic determinant of the monoclonal dys-1 Ab. This dys-1 epitope is located in the mid-rod region between amino acids 1181 and 1388, which correspond to the exons 27 to 30 (Fig. 2). The genetic defect appears to be located on exon 29 as SSCP analysis of the related exons 27–30 resulted in a polymorphic banding pattern only in this exon. A mutation could be a possible cause for protein and/or mRNA instability leading to a reduced expression of an eventually semi-functional dystrophin protein in cardiac and skeletal muscle. Disruption of the dys-1 epitope may be caused by a pointmutation leading to a conserved amino acid exchange or an alternative splicing resulting in a small deletion of dystrophin mRNA.

The pathogenesis of X-linked DCM in patients with phenotype A may either be explained by a reduced or lacking expression of dystrophin in the myocardium or by a disturbed interaction of a mutated protein with actin or dystrophin associated proteins of the myocardial sarcolemma. The first hypothesis can be rejected in our family since Western blot, and immunohistochemistry clearly showed presence of dystrophin in both cardiac and skeletal muscle. The second hypothesis may be more relevant for our family. Dystrophin interacts with actin and dystrophin-associated glycoproteins of the sarcolemma. Conformational changes of the rod region of dystrophin may profoundly affect this interaction and cause by itself membrane instability.

Further analysis of the mutated dystrophin gene and the dystrophin-associated proteins in this family may improve our understanding of the causal relationship of dystrophin mutation and DCM and perhaps give an explanation for the predominant cardiac involvement due to this mutation.

Linkage analysis performed in other DCM families of our registry may lead to the identification of new genes and mutations involved in the molecular pathogenesis of this inherited disorder.

References

1. Ahn AH, Kunkel LM (1993) The structural and functional diversity of dystrophin. Nature Genet 3: 283–291
2. Bowles KR, Gajarski R, Porter P, Goytia V, Bachinski L, Roberts R, Pignatelli R, Towbin JA (1996) Gene mapping of familial autosomal dominant dilated cardiomyopathy to chromosome 10q21-23. J Clin Invest 98: 1355–1360
3. Chamberlain JS, Gibbs RA, Ranier JE, Nguyen PN, Caskey CT (1988) Deletion screening of the Duchenne muscular dystrophy locus via multiplex DNA amplification. Nucleic Acids Res 16: 11141–11156
4. Church GM, Gilbert W (1984) Genomic sequencing. Proc Natl Acad Sci (USA) 81: 1991–1995
5. Clemens PR, Fenwick RG, Chamberlain JS, Gibbs RA, De Andrade M, Chakraborty R, Caskey C (1991) Carrier detection and prenatal diagnosis in Duchenne and Becker muscular dystrophy families, using dinucleotide repeat polymorphisms. Am J Hum Genet 49: 951–960
6. Codd MB, Sugrue DD, Gersh BJ, Melton LJ 3d (1989) Epidemiology of idiopathic dilated and hypertrophic cardiomyopathy. A population-based study in Olmsted County, Minnesota, 1975–1984. Circulation 80: 564–572
7. D'Adamo P, Fassone L, Gedeon A, Janssen EA, Bione S, Bolhuis PA, Barth PG, Wilson M, Haan E, Orstavik KH, Patton MA, Green AJ, Zammarchi E, Donati MA, Toniolo D (1997) The X-linked gene G4.5 is responsible for different infantile dilated cardiomyopathies. Am J Hum Genet 61: 862–867
8. Durand JB, Bachinski LL, Bieling LC, Czernuszewicz GZ, Abchee AB, Yu QT, Tapscott T, Hill R, Ifegwu J, Marian AJ et al. (1995) Localization of a gene responsible for familial dilated cardiomyopathy to chromosome 1q32. Circulation 92: 3387–3389
9. Feener CA, Boyce FM, Kunkel LM (1991) Rapid detection of CA polymorphisms in cloned DNA: application to the 5´ region of the dystrophin gene. Am J Hum Genet 48: 621–627
10. Feinberg AP, Vogelstein B (1983) A technique for radiolabeling DNA restriction endonuclease fragments to high specific activity. Anal Biochem 132: 6–13
11. Franz WM, Cremer M, Herrmann R, Grünig E, Fogel W, Scheffold T, Goebel HH, Kircheisen R, Kübler W, Voit T, Katus HA (1995) X-linked dilated cardiomyopathy. Novel mutation of the dystrophin gene. Ann N Y Acad Sci 752: 470–491
12. Fuster V, Gersh BJ, Giuliani ER, Tajik AJ, Brandenburg RO, Frye RL (1981) The natural history of idiopathic dilated cardiomyopathy. Am J Cardiol 47: 525–531
13. Gibson F, Walsh J, Mburu P, Varela A, Brown KA, Antonio M, Beisel KW, Steel KP, Brown SD (1995) A type VII myosin encoded by the mouse deafness gene shaker-1. Nature 374: 58–59
14. Grünig E, Tasman JA, Kücherer H, Franz WM, Kübler W, Katus HA (1998) Frequency and phenotypes of familial dilated cardiomyopathy. J Am Coll Cardiol 31: 186–194
15. Kass S, MacRae C, Graber HL, Sparks EA, McNamara D, Boudoulas H, Basson CT, Baker PB 3rd, Cody RJ, Fishman MC et al. (1994) A gene defect that causes conduction system disease and dilated cardiomyopathy maps to chromosome 1p1-1q1. Nat Genet 7: 546–551
16. Keeling PJ, Gang Y, Smith G, Seo H, Bent SE, Murday V, Caforio AL, McKenna WJ (1995) Familial dilated cardiomyopathy in the United Kingdom. Br Heart J 73: 417–421
17. Kitaoka H, Kameoka K, Suzuki Y, Sasaki E, Majima M, Takada K, Katagiri H, Oka Y, Ohsawa N (1995) A patient with diabetes mellitus, cardiomyopathy, and a mitochondrial gene mutation: confirmation of a gene mutation in cardiac muscle. Diabetes Res Clin Pract 28: 207–212
18. Komajda M, Jais JP, Reeves F, Goldfarb B, Bouhour JB, Juillieres Y, Lanfranchi J, Peycelon P, Geslin P, Carrie D et al. (1990) Factors predicting mortality in idiopathic dilated cardiomyopathy. Eur Heart J 11: 824–831
19. Krajinovic M, Pinamonti B, Sinagra G, Vatta M, Severini GM, Milasin J, Falaschi A, Camerini F, Giacca M, Mestroni L (1995) Linkage of familial dilated cardiomyopathy to chromosome 9. Heart Muscle Disease Study Group. Am J Hum Genet 57: 846–852
20. Kunkel LM (1985) Analysis of deletions in DNA from patients with Becker and Duchenne Muscular dystrophy. Nature 322: 73–77
21. Lathrop GM, Lalouel JM, Julier C, Ott J (1984) Strategies for multilocus linkage analysis in humans. Proc Natl Acad Sci (USA) 81: 3443–3446
22. Mao Y, Cremer M (1989) Detection of Duchenne muscular carriers by dosage analysis using the DMD cDNA clone 8. Hum Genet 81: 193–195
23. Messina DN, Speer MC, Pericak-Vance MA, McNally EM (1997) Linkage of familial dilated cardiomyopathy with conduction defect and muscular dystrophy to chromosome 6g23. Am J Hum Genet 61 (4): 909–917
24. Michels VV, Moll PP, Miller FA, Tajik AJ, Chu JS, Driscoll DJ, Burnett JC, Rodeheffer RJ, Chesebro JH, Tazelaar HD (1992) The frequency of familial dilated cardiomyopathy in a series of patients with idiopathic dilated cardiomyopathy. N Engl J Med 326: 77–82
25. Muntoni F, Cau M, Ganau A, Congiu R, Arvedi G, Mateddu A, Marrosu MG, Cianchetti C, Realdi G, Cao A, Melis MA (1993) Brief report: Deletion of the dystrophin muscle-promoter region associated with X-linked dilated cardiomyopathy. N Engl J Med 329: 921–925

26. Olson TM, Keating MT (1996) Mapping a cardiomyopathy locus to chromosome 3p22-p25. Clin Invest 97: 528–532
27. Olson TM, Michels VV, Thibodeau SN, Tai YS, Keating MT (1998) Actin mutations in dilated cardiomyopathy, a heritable form of heart failure. Science 280: 750–752
28. Oudet C, Heilig R, Mandel J (1990) An informative polymorphism detectable by polymerase chain reaction at the 3' end of the dystrophin gene. Hum Genet 84: 283–285
29. Ray PN, Belfall B, Duff C, Logan C, Kean V, Thompson MW, Sylvester JE, Gorski JL, Schmickel RD, Worton RG (1985) Cloning of the breakpoint of an X;21 translocation associated with Duchenne muscular dystrophy. Nature 318: 672–675
30. Richardson P, McKenna W, Bristow M, Maisch B, Mautner B, O'Connell J, Olsen E, Thiene G, Goodwin J, Gyarfas I, Martin I, Nordet P (1996) Report of the 1995 World Health Organization/International Society and Federation of Cardiology Task Force on the Definition and Classification of cardiomyopathies. Circulation 93: 841–842
31. Santorelli FM, Mak SC, El-Schahawi M, Casali C, Shanske S, Baram TZ, Madrid RE, DiMauro S (1996) Maternally inherited cardiomyopathy and hearing loss associated with a novel mutation in the mitochondrial tRNA(Lys) gene (G8363A). Am J Hum Genet 58: 933–939
32. Shoeffner JM, Wallace DC (1992) Heart disease and mitochondrial DNA mutation. Heart Dis Stroke 235–241
33. Suomalainen A, Paetau A, Leinonen H, Majander A, Peltonen L, Somer H (1992) Inherited idiopathic dilated cardiomyopathy with multiple deletions of mitochondrial DNA. Lancet 340: 1319–1320
34. Sunnerhagen KS, Bhargava V, Shabetai R (1990) Regional left ventricular wall motion abnormalities in idiopathic dilated cardiomyopathy. Am J Cardiol 65: 364–370
35. Thompson MW, Ray PN, Belfall B, Duff C, Oss I, Worton RG (1986) Linkage analysis of polymorphisms within the DNA fragment XJ cloned from the breakpoint of an X;21 translocation associated with X-linked muscular dystrophy. J Med Genet 23: 548–558
36. Towbin JA, Hejtmancik F, Brink P, Gelb B, Zhu XM, Chamberlain JS, McCabe ERB, Swift M (1993) X-linked dilated cardiomyopathy: Molecular genetic evidence of linkage to the Duchenne muscular dystrophy (dystrophin) gene at the Xp21 locus. Circulation 87: 1854–1865
37. Verellen-Dunoulin C, Freund M, De Meyer K, Caterre C, Frederick J, Thompson MW, Markovic VO, Wartan RG (1984) Expression of an X-linked muscular dystrophy in a female due to translocation involving Xp21. Hum Genet 67: 115–119
38. Wallis DE, O'Connell JB, Henkin RE, Costanzo-Nordin MR, Scanlon PJ (1984) Segmental wall motion in cardiomyopathy: A common finding and good prognostic sign. J Am Coll Cardiol 4: 674–681
39. Weil D, Blanchard S, Kaplan J, Guilford P, Gibson F, Walsh J, Mburu P, Varela A, Levilliers J, Weston MD et al. (1995) Defective myosin Ia gene responsible for Usher syndrome type 1b. Nature 374: 60–61
40. Zeviani M, Gellera C, Antozzi C, Rimoldi M, Morandi L, Villani F, Tiranti V, DiDonato S (1991) Maternally inherited myopathy and cardiomyopathy: Association with mutation in mitochondrial DNA tRNA $^{Leu(UUR)}$. Lancet 338: 143-147

Author's address:
Dr. Wolfgang-Michael Franz
Medizinische Klinik II
Medical University of Luebeck
Ratzeburger Allee 160
D-23538 Luebeck, Germany
E-mail: franz@medinf.mu-luebeck.de

Distinct phenotype patterns of Ca^{2+} handling proteins in end-stage failing human hearts

B. Pieske, W. Schillinger, S. Dieterich, L. S. Maier, G. Hasenfuss, J. Prestle

Zentrum Innere Medizin, Abteilung Kardiologie und Pneumologie,
Georg-August-Universität Göttingen, Germany

Abstract

Downregulation of SR Ca^{2+}-ATPase (SERCA2a) and upregulation of Na$^+$/Ca^{2+}-exchanger (NCX1) is regarded to be relevant for altered systolic and diastolic performance of the failing human heart. We tested the hypothesis that large variations in the degree of altered expression of these proteins exist between failing hearts, determining the extent of impaired contractile function. Furthermore, we evaluated whether differences in protein expression can also be observed in different regions of individual hearts.

We observed a blunted force-frequency response and a significant downregulation of SERCA2a in end-stage failing human myocardium. However, there was a wide variation in force-frequency behavior (with some failing hearts showing even a preserved positive force-frequency relation) and a wide variation in SERCA2a protein expression in these hearts. There was a close correlation between the degree of altered force-frequency response and reduced SERCA2a expression. Furthermore, average diastolic contractile behavior was significantly disturbed in end-stage failing myocardium, but NCX1 protein was significantly upregulated. Again, there was a wide variation in distolic force-frequency behavior and the degree of increased NCX1 expression, but a significant inverse correlation between the extent of diastolic dysfunction and NCX1 upregulation existed. In individual failing hearts, a transmural gradient within the left ventricular free wall existed for the expression of both SERCA2a and atrial natriuretic peptide (ANP), but not for NCX1.

In conclusion, average force-frequency behavior is blunted in human heart failure, associated with reduced expression of SERCA2a and increased expression of NCX1. However, large variations in the degree of altered expression of these proteins determine the extent of systolic and diastolic dysfunction of individual hearts. Furthermore, transmural gradients for SERCA2a, but not for NCX1 were observed within the same hearts, making a coordinate regulation of these proteins unlikely.

Introduction

Frequency-potentiation of contractile force represents a major physiological mechanism for regulation of cardiovascular function (6, 9, 24). However, this positive force-frequency relation in nonfailing myocardium is blunted or even inverse in end-stage failing human hearts (20, 24). The altered force-frequency behavior in heart failure was recently related to disturbed intracellular Ca^{2+} handling (24).

Several groups have reported a decrease in SR Ca^{2+}-ATPase on mRNA and protein levels in failing human myocardium, which was associated with reduced SR Ca^{2+} uptake (12, 16, 17). Furthermore, increased expression of the sarcolemmal Na^+/Ca^{2+}-exchanger on mRNA and protein levels was reported in end-stage failing hearts (31). In consequence, it was speculated that reduced intracellular Ca^{2+} transients and contractile force result from reduced SR Ca^{2+} reuptake and enhanced transsarcolemmal Ca^{2+} elimination in failing human hearts (24, 29). This might become even more prominent at higher heart rates, where diastole, i.e., time for Ca^{2+} reuptake to the SR, shortens, resulting in the negative force-frequency relationship in failing human myocardium.

However, despite this attractive model for altered excitation-contraction processes in end-stage failing human myocardium, large variations in contractile behavior between individual end-stage failing hearts can be observed (26). Furthermore, large variations in the regulation of proteins relevant for Ca^{2+} handling seem to occur, and a direct correlation between the degree of downregulation of SR Ca^{2+} pump proteins and the severity of contractile dysfunction at higher stimulation rates was observed (10).

In addition to pronounced systolic contractile dysfunction, diastolic dysfunction may be present in human heart failure, possibly due to delayed decline of intracellular Ca^{2+} transients and increased diastolic Ca^{2+} levels (4). However, altered diastolic function is not consistently encountered, even if severe systolic dysfunction is observed (22). Diastolic Ca^{2+} levels and mechanical performance critically depend on the activity of cytosolic Ca^{2+} elimination mechanisms, which are dominated by Ca^{2+} reuptake to the SR and trans-sarcolemmal Ca^{2+} elimination via NCX1 (3).

Therefore, the goal of the present study was to determine whether differences in protein expression patterns for the Na^+/Ca^{2+}-exchanger and the SR Ca^{2+}-ATPase exist in end-stage failing human hearts, which might determine the large variations in systolic and diastolic contractile behavior. Furthermore, we tested the hypothesis that regional differences in gene expression patterns can also be observed within individual failing hearts.

Materials and methods

Human myocardium

Studies were perfomed in left ventricular human myocardium from 21 patients with end-stage heart failure (NYHA IV) and from 9 brain dead multiorgan donors whose hearts could not be used for transplantation for technical reasons. The mean ejection fraction in the heart failure group was 21 ± 3 %; multiorgan donors had a normal left ventricular function and no history of heart disease. The study was reviewed and approved by the Ethical Committee of the University Clinics of Freiburg.

Muscle strip preparation

Immediateley after explantation, a part of the left or right ventricle was excised and submerged in an oxygenated (95 % O_2, 5 % CO_2, pH 7.4) cardioplegic solution and transported to the laboratory at ~10 °C. Thin muscle strips or trabeculae were dissected under microscopic control from the endocardial layer as described previously, mounted to an isometric force transducer in a muscle chamber, and superfused with tyrode's solution (2.5 mM Ca^{2+}, 37 °C). After a short equilibration period, muscles were electrically stimulated (field stimulation; voltage 20 % above threshold), and gradually stretched until maximal isometric twitch tension was reached. The force-frequency relationship was evaluated by stepwise increasing stimulation rate from a basal stimulation frequency of 0.5 Hz to 1.0, 1.5, 2.0, 2.5, and 3.0 Hz. At each stimulation rate, developed twitch force as well as active systolic and diastolic twitch tension were evaluated. Developed force is the active force developed during the isometric twitch. Diastolic force is the lowest force value during each stimulus interval. Average cross-sectional area of the muscle strips, calculated as the ratio of blotted muscle weight to muscle length, was 0.34 ± 0.04 mm^2 (no differences between groups).

Quantification of Na$^+$/Ca^{2+}-exchanger and SR Ca^{2+}-ATPase protein levels

Preparation of cardiac tissue homogenates

Samples of the ventricular free wall were taken immediateley after explantation, frozen in liquid nitrogen, and stored at –80 °C until use. For determination of Na$^+$/Ca^{2+}-exchanger and SR Ca^{2+}-ATPase protein levels in different hearts, transmural samples from the left or right free ventricular wall were obtained. For determination of transmural variations in mRNA expression within the same heart, samples from the endocardial layers and the epicardial layers of the left ventricle were dissected.

About 100 mg of myocardium was thawed in a ninefold volume of ice-cold 20 mmol/L Na-HEPES, pH 7.4, 4mmol/L EGTA, 0.1 mmol/L Leupeptin, 0.3 mmol/L PMSF, and 0.15 μmol/L Aprotinin. Homogenization was performed at 4 °C for 8 × 15 s by use of a Polytron-Homogenizer PT-K (Brinkman Instruments), followed by 15 strokes of a glass homogenizer. The protein contractions were determined in triplicate according to Lowry. Aliquots of the homogenates were frozen in liquid nitrogen and stored at –80 °C until use.

Western blot analysis

Experiments were performed as described previously (17, 31). Briefly, equal amounts of protein from all samples were subjected to SDS-PAGE and blotted to nitrocellulose. The blots were blocked in 5 % nonfat milk dissolved in TBS (20 mmol/L Tris-Cl, pH 7.4, 150 mmol/L NaCl), then probed for 2 h with an antibody to Na$^+$/Ca^{2+}-exchanger diluted 1:3000 in TBS, containing 1 % bovine serum albumin and 0.1 % TWEEN-20, or with antibodies to SR Ca^{2+}-ATPase (1:10000), and calsequestrin (1:2000), respectively. Then, the membranes were incubated for 1 h with a peroxidase-labeled secondary antibody (Amersham Buchler Ltd.). Immunoreactive bands were visualized utilizing a chemoluminescence kit (Amersham Buchler Ltd.) and exposure to a Kodak X-ray film. Specific bands were seen at 120 kDa, 70 kDa, and 40 kDa with the Na$^+$/Ca^{2+}-exchanger antibody, at ~110 kD with the SR Ca^{2+}-ATPase antibody, and at 53 kD with the calsequestrin antibody. The calsequestrin data were used as an internal standard to normalize the SERCA 2a and NCX1 data.

Northern blot analysis

Tissue (100–150 mg) was ground in liquid nitrogen and homogenized in lysis buffer RTL (Qiagen) using a FP 120 Fast Prep™ Cell Disruptor (Savant Instruments). Total RNA was extracted using RNeasy-Mini Kit (Qiagen) according to the manufacturer's instructions. Seven μg total RNA per lane were size-fractionated on a 0.7 mol/L formaldehyde/1 % agarose gel, transferred to nylon membrane (Duralon-UV™, Stratagene) by overnight capillary blotting, and fixed by UV irradiation. Hybridization was performed using Quick-Hyb Hybridization Solution (Stratagene) for 2 h at 68 °C. Blots were probed with a 0.57 kb Xbal/Xhol cDNA fragment of the human SERCA2a gene, a 0.65 kb EcoRI/PstI cDNA fragment of the human NCX1 gene, and a 0.58 kb Pstl/Pstl cDNA fragment of the rat ANP gene. Specific DNA probes for detection of glyceraldehyde-3-phosphate dehydrogenase (GAPDH) transcripts were generated by polymerase chain reaction (PCR). DNA probes were labeled with [^{32}P]dCTP by random priming (DNA-Labelling Kit, Pharmacia Biotech) and unbound radioactivity was removed by spin columns. Blots were washed 2×10 min in 2XSSC/0.1 % SDS at room temperature and 1×30 min in 0.1XSSC/0.1 % SDS at 60 °C. After autoradiography, specific signals were quantified by two dimensional laser densitometry. The GAPDH data were used as an internal standard to normalize the SERCA2a, Na^+/Ca^{2+}-exchanger, and ANP data.

Quantification of immunoreactive bands

Band densities were evaluated using a 2202 Ultrascan laser densitometer (LKB). Since several blots had to be performed for quantificating each protein in all samples, one heart was used as a reference on all blots. Na^+/Ca^{2+}-exchanger and SR Ca^{2+}-ATPase protein levels were normalized to calsequestrin protein levels to account for differences in connective tissue content. Each individual value respresents the mean of two independent determinations. A series of blots was preceded by checking linearity of the assay by plotting different amounts of proteins to corresponding densitrometric units.

Statistical analysis

Data are expressed as mean ± SEM. Comparison of force values at different stimulation rates were performed by repeated measures ANOVA, followed by Student-Newman-Keuls test. Differences between protein levels or force values of the different groups were tested for significance by one way ANOVA followed by Student-Newman-Keuls Test, or by Kruskal-Wallis one way ANOVA on ranks followed by Dunn's test. Correlations were examined by linear or non-linear regression analysis or by muliple regression analysis, if appropriate. A value of $p < 0.05$ was accepted as statistically significant.

Results

Influence of stimulation rate on force-frequency behavior

Figure 1 depicts the influence of increases in stimulation rate on force of contraction in nonfailing and end-stage failing human myocardium. Individual experiments from 9 non-failing and 20 end-stage failing human hearts are shown. On average, force of contraction increases at higher stimulation rates in nonfailing tissue (positive force-frequency relationship), but decreases in end-stage failing myocardium (negative force-frequency relationship). However, there is a large variation in force-frequency behavior from heart to heart: while the force-frequency relationship is relativeley flat in some preparations from nonfailing hearts, it can be quite preserved in some end-stage failing hearts. We have recently shown that the altered force-frequency behavior in failing human myocardium is related to paralell changes in intracellular Ca^{2+} transients (24) and SR Ca^{2+} content (25).

Variability of SR Ca^{2+}-ATPase protein expression between end-stage failing hearts

Since both SR Ca^{2+} content and intracellular Ca^{2+} transients critically depend on the capacity of SR Ca^{2+} reuptake mechanisms, we determined the protein expression of SR Ca^{2+}

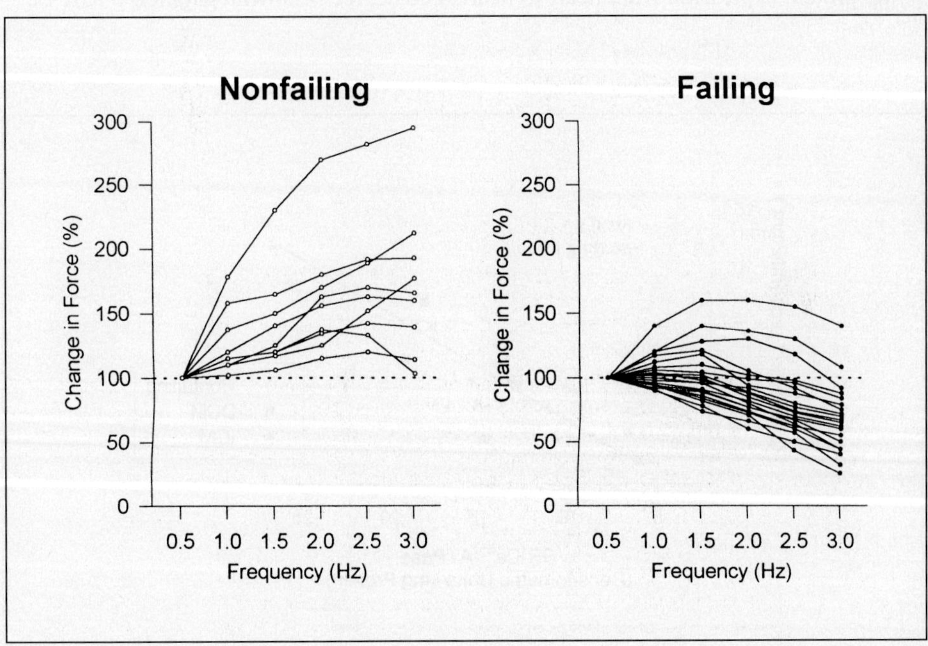

Fig. 1. Force-frequency behavior in isolated human nonfailing (left; n = 9) and end-stage failing (right; n = 20) myocardium. Each line represents one experiment from one nonfailing or failing heart. Developed active force is plotted versus stimulation frequency. Data adapted from (26).

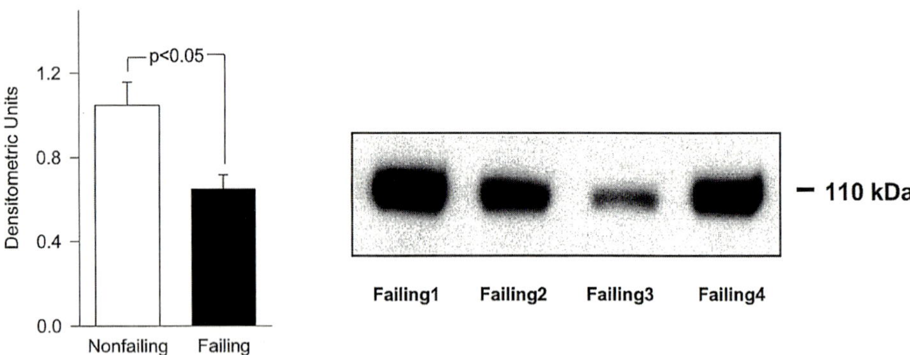

Fig. 2. Left: bar graphs showing average SERCA2a protein levels (normalized to calsequestrin; densitometric units) in nonfailing (n = 8) as compared to failing (n = 14) human myocardium. Right: representative Western blots showing immunochemical detection of SERCA2a in left ventricular myocardium from 4 failing human hearts. A single immunoreactive band at about 110 kDa was detected.

ATPase in both types of myocardium. The results are shown in Fig. 2. As becomes evident from the left part of the figure, protein expression of SR Ca^{2+} ATPase is significantly reduced in myocardium from end-stage failing hearts. However, as shown by 4 representative blots from 4 end-stage failing hearts (right side of Fig. 2), there is a large variation in SR Ca^{2+} pump protein expression from heart to heart. The degree of downregulation of SR Ca^{2+}-

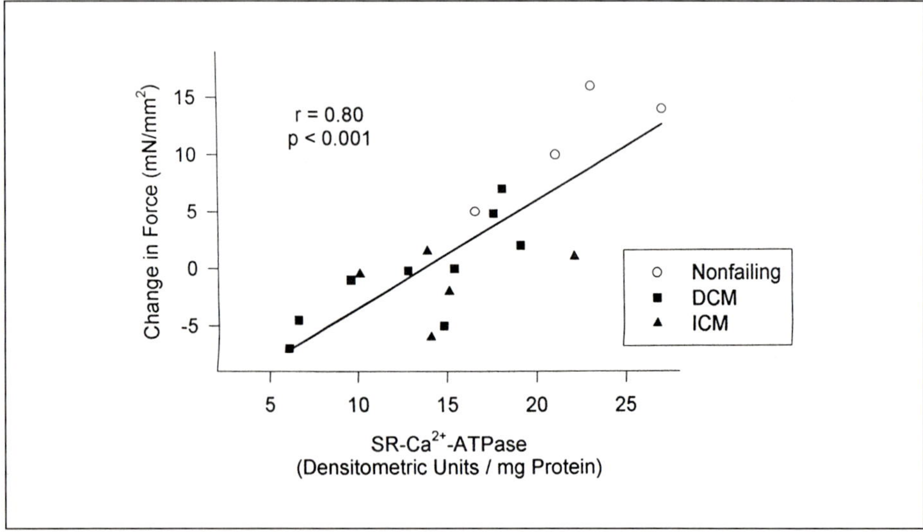

Fig. 3. Relation between the change in isometric twitch force after an increase in stimulation frequency from 0.5 to 2.0 Hz and protein levels of SR Ca^{2+}-ATPase. Functional and biochemical measurements were performed in myocardium from the same area of individual hearts. Adapted from (10).

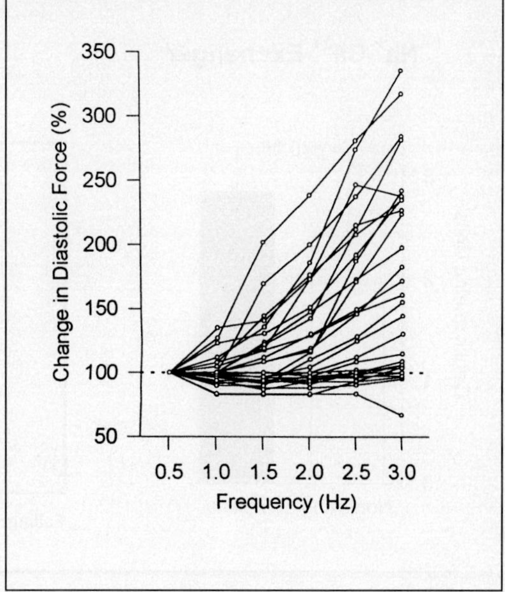

Fig. 4. Influence of stimulation frequency on diastolic tension in individual muscle strips (n = 28) from 28 failing human hearts. Each line represents contractile behavior of one muscle strip fom one heart.

ATPase proteins did not correspond to any of the clinical or hemodynamic parameters of the patients prior to transplantation. However, as depicted in Fig. 3, there was a close correlation between the degree of altered contractile function upon increases in stimulation rate and the severity of reduced protein expression of SR Ca^{2+}-ATPase in failing human hearts.

Variability of Na$^+$/Ca^{2+}-exchange protein expression between end-stage failing hearts

In addition to reduced SR Ca^{2+}-ATPase levels, protein expression of the Na$^+$/Ca^{2+}-exchanger may be increased in heart failure (31). Since Na$^+$/Ca^{2+}-exchange is the major transsarcolemmal Ca^{2+} elimination mechanism, we tested the hypothesis that its expression in individual end-stage failing hearts (with impaired SR Ca^{2+} reuptake) determines diastolic contractile behavior. Figure 4 demonstrates the influence of increasing stimulation rates on diastolic force-frequency behavior in 28 muscle strip preparations from 28 end-stage failing human hearts. As compared to nonfailing myocardium (with only minor changes in diastolic tension at increasing stimulation rates; (24)), there was a large variation in diastolic contractile behavior in end-stage failing human myocardium: while in some hearts, increasing stimulation rates did not affect diastolic tension, severe diastolic dysfunction was observed in muscle preparations from other end-stage failing hearts. Figure 5 (left) shows a significant upregulation of Na$^+$/Ca^{2+}-exchanger protein levels in end-stage failing myocardium from the 28 hearts which were functionally characterized as compared to nonfailing myocardium (n = 7). However, there was a large variation in the degree of upregulation of the Na$^+$/Ca^{2+}-exchanger from heart to heart. This becomes evident from 4 representative blots from 4 end-stage failing hearts on the right hand side of Fig. 5. To test whether protein expression determines diastolic function, individual protein expression of Na$^+$/Ca^{2+}-

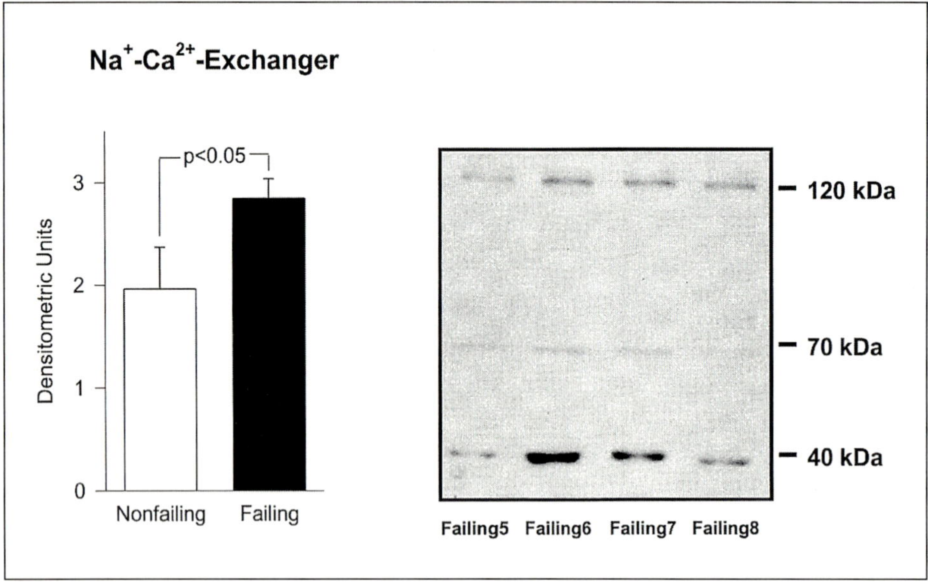

Fig. 5. Left: bar graphs showing average NCX1 protein levels (normalized to calsequestrin; densitometric units) in nonfailing (n = 7) as compared to failing (n = 28) human myocardium. Right: representative Western blots showing immunochemical detection of NCX1 in left ventricular myocardium from 4 failing human hearts.

exchanger from each heart was plotted against the degree of diastolic dysfunction at increasing stimulation rates in the isolated myocardium from the corresponding heart. As can be seen from Fig. 6, there was a close inverse relationship between protein levels of the Na$^+$/Ca^{2+}-exchanger (normalized to calsequestrin) and the frequency-dependent rise in diastolic tension when stimulation rate was increased from 0.5 to 3.0 Hz.

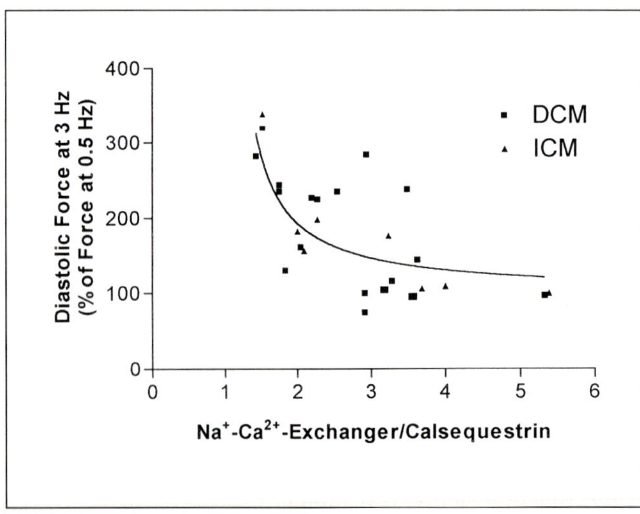

Fig. 6. Graph showing the relationship between protein levels of Na$^+$/Ca^{2+}-exchanger (normalized to calsequestrin) and the change in diastolic force upon an increase in stimulation frequency from 0.5 to 3.0 Hz given in percent of the diastolic force value at 0.5 Hz. Non-linear regression analysis yielded r = 0.74; p < 0.0001; n = 28.

Fig. 7. Representative Northern blots showing mRNA expression of SR Ca^{2+}-ATPase (SERCA2a), Na$^+$/Ca^{2+}-exchanger (NCX1), atrial natriuretic peptide (ANP), and glyceraldehyde-3-phosphate dehydrogenase (GAPDH) in subepicardium (epi) and subendocardium (endo) in the left ventricular wall from an end-stage failing human heart.

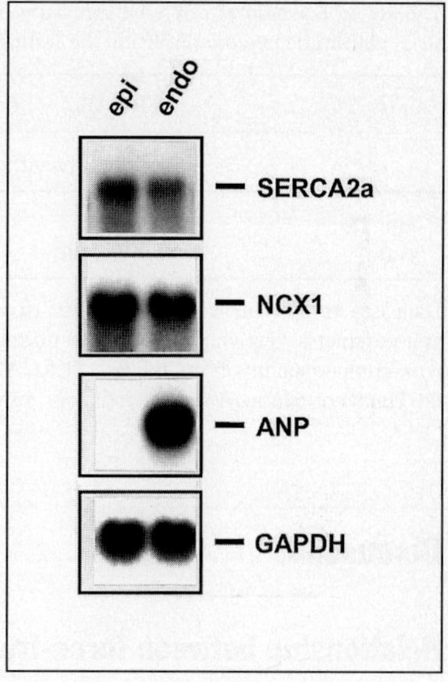

Transmural gradients of SR Ca^{2+}-ATPase and Na$^+$/Ca^{2+}-exchanger in failing hearts

To test whether variations of gene expression of Ca^{2+} handling proteins in failing hearts may also occur within different regions of the same heart, mRNA levels for SR Ca^{2+}-ATPase and Na$^+$/Ca^{2+}-exchanger were investigated in samples from the epicardial and the endocardial region of the left ventricular free wall of 8 end-stage failing hearts. In addition, mRNA levels of ANP as a marker for wall stress were investigated. Figure 7 shows representative Northern blots representing hybridization signals for SR Ca^{2+}-ATPase, Na$^+$/Ca^{2+}-exchanger, atrial natriuretic peptide, and glyceraldehyde-3-phosphate dehydrogenase (GAPDH) mRNA from the epicardial (epi) and the endocardial (endo) region of an end-stage failing heart. It becomes evident that mRNA expression of SR Ca^{2+}-ATPase is markedly reduced in the endocardial as compared to the epicardial region, while no difference is observed for Na$^+$/Ca^{2+}-exchanger or GAPDH. In contrast, ANP mRNA expression is highly upregulated in the endocardial as compared to the epicardial region. On average, SR Ca^{2+}-ATPase mRNA was significantly reduced by 24 ± 6 % in endo relative to epi (p < 0.05) in 8 end-stage failing hearts. In contrast, there was no significant difference in mRNA levels for SERCA2a between epicardial and endocardial myocardium from 4 non-failing human hearts. Interestingly and in contrast to transmural regulation of SERCA2a, there were no differences in Na$^+$/Ca^{2+}-exchanger mRNA levels between epicardial end endocardial regions in these hearts. The most pronounced differences between epi and endo were found for ANP expression. The expression level for ANP mRNA in epi reached only 4 ± 1 % (n = 8; p < 0.01) of that in endo. This pronounced upregulation of ANP mRNA in endo was not observed in nonfailing human myocardium: in 4 nonfailing hearts, no ANP mRNA expression could be detected in either epi or endo by means of Northern blot analysis. Average values for transmural mRNA expression of SERCA2a, Na$^+$/Ca^{2+}-exchanger, and ANP are summarized in Table 1. Similar results were obtained by using calsequestrin mRNA levels as a standard to normalize the SR Ca^{2+}-ATPase, NCX1, and ANP data.

Tabelle 1. Transmural mRNA expression of SR-Ca^{2+}-ATPase (SERCA2a), Na$^+$-Ca^{2+}-exchanger (NCX1), and atrial natriuretic peptide (ANP) in the failing human heart

	SERCA2a	NCX1	ANP
	relative arbitrary units (normalized to GAPDH)		
epi	1	1	0.04 ± 0.01*
endo	0.76 ± 0.06*	1.01 ± 0.17	1

Data are expressed as $\pm$ SEM. *$P < 0.05$ (n = 8; 5 DCM, 3 ICM). Overall group differences were first assessed by non-parametric-one-way ANOVA for normalized data. When a significant difference was found, multiple pairwise comparison involving the epi (SERCA2a, NCX1) or endo (ANP) group as a reference were performed with the Dunn correction. Abbreviations: epi, subepicardial; endo, subendocardial

Discussion

Relationship between force-frequency behavior and expression of SERCA2a

Disturbed function of the SR seems to play a predominant role for altered systolic perfomance of the failing human heart. Under physiological conditions, Ca^{2+} released from the SR is the major source of activator Ca^{2+} at the level of the contractile proteins (29). However, we have recently shown that both intracellular Ca^{2+} transients (24) and SR Ca^{2+} release (25) are significantly reduced in failing as compared to nonfailing myocardium at increasing stimulation rates, resulting in the negative force-frequency relationship. There is considerable evidence that disturbed Ca^{2+} homeostasis results from a decreased capacity of the SR to accumulate Ca^{2+} (10, 12, 24) possibly related to decreased expression of SERCA2a. In addition, altered SERCA2a protein function and increased inhibition of SERCA2a pump function by phospholamban may play a role. With respect to SERCA2a expression, reduced mRNA levels have been demonstrated in failing human myocardium of different etiologies (13, 16, 30). In contrast, while a reduced SERCA2a pump activity was consistently observed, reduced SERCA2a expression at the protein level remains a matter of debate. While a significant reduction in SERCA2a protein in end-stage failing human hearts of different etiologies has been described by several authors (10, 17, 31), this could not be observed by others (13, 20, 30).

In this study, we demonstrate a wide variation in force-frequency behavior in end-stage failing human myocardium. While average force frequency behavior was severely altered, both end-stage failing hearts showing a preserved positive force-frequency relation and end-stage failing hearts with a steep negative force-frequency relation could be observed (4, 26, this study). Interestingly, a similar degree of variation could be observed for protein expression of SERCA 2a between failing hearts. The latter may have contributed to the lack of significance in reduced SERCA2a protein levels in some studies (20, 30). However, most importantly, there was a clear correlation between the extent of downregulation of SERCA2a protein levels and altered force-frequency behavior. This indicates that though a wide variation in SERCA2a protein expression exists between different end-stage failing human hearts, SERCA2a levels determine systolic contractile function of failing human myocardium. Assuming a causal relation between the expression of SERCA2a and developed force of contraction, this causal relation may be explained by the following mechanisms: in hearts with a higher expression of SERCA2a, higher stimulation rates with increased transsarcolemmal Ca^{2+} influx (due to frequency-dependent upregulation of Ca^{2+}

transients (27) and increased Ca^{2+} influx per unit of time) result in increased Ca^{2+} loading and release from the SR. In myocardium with a lower expression of SERCA2a protein, the decrease in twitch tension at higher stimulation rates may be the consequence of a reduced time for Ca^{2+} reuptake to the SR, resulting in SR Ca^{2+} depletion due to reduced Ca^{2+} transport capacity.

Relationship between diastolic function and expression of Na$^+$/Ca^{2+}-exchanger

This study demonstrates that while average NCX1 protein expression is significantly increased in end-stage heart failure, a large variation in the degree of upregulation of this protein exists between different failing hearts. In the same hearts, there was a wide variation in diastolic force-frequency behavior, but a clear correlation between preserved diastolic function and increased NCX1 could be observed: the degree of rise in diastolic force at high stimulation rates was inversely related to protein expression of NCX1.

Diastolic function of the heart depends on passive elastic properties of the myocardium as well as on active diastolic force generation due to Ca^{2+} activation of contractile proteins (15, 32). Beat-to-beat regulation of diastolic Ca^{2+} occurs predominantly by SR Ca^{2+} reuptake and transsarcolemmal Na$^+$/Ca^{2+}-exchange (2, 3). In addition, Ca^{2+} uptake by mito-chondria may contribute to control of diastolic Ca^{2+} (19). The present finding of the close correlation between preserved diastolic function and increased expression of NCX1 supports the hypothesis that an increase in protein levels of NCX1 represents an important mechanism for regulation of diastolic Ca^{2+} elimination and diastolic function in the failing human myocardium. If protein levels reflect transport function, this may suggest that transsarcolemmal Ca^{2+} elimination is increased relative to Ca^{2+} uptake by the SR, especially since SERCA2a protein expression is reduced in failing hearts. Accordingly, by directly assessing intracellular Ca^{2+} handling using the photoprotein aequorin, Schlotthauer et al. (29) recently described a pronounced increase in transsarcolemmal Ca^{2+} cycling relative to intracellular Ca^{2+} turnover in failing as compared to nonfailing human hearts. Furthermore, NCX1 is the physiological competitor of SERCA2a for cytosolic Ca^{2+} elimination. There-fore, increased NCX1 and reduced SERCA2a activity could both result in a reduced SR Ca^{2+} content in failing human myocardium. Using rapid cooling contractures, we could indeed demonstate a stimulation-rate dependent decline in SR Ca^{2+} content underlying the inverse force-frequency relationship in failing human myocardium (25). Taken together, both the decline in SERCA2a expression and the increase in NCX1 expression may contribute to a gradual decline in SR Ca^{2+} content at higher heart rates, where diastole, i.e., the time for Ca^{2+} reuptake to the SR, shortens. In failing hearts with reduced SERCA2a, but unaltered NCX1 levels, both systolic and diastolic dysfunction may occur. In contrast, failing hearts showing increased NCX1 expression in concert with reduced SERCA2a may demonstrate reduced sytolic force generation, but relatively well preserved diastolic function at the expense of increased transsarcolemmal Ca^{2+} cycling. The latter, however, is energetically unfavorable due to the different Ca^{2+}/ATP transport stoichometry of SERCA2a (2:1) vs. NCX1 (1:1, since 1 mol ATP is required for 3 moles of Na$^+$ transported via Na$^+$/K$^+$-ATPase).

Transmural gradients of SR Ca^{2+}-ATPase and ANP in individual failing human hearts

In addition to differences in protein expression between nonfailing and failing human myocardium and distinct phenotype patterns in failing hearts, we could also demonstrate regional variations of Ca^{2+} handling proteins within the same failing hearts. We observed a significant transmural gradient for SR Ca^{2+}-ATPase mRNA expression from epicardial to endocardial layers. A transmural gradient was also observed for ANP (which was predominantly expressed in endocardial regions), but not for the Na^+/Ca^{2+}-exchanger.

As calsequestrin and GAPDH mRNA levels were similar across the left ventricular free wall, this argues against marked structural changes, i.e., myocyte loss, underlying the observed transmural gradients for SR Ca^{2+}-ATPase. Another possible factor involved in the downregulation of SR Ca^{2+}-ATPase in the endo- as compared to the epicardial region is increased wall stress. Wall stress rises in heart failure (23), and a steep transmural wall stress gradient was observed in end-stage failing hearts (18, 34). Wall stress is a major determinant for ventricular secretion of ANP (11, 28). Accordingly, ANP expression was highly upregulated in endocardial as compared to epicardial muscular layers in these failing hearts. Therefore, one may speculate that a reciprocal correlation between wall stress and SERCA2a expression may account for its overall downregulation in transmyocardial sections from failing hearts (10, 17), which result predominantly from a loss of SR Ca^{2+}-ATPase pump proteins at the endocardial level (this study). However, Na^+/Ca^{2+}-exchanger expression is upregulated in failing as compared to nonfailing myocardium (this study; 7, 31), but no transmural gradients for Na^+/Ca^{2+}-exchanger were observed in the present study. Therefore, mechanisms different from those regulating SERCA 2a expression may underly gene expression of Na^+/Ca^{2+}-exchanger.

Which molecular changes may be responsible for the differences in protein expression in failing human myocardium?

In the present study, differences in phenotype patterns could not be related to differences in etiologies of underlying cardiac diseases (ischemic versus idiopathic dilated cardiomyopathy) or to clinical or hemodynamic parameters obtained prior to transplantation. The finding of a relative increase in NCX1 over SERCA2a protein expression in failing myocardium is in accordance with a previous study on mRNA levels (31). This may suggest that these changes occur at a transcriptional level. Increased expression of NXC1 and decreased expression of SERCA2a reflects the fetal type of expression of Ca^{2+} cycling proteins (5, 14, 33). While decreased expression of SERCA2a was observed in many animal models of myocardial hypertrophy and failure, the finding of increased expression of NCX1 is less consistent (1, 8). This may suggest that regulation of expression of these Ca^{2+} transporters occurs by different and independent signals. This is further supported by the finding of the present study, where SERCA2a, but not NCX1 expression, is decreased in the endocardial as compared to the epicardial regions of failing human hearts.

In summary, discrimination of failing myocardium according to differences in systolic or diastolic function allows the identification of individual phenotypes with preserved or altered expression of both SERCA2a and NCX1. While the extent of downregulation of SERCA2a may predominantly determine systolic dysfunction due to reduced SR Ca^{2+} reaccumulation, NCX1 upregulation can prevent diastolic Ca^{2+} overload and relaxation abnormalities. The relative expression of SERCA2a and NCX1 may ultimately determine the degree of systolic and diastolic contractile dysfunction. However, since transmural gradients for SERCA2a, but not for NCX1 were observed, no coordinate regulation of the two Ca^{2+} cycling proteins seems to occur in failing human hearts.

References

1. Arai M, Matsui H, Periasamy M (1994) Sarcoplasmic reticulum gene expression in cardiac hypertrophy and heart failure. Circ Res 74: 555–564
2. Barry WH, Bridge JHB (1993) Intracellular calcium homeostasis in cardiac myocytes. Circulation 87: 1806–1815
3. Bassani JWM, Bassani RA, Bers DM (1994) Relaxation in rabbit and rat cardiac cells: Species-dependent differences in cellular mechanisms. J Physiol 476: 279–293
4. Beuckelmann DJ, Näbauer M, Erdmann E (1992) Intracellular calcium handling in isolated ventricular myocytes from patients with terminal heart failure. Circulation 85: 1743–1750
5. Boerth SR, Zimmer DB, Artman M (1994) Steady-state mRNA levels of the sarcolemmal Na⁺/Ca²⁺-exchanger peak near birth in developing rabbit and rat hearts. Circ Res 74: 354–359
6. Feldman MD, Alderman JR, Aroesty JM, Royal HD, Fergusin JJ, Owen RM, Grossman W, McKay RG (1988) Depression of systolic and diastolic myocardial reserve during atrial pacing tachykardia in patients with dilated cardiomyopathy. J Clin Invest 82: 1661–1669
7. Flesch M, Schwinger RH, Schiffer F, Frank K, Südkamp M, Kuhn-Regnier F, Arnold G, Böhm M (1996) Evidence for functional relevance of an enhanced expression of the Na⁺/Ca²⁺-exchanger in failing human myocardium. Circulation 94: 992–1002
8. Hasenfuss G (1998) Alterations of calcium-regulatory proteins in heart failure. Cardiovasc Res 37: 279–289
9. Hasenfuss G, Holubarsch C, Hermann HP, Astheimer K, Pieske B, Just H (1994) Influence of the force-frequency relationship on haemodynamics and left ventricular function in patients with non-failing hearts and in patients with dilated cardiomyopathy. Eur Heart J 15: 164–170
10. Hasenfuss G, Reinecke H, Studer R, Meyer M, Pieske B, Holtz J, Holubarsch Ch, Posival H, Just H, Drexler H (1994) Relation between myocardial function and expression of sarcoplasmic reticulum Ca²⁺-ATPase in failing and nonfailing human myocardium. Circ Res 75: 434–442
11. Kinnunen P, Vuolteenaho O, Martilla M, Ruskoaho H (1993) Mechanisms of atrial and brain natriuretic peptide release from rat ventricular myocardium: effect of stretching. Endocrinology 132: 1961–1970
12. Limas CJ, Olivari MT, Goldenberg IF, Levine TB, Benditt DG, Simon A (1987) Calcium uptake by cardiac sarcoplasmic reticulum in human dilated cardiomyopathy. Cardiovasc Res 21: 601–605
13. Linck B, Boknik P, Eschenhagen T, Müller FU, Neumann J, Nose M, Jones LR, Schmitz W, Scholz H (1996) Messenger RNA expression and immunological quantification of phospholamban and SR-Ca²⁺-ATPase in failing and nonfailing human hearts. Cardiovasc Res 31: 625–632
14. Lompré AM, Lambert F, Lakatta EG, Schwartz K (1991) Expression of sarcoplasmic reticulum Ca²⁺ ATPase and calsequestrin genes in rat heart during ontogenic development and aging. Circ Res 69: 1380–1388
15. Lorell BH, Grossmann W (1987) Cardiac hypertrophy: the consequences for diastole. J Am Clin Cardiol 95: 1189–1193
16. Mercadier JJ, Lompre AM, Duc P, Boheler KR, Fraysse JB, Wisnewsky C, Allen PD, Komajda M, Schwartz K (1990) Altered sarcoplasmic reticulum Ca²⁺-ATPase gene expression in the human ventricle during end-stage heart failure. J Clin Invest 85: 305–309
17. Meyer M, Schillinger W, Pieske B, Holubarsch C, Heilmann C, Posival H, Kuwajima G, Mikoshiba K, Just H, Hasenfuss G (1995) Alterations of sarcoplasmic reticulum proteins in failing human dilated cardiomyophty. Circulation 92: 778–784
18. Mirsky I (1973) Ventricular and arterial wall stress based on large deformation analysis. Biophys J 13: 1141–1159
19. Miyata H, Silverman HS, Sollott SJ, Lakatta EG, Stern MD, Hansford RG (1991) Measurement of mitochondrial free Ca²⁺ concentration in living single rat cardiac myocytes. Am J Physiol 261: H1123–H1134
20. Movesian MA, Karimi M, Green K, Jones LR (1994) Ca²⁺-transporting ATPase, phospholamban, and calsequestrin levels in nonfailing and failing human myocardium. Circulation 90: 653–657
21. Mulieri LA, Hasenfuss G, Leavitt B, Allen PD, Alpert NR (1992) Altered myocardial force-frequency relation in human heart failure. Circulation 85: 1743–1750
22. Mulieri LA, Leavitt B, Hasenfuss G, Allen PD, Alpert NR (1992) Contraction-frequency dependence of twitch and diastolic tension in human dilated cardiomyopathy (Tension-frequency-relation in cardiomyopathy). Bas Res Cardiol
23. Opie LH (1991) The Heart: Physiology and Metabolism. New York; NY; Raven Press
24. Pieske B, Kretschmann B, Meyer M, Holubarsch C, Weirich J, Posival H, Minami K, Just H, Hasenfuss G (1995) Alterations in intracellular calcium handling associated with the inverse force-frequency relation in human dilated cardiomyophathy. Circulation 92: 1169–1178
25. Pieske B, Maier LS, Weber T, Bers DM, Hasenfuss G (1997) Alterations in sarcoplasmic reticulum Ca²⁺ content in myocardium from patients with heart failure. Circulation 96 (Suppl I) 199
26. Pieske B, Sütterlin M, Schmidt-Schweda S, Minami K, Meyer M, Olschewski M, Holubarsch C, Just H, Hasenfuss G (1996) Diminished post-rest potentiation of contractile force in human dilated cardiomyophaty. J Clin Invest 98: 764–776

27. Piot C, Lemaire S; Albat B, Seguin J, Nargeot J, Richard S (1996) High frequency-induced upregulation of human cardiac calcium currents. Circulation 93: 120–128
28. Ruskoaho H, Leskinen H, Taskinen JMP, Mäntymaa P, Leppäluoto OVJ (1997) Mechanism of mechanical load-induced atrial natriuretic peptide secretion: role of the endothelin, nitric oxide, and angiotensin II. J Mol Med 75: 876–885
29. Schlotthauer K, Schattmann J, Bers DM, Maier LS, Schütt U, Minami K, Just H, Hasenfuss G, Pieske B (1998) Frequency-dependent changes in contribution of SR Ca^{2+} to Ca^{2+} transients in failing human myocardium assessed with ryanodine. J Mol Cell Cardiol 30: 1285–1294
30. Schwinger RH, Böhm M, Schmidt U, Karczewski P, Bavendiek U, Flesch M, Krause EG, Erdmann E (1995) Unchanged protein levels of SERCA II and phospholamban but reduced Ca^{2+} uptake and Ca^{2+}-ATPase activity of cardiac sarcoplasmic reticulum from dilated cardiomyophaty patients compared with patients with nonfailing hearts. Circulation 92: 3220–3228
31. Studer R, Reinecke H, Bilger J, Eschenhagen T, Böhm M, Hasenfuss G, Just H, Holtz J, Drexler H (1994) Gene expression of the cardiac Na^+/Ca^{2+}-exchanger in end-stage human heart failure. Circ Res 75: 443–453
32. Sys SU, Brutsaert DL (1995) Diagnostic significance of impaired LV systolic relaxation in heart failure. Circulation 92: 3377–3380
33. Vetter R, Studer R, Reinecke H, Kolar F, Ostadalova I, Drexler H (1995) Reciprocal changes in the postnatal expression of the sarcolemmal Na^+/Ca^{2+}-exchanger and SERCA2a in rat heart. J Mol Cell Cardiol 27; 8: 1689–1701
34. Yin FCP (1981) Ventricular wall stress. Circ Res 49: 829–842

Author's address:
PD Dr. Burkert Pieske
Georg-August-Universität Göttingen
Zentrum Innere Medizin
Abteilung Kardiologie und Pneumologie
Robert-Koch-Str. 40
37075 Göttingen, Germany
email: pieske@med.uni-goettingen.de

Apoptosis in the overloaded myocardium: potential stimuli and modifying signals

H. Schumann, H. Heinrich,* B. Bartling, D. Darmer, J. Holtz

Institut für Pathophysiologie, Medizinische Fakultät, Martin-Luther-Universität Halle-Wittenberg, Halle, Germany

Abstract

Distension-induced apoptosis of cardiomyocytes has been proposed as a mechanism for the progression from overload-induced cardiac hypertrophy to terminal heart failure with dilative remodeling, since extreme distension of myocardial preparations in vitro or of isolated myocytes in culture induces apoptosis. Furthermore, a very low number of apoptotic myocytes, disseminated in nonischemic myocardial areas of overloaded hearts, is demonstrable in experimental models and in explanted human myocardium. Hemodynamic unloading of terminally failing human hearts by ventricular assist devices reduces the amount of apoptotically cleaved DNA in myocardial extraxts and time-dependently renormalizes the myocardial expression of potentially proapoptotic signal molecules from the apoptotic machinery. While a cellular mechanism for distension-induced myocyte apoptosis in situ is not established, a tentative working hypothesis for the induction of apoptosis in overloaded, nonischemic myocardium postulates the combined actions of impaired mitochondrial function, exaggerated neuroendocrine activity, cytosolic calcium overload, and attenuated survival signals from cytoskeleton, from gp130 containing receptors, and from IGF-1. However, it is not yet possible to derive a rate of myocyte loss from the reported figures of apoptotic myocyte nuclei in overloaded myocardium. Therefore, the causal role of demonstrable myocyte apoptosis in terminal hear failure is unknown.

Introduction

Apoptosis, the "cellular suicide" or "programmed cell death", of cardiomyocytes is associated with the physiological pre- and perinatal organogenesis of the heart as well as with the patho-physiological myocardial dysfunction in myocarditis, cardiac allograft rejection, arrhythmogenic right ventricular dysplasia, acute myocardial infarction, and overload cardiomyopathy (for recent reviews see (11, 29, 91, 106, 150, 175)). Based on theoretical considerations, it was proposed in 1994 that distension-induced cardiomyocyte apoptosis is the mechanism causing the transition from compensated cardiac pressure overload to ouvert heart failure (24). This speculative proposal triggered great interest, since it contained an attractive theoretical concept for the progressive vicious cycle of cardiac failure,

* Supported by a stipendium from the Deutsche Herzstiftung

Table 1. Overload-induced apoptosis of cardiomyocytes in ventricular myocardium

Experiment or intervention	Observation	Reference
Severe overstretching of rat papillary muscles *in vitro*	21-fold increase in apoptotic cardiomyocytes (identified by TUNEL[a] positive nuclei)	(37)
Stretching of isolated adult rat cardiomyocytes, cultured on distensible membranes	Angiotensin II-mediated cardiomyocyte apoptosis via p53 activation	(134)
Experimental cardiac pressure overload in rats	Ventricular cardiomyocyte apoptosis demonstrable during the first 7 days after overload induction	(265)
Transition from stable, compensated overload hypertrophy to heart failure in spontaneously hypertensive rats or mice	Increased occurrence of apoptotic ventricular cardiomyocytes in comparison with normotensive animals	(81, 142, 56)
Experimental myocardial infarction due to coronary ligation in mice or rats	Apoptosis of cardiomyocytes, scattered in the viable ventricular myocardium remote from the ischemic area	(36, 140)
Ventricular tissue samples from autopsies of patients deceased from acute myocardial infarctions	cardiomyocyte apoptosis in the surviving myocardium remote from the infarcted area	(190, 234)
Ventricular samples from explanted, terminally failing human hearts (dilative cardiomyopathy as well as ischemic heart disease (noninfarcted areas) and from nonfailing donor hearts, not used for transplantation	20-fold cardiomyocyte apoptotic index in failing vs. donor hearts; 0.24% apoptotic cardiomyocytes in failing, 0.01% in donor hearts; enhanced "DNA ladder" formation in failing hearts;	(174) (189) (240)
Ventricular samples from terminally failing human ventricles, obtained during installation of a ventricular assist device (VAD) and, following VAD-induced hemodynamic unloading of 5 – 26 weeks duration, from the same ventricles during heart transplantation	reduction in ventricular apoptosis (DNA ladder formation) under VAD-induced hemodynamic unloading in the majority of patients	(12)

[a]TUNEL (= terminal uridine nick end labeling), a technique for identification of apoptotic nuclei by DNA labeling of apoptotically fragmented DNA. Unless otherwise stated, identification of cardiomyocyte apoptosis in all studies from the table was obtained by variations of DNA nick end labeling techniques.

driven by compensatory enhancement of cardiac load and further load-induced myocyte losses.

Meanwhile, important experimental and clinical data, consistent with this concept, have been obtained (Table 1). These *in vitro* and *in vivo* data support the existence of distension-associated apoptosis of cardiomyocytes in failing myocardium. However, these data cannot establish whether and to what extent the demonstrable apoptosis of a rather small number of myocytes causally contributes to the failure of the overloaded myocardium *in vivo*.

A number of other important aspects of this speculative concept are also unresolved: a causal relation between overload-induced myocyte distension and apoptosis of these distended myocytes is far from being proven. For the induction of myocardial apoptosis by overstretching of papillary muscle *in vitro* (Table 1), a degree of myocyte distension has to be applied, which is unlikely to occur *in vivo*. The demonstration of myocyte apoptosis in myocardial areas of presumably enhanced wall stress in experimental and clinical *ex vivo* analyses (Table 1) cannot exclude that additional factors contributed to the induction of apoptosis, such as augmented neuroendocrine activity (see below). Similarly, the reduction of myocardial apoptosis in response to hemodynamic unloading by ventricular assist devices in patients with terminal heart failure (12), which is associated with reduced ventricular distension, is also accompanied by altered peripheral perfusion, altered systemic

Table 2. Viral and human endogenous inhibitors of apoptosis

Group	Viral inhibitor	Human homologs	Motif	Mode of apoptosis inhibition
1)	vFLIP (268) BORFE2 (282) MC159, E8 (99, 20)	FLIP (101) =I-FLICE, MRIT, Usurpin, CASH, casper,	DED, proteolytic inactive caspase-like domain CLARP, FLAME-1	Blocking of the formation of an active DISC, interaction with FADD and/or caspase-8
3)	African swine fever virus Bcl-2 homolog (220) E1B 19K protein (212, 282)	Bcl-2 protein family	BH domains	Interaction of pro- and antiapoptotic proteins, block of mitochondrial PT, cytochrome c release
4)	Baculovirus Op-IAP, Cp-IAP (43, 49)	NAIP (224) XIAP = MIHA = hILP hIAP1 = MIAB = c-IAP2 hIAP2 = MIHC = c-IAP1 (144) survivin (5)	BIR, RING finger	With the exception of NAIP, interaction and inhibition of activation of caspase-3 and -7 (55, 225), downstream of mitochondrial events (60); c-IAP2 is involved in NF-kB activation (39)
4)	p35 (17) CrmA (214)	a not jet identified endogenous heat-labile ICE-inhibitor found in SMC (237)	Serpin superfamily	Inhibition of proteolytic activity of caspases
5)	HPV typ16/18 E6 protein (E7), HCV core protein, HBC encoded x antigen, HAV protein E1B 55kDa, HHV 6 ORF-1, human cytomegalovirus mtr II oncoprotein, EBV oncogene LMP1, group c adenovirus E4orf6 (273)	mdm2	p53-binding motif	Binding, inactivation and ubiquitin-dependent degradation of p53
6)	Unknown	CAD/ICAD-system (62, 232)		ICAD (=DFF 40) blocks DNase activity of CAD and its translocation into the nucleus, ICAD cleavage by caspases

Abbreviations: FLIP: FLICE inhibitory protein; FLAME: FADD-like anti-apoptotic molecule that regulates Fas/TNFR1-induced apoptosis; CLARP: caspase like apoptosis regulatory protein; IAP: inhibitor of apoptosis protein; DED: death effector domain; BIR: baculoviral IAP repeat; BH: Bcl-2 homologous domains; PT: permeability transition; Crm: cytokine response modifier; CAD: caspase activated deoxyribonuclease; ICAD: inhibitor of CAD; DFF: DNA fragmentation factor

activation of inflammation, and normalized neuroendocrine activity. Furthermore, we cannot yet quantify the degree of apoptotic cardiomyocyte losses in a failing heart. While the nuclear morphology of myocytes undergoing apoptosis and the techniques for their identification are well established (for details see (91)), we do not know exactly the duration of the apoptotic death of a myocyte in the failing heart and therefore cannot calculate rates of apoptotic cell losses. Furthermore, the cellular composition of failing human myocardium is not only determined by the rate of myocyte losses, but also by the rate of myocyte proliferation (113). The classical dogma of a complete block of the cell cycle in terminally differentiated myocytes of the adult myocardium is presently challenged: recently, it could be demonstrated by confocal microscopy that true myocyte mitoses and myocyte proliferations, not only augmentations of myocyte polyploidy, do occur in adult human myocardium and even more so in terminally failing human ventricles (113), similarly as in human brain cortex (64). This means that an apoptotic "melting rate" of failing myocardium cannot be obtained from reported figures of apoptosis-positive myocyte nuclei in failing hearts (Table 1).

Nonwithstanding these open questions, efforts to unravel the incompletely understood program of apoptosis in overloaded cardiac myocytes appears worth while. Many potential sites for specific interventions into the apoptotic program by endogenous signals or by exogenous molecules are known (Table 2), mainly from studies on cells of the immune system or from tumors (for reviews see (10, 76, 267, 273)). In the myocardium, myocyte losses due to coronary occlusion and due to ischemia/reperfusion can be reduced or at least retarded by several specific interventions, which interfere with the apoptotic program (for review see (11)). This susceptibility to antiapoptotic interventions illustrates that ischemia associated myocyte necrosis contains important apoptotic steps (although features of necrosis or oncosis are clearly demonstrable in this mixed form of ischemic myocyte death (11, 32, 108)). It remains to be demonstrated whether antiapoptotic interventions similarly might affect the occurrence of myocyte apoptosis in the overloaded, failing myocardium and whether such interventions really do modify the progression of overload-induced heart failure. Furthermore, ongoing research asks whether there is an attenuation of myocyte apoptosis under established forms of heart failure therapy and whether this attenuation contributes to the established protective actions of those therapies.

Elements of the apoptotic program

A high number of recent excellent reviews on various aspects of the rapidly growing field of apoptosis has been published within the last 18 months (1, 9, 65, 91, 105, 150, 207, 216, 238, 269), stressing the highly conserved nature of the central apoptotic machinery, but also the great variability and versatility in the induction and control of the program in different cell types. Therefore, a strongly simplified, general scheme is given in Fig. 1 as a basic skeleton of the central machinery.

Caspases

The final steps of this machinery are executed by a cascade of strictly specific proteases. They are called *caspases* (for *c*ysteine-containing *asp*artic acid proteases), since all 13

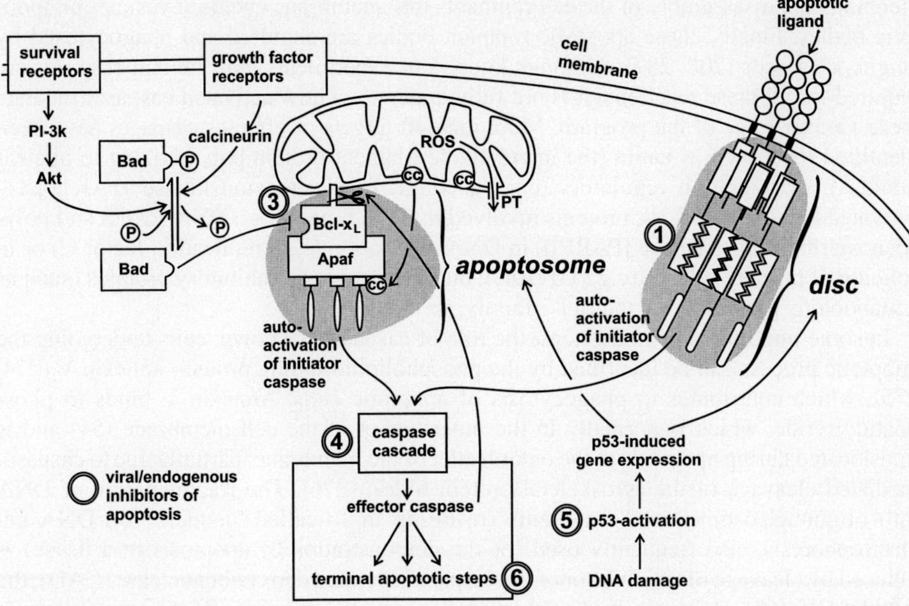

Fig. 1. Signal elements of the apoptotic program and inhibitory interaction sites of viral apoptosis inhibitors and of their endogenous homologs.
The activated cascade of caspases triggers the terminal apoptotic steps of the program with nuclear DNA degradation, degradation of cytoskeleton and cytosol, membrane phospholipid translocation and formation of apoptotic bodies (cytosolic remnants surrounded by altered membranes). Caspase activation is started by autoactivation of initiator caspases, resulting from oligomerization of the initiator caspases at mitochondrial apoptosomes or at "death inducing signal complexes" (disc) at the cytosolic death domains of receptors from the TNF receptor family. Signal transduction from survival receptors causes phosphorylation of the proapoptotic protein Bad, calcineurin activation by growth factor signaling dephosphorylates Bad. Dephosphorylated Bad induces caspase activation via several mechanisms, e.g.: by complexing and inactivating the antiapoptotic Bcl-x$_L$.
The numbers in double circles denote goups of inhibitors listed in Table 2.

Abbreviations: PI-3k: phosphatidylinositol-3 kinase; Bad: Bcl-associated death inducer; Apaf: apoptosis protease activating factor; ROS: reactive oxygen species; CC: cytochrome c; PT: permeability transition pore; disc: death inducing signaling complex.

caspases so far identified in mammals (3) have a cysteine in their active center and an absolute requirement for cleavage after aspartic acid. The last four amino acids N-terminal to the cleavage site of substrates as recognition motifs as well as some tertiary structural elements of substrates are specific for individual caspases, explaining their different biological functions (269). All caspases are constitutively expressed as proenzymes with 3 domains: a N-terminal regulatory prodomain, a large ($\approx$ 20 kD) subunit, and a small subunit ($\approx$ 10 kD). Activation of the procaspases requires proteolytic cleavage between these domains and heterodimerization to a tightly associated tetramer, consisting of two large and two small subunits with two independent catalytic sites. Caspases can be grouped into *initiator* caspases with large prodomains, activated by binding of distinct structural motifs of their prodomains to various proapoptotic signal complexes, and into *effector* caspases with short prodomains and very high enzymatic activity (269, 270).

Activated effector caspases induce the terminal events of the apoptotic program, including DNA fragmentation and chromatin condensation, cytosol proteolysis and cell shrinkage, translocation of membrane phospholipids to the outer membrane leaflet, membrane blebbing, and disassembly of the cell remnants into membrane enclosed vesicles or apoptotic bodies. Finally, these apoptotic remnant bodies are engulfed and phagocytosed by neighboring cells (208, 287). Although knock-out experiments indicate that caspases are required for all these reactions, it is not fully understood how activated caspases mediate these various steps of the program. More than 40 targets of effector caspases have been identified (50), such as lamin (the intermediate filament protein polymerizing to nuclear laminas), cytoskeleton regulators (e.g., gelsolin, focal adhesion kinase [FAK], p21-activated kinase 2 [PAK2]), proteins involved in DNA repair (e.g., DNA-PKCS and poly-adenosylribose-polymerase [PARP]), in DNA replication (e.g., replication factor C) or in splicing of primary mRNA (e.g., U1-70K), but also apoptosis-inhibitory proteins (such as antiapoptotic proteins from the Bcl-2 family, see below).

In some important apoptotic steps, the role of caspases is known: cells undergoing the apoptotic process can be identified by the phospholipid-binding protein annexin V (274, 275), which contributes to phagocytosis of apoptotic cells. Annexin V binds to phosphatidylserine, which is normally in the inner leaflet of the cell membrane (54) and is translocated during apoptosis to the outer leaflet of the membrane, partially due to caspase-mediated cleavage of the cytoskeletal protein fodrin (276). The fragmentation of DNA into oligonucleosome-sized fragments (resulting in so-called "ladders" on DNA gel electrophoresis, also frequently used for the demonstration of apoptosis in a tissue) is induced by cleavage of an inhibitor of the caspase-activated deoxyribonuclease (CAD), the I^{CAD}/DFF45 (62). However, it is not known how much activation of effector caspases is necessary for pushing a cell beyond the point of no return within the deadly program and which apoptotic reaction is the critical step. Probably, such a step is different in a cultured cell without intercellular contacts or in a cell within a tissue, surrounded by other cells starting the apoptotic phagocytosis.

Similarly as in other complex proteolytic systems, the caspase cascade is regulated by a combination of inhibitor and activator processes (269). The initiator caspases have the potential of autoactivation, which is stimulated by complexing the regulatory prodomain of the initiator caspases to one of the two important apoptosis-regulating complexes in cells: the cytosolic complexes on the death receptors of the cell membrane or the so-called "apoptosomes", anchored by antiapoptotic proteins of the Bcl-2 family to the outer mitochondrial membrane (see Fig. 1).

Death receptors

These receptors are structurally similar type I transmembrane proteins belonging to the TNF receptor family (238). They have 2 to 4 imperfect repeats of 40 amino acid domains with 6 cysteine residues, and they contain an homologous cytoplasmic domain, which is called "death domain", since it mediates the transmission of the apoptotic signal (173, 264). The activation of these receptors occurs by a family of type II transmembrane proteins, which act in a trimeric form (Fig. 1), inducing trimerization of their cognate receptors. This trimerization is the critical step, which results in activation of an initiator caspase by complexing its regulatory prodomain to the death domains of the receptor trimers, with the help of one or two adapter molecules (Fig. 1). This association at the death domain complexes brings the initiator procaspases (which have a very low, but detectable catalytic activity) into close proximity, allowing for intermolecular autoproteolytic activation of the procaspase, until the activated caspases can activate downstream caspases and the whole cascade. This receptor activation by trimerization is most effectively induced by their cognate ligands, when these ligands are inserted in the cell membrane of immune cells (but several death recep-

Table 3. "Death domain"-containing receptors of the TNF receptor family

Ligand	Receptor	Competitive antagonists
FasL	Fas = CD95 = Apo1 (9)	sFas: 5 soluble Fas isoforms by alternative splicing; DcR3: secreted FasL-binding protein with homology to extracellular domains of the TNF receptor family (203); sFas isoforms are expressed in normal human myocardium, but are downregulated in failing hearts (240)
TNFα	TNF-RI = CD120a = p55 (159)	sTNF-RI (generated by proteolytic cleavage of membrane receptor TNF-RI) (159)
TRAIL = Apo2L (204)	DR4 = TRAIL-R1 DR5 = TRAIL-R2 = TRICK2 (236, 242, 247)	TRAIL-binding membrane receptors without or with incomplete intracellular signal transducing domain = decoy receptors (195) DcR1 = TRID = TRAIL-R3 = LIT DcR2 = TRUNDD
Apo3L = TWEAK (38, 154, 155)	DR3 = LARD (243)	11 isoforms by alternative splicing; some of them soluble receptors (243)
?	DR6 (194)	2 isoforms by alternative splicing

Abbreviations: Fas: FS7-associated cell surface antigen; FasL: Fas ligand; DcR: decoy receptor; TNF: tumor necrosis factor; DR: death receptor; TRAIL: TNF-related apoptosis-inducing ligand; TRICK: TRAIL receptor inducer of cell killing; TRID: TRAIL receptor without an intracellular domain; LIT: Lymphocyte inhibitor of TRAIL; TRUNDD: TRAIL receptor with truncated death domain; TWEAK: TNF releated with weak ability to induce cell death; LARD: Lymphoid associated receptor with death domain.
Note that a nerve growth factor receptor also contains a cytosolic death domain, but is not a member of the TNF receptor family.

tor ligands occur also at cells outside the immune system). Table 3 lists the death domain-containing receptors of the TNF receptor family, their cognate ligands, and the competitive antagonists of these receptors. Most ligands of Table 3 exist also as soluble forms, cleaved from their membranes by specific metalloproteases (238), and they can activate their receptors also as soluble ligands, but with less efficacy. Furthermore, death receptor oligomerization with activation of caspases is also possible without interaction with their ligands, for instance under irradiation, which directly oligomerizes death receptors (238). The death receptor activation by ligands not only results in caspase activation, but also in the stimulation of other functions not directly related to cell death. Such caspase unrelated signals are activation of sphingomyelinase with formation of ceramide, activation of ceramide-activated protein kinase (CAPK), phosphorylation of Raf-I and other kinase cascades, the activation of $NF_{\kappa B}$, the activation of phospholipase C, and the recruitment of pathways involving the stress-activated c-Jun N-terminal kinase (JNK) (9, 238, 266).

The receptor-mediated caspase activation is regulated and modulated at several levels: at the interaction between ligands and receptors by competitive antagonists (Table 3), at the binding of receptor death domains with adapter molecules, and/or at the interaction between adapter molecules and activator caspase prodomains (Fig. 1). At the level of ligand-receptor interaction, cells can form competitive antagonists as soluble receptors (by enzymatic cleavage of receptors or by alternative splicing of receptor RNA) or as decoy receptors, competing with the cognate death receptor for the activating ligand (Table 3).

Antiapoptotic inhibitor proteins, competing for the interaction site of adapter molecules with the regulatory prodomain of initiator caspases (the death effector domain, see Fig. 1), are called ADEDs (antiapoptotic death effector domain proteins). Molecules such as FLIP/

FLAME (see Table 2) belong to this class of regulator proteins. Interestingly, ongoing research (not yet published) indicates that the activity/availability of ADEDs for inhibition of apoptotic signal transduction at this level can be regulated by certain cytokine receptors.

Mitochondrial apoptosomes

The major regulator of the caspase cascade activation during the induction of apoptosis is a protein complex or "apoptosome" at the outer mitochondrial membrane (93). This complex consists of cytosolic proteins of the Bcl-2 family, which are anchored in the outer mitochondrial membrane (such as, Bcl-2 or Bcl-x$_L$) and keep the apoptosome attached to the outer membrane of the mitochondrion, as long as there is no activation of apoptosis. Other important elements of the apoptosome are APAF-1 (for apoptosis protease activating factor), the mammalian homolog of the proapoptotic factor CED-4 of C. *elegans* (301) and mitochondria-associated initiator caspases such as procaspase-9 or APAF-3 (139). Autoactivation of the initiator caspases in the apoptosome is required for triggering apoptosis from these mitochondrial apoptosomes, and this is achieved by several proteins and factors released from the intermembrane space of the mitochondria into the cytosol. Surprisingly, one of such released mitochondrial proteins necessary for triggering the cascade was identified as the mature heme-containing form of cytochrome c (120, 121, 145). Other released proteins in the apoptosome, probably contributing to the cascade activation are initiator caspases and another mitochondrial protein with proteolytic activity, AIF (apoptosis-inducing factor (256, 298)). Finally, the apoptotic, caspase activating interaction of these released mitochondrial factors requires the presence of ATP released into the cytosol. While the exact mechanism causing the release of proapoptotic signal proteins from the mitochondria is not yet clear, there is general agreement that a collapse of the membrane potential of the inner mitochondrial membrane is associated with and involved in the mitochondrial release of apoptotic proteins (297, 300). Antiapoptotic proteins of the Bcl-2 family (mainly Bcl-x$_L$, Bcl-2 and Mcl-1) proved to prevent this collapse of the mitochondrial membrane potential, the release of proapoptotic mitochondrial signal proteins, and the activation of the caspase cascade (169, 259). Probably, the factors released from the mitochondrial intermembrane space are required for releasing APAF-1 from the antiapoptotic Bcl proteins, changing APAF-1 into an apoptosis promoting factor. Furthermore, activated effector caspases cleave Bcl-x$_L$/Bcl-2 from their anchorage at the outer mitochondrial membrane, and these cleavage products of Bcl-x$_L$/Bcl-2 appear to act proapoptotically, further potentiating the activation of the cascade (Fig. 1).

This association of mitochondrial apoptotic signal release with the mitochondrial membrane potential puts the regulation of this mitochondrial membrane potential into the center of apoptosis research. The general assumption is that in all eukaryotic cells, apoptosis can be induced by release of mitochondrial factors. In agreement with this assumption, release of cytochrome c from mitochondria is demonstrated in the failing human heart with ongoing myocyte apoptosis as well as in cultured cardiomyocytes under various apoptotic stimuli *in vitro* (22, 118). Disturbances of this mitochondrial membrane potential regulation due to oxidative stress, cytosolic Ca^{2+} overload and/or advanced age may be important determinants of apoptosis susceptibility (see Mitochondrial dysfunction and apoptosis section). Furthermore, the antiapoptotic function of Bcl-x$_L$, Bcl-2 or Mcl-1 in the mitochondrial apoptosome can be modulated by heterocomplexation with proapoptotic Bcl proteins such as Bax or Bad, which abolish the protective function of Bcl-x$_L$ and congeners. Phosphorylation of Bad by survival factors (see Mitochondrial dysfunction and apoptosis section) helps to keep the protective potential of Bcl-x$_L$/Bcl-2/Mcl-1 in function, dephosphorylation of Bad by the phosphatase calcineurin acts in the opposite direction (see Enhanced neuroendocrine activity as promoter of cardiomyocyte apoptosis section). Finally, interaction of apoptosis-inducing death domain receptor complexes and mitochondrial apoptosomes is mediated by signals, which have been called CAF (caspase activating factor) (254) or CIF (cytochrome c efflux-inducing factor) (82, 83) and may be identical with or closely related to the Bcl protein Bid (77).

The cellular expression of many elements in the mitochondrial apoptosomes or in the death-inducing signal complexes at the death domain-containing receptors of the cell membrane is under the regulation of tumor suppressor genes such as p53 (Fig. 1). This regulation by p53 activation, which occurs in response to DNA damage and to several other forms of cellular damage, is considered as very important in tumor biology and will not be considered here, although p53 activation has been observed in cardiomyocytes under hypoxia (149) or acute stretching (134).

Apoptotic elements in cardiomyocytes

As any other eukaryotic cell type, the cardiomyocyte contains the complete apoptotic program, and this program contributes to the adjustment of the cellular stoichiometry of the heart during embryonic organogenesis (106, 107). Therefore, it is no surprise that key steps of the apoptotic program, such as oligonucleosome-sized DNA fragmentation, caspase-3 activation, translocation of phosphatidylserine to the outer leaflet of the cell membrane, collapse of the mitochondrial cell membrane, release of cytochrome c into the cytosol, and caspase-3 mediated cleavage of Bcl-x$_L$ have been observed in isolated cardiomyocytes or in intact myocardium (for reviews see (29, 91, 150)). Furthermore, cardiomyocyte death induced by ischemia/reperfusion demonstrates several steps of the apoptotic program and appears to be a variable mixture of regulated activation of the apoptotic program and of a necrotic collapse of any cellular regulation (11, 32). While the existence of the program and its activation in response to cellular damage is common in all cell types, organ-specific features of the program appear to consist of quantitative variabilities in the basal expression of many different effector and signal molecules of the program. At the level of proteins, such quantitative data are not yet available for myocardium or for any other organ. At the level of message concentration, the predominantly expressed antiapoptotic *bcl-2* genes in the myocardium are *bcl-x$_L$* and *mcl-1*; among the death domain-containing receptors, the myocardial mRNA abundance (preferentially in myocytes) is TNF-R1 > DR6 > TRAIL receptors > Fas (data from our laboratory), but these data must not necessarily indicate the regulatory relevance of these genes for the induction of the apoptotic program in the heart. From research in cells from tumors and from the immune system, a dominant role of death domain-containing receptors and their activation by their cognate receptors (see Table 3) in the activation of apoptosis has emerged. This might be quite different in other cell types. Although most of the death domain-containing receptors are expressed in the myocardium, partially at a rather substantial level of mRNA concentration, as mentioned above, we do not yet see any convincing evidence for an apoptosis-triggering role of these receptors in the intact myocardium *in vivo*.

This apparent discrepancy is best illustrated for the TNF receptor type I (TNF-RI) in the heart: the heart is a TNF-producing organ, the cardiomyocytes contribute to this local production, they contain measurable quantities of TNF-RI, and they respond with apoptosis to the exposure to TNF under culture conditions (for review see (159)). Cardiac overexpression of TNF causes cardiac failure with signs of·apoptosis in mice; and in patients with terminal heart failure, enhanced expression of the autocrine myocardial TNF system and systemic activation of the TNF system are demonstrable together with significant myocyte apoptosis, suggesting a causal relation between TNF activation and myocardial apoptosis (159). However, this postulated relation could not be confirmed: chronic infusion of TNF, resulting in pathophysiologically relevant plasma concentrations of TNF, caused depressed cardiac function and dilatative ventricular remodeling, but not clear signs of enhanced myocyte apoptosis (28). This result pushes other components of the signal transduction of TNF-RI besides caspase activation, such as ceramide formation, NF-κB activation, and activation of cysteine proteases or protein kinases into the focus of interest (266). For the myocyte apoptosis in the overloaded myocardium, we hypothesize that the integrated effect of disturbances in mitochondrial function and in cytosolic Ca^{2+} homeostasis, enhanced activation of receptors of the neuroendocrine activity and alterations in the regulation of myocardial survival factors are relevant for the activation of the death program. Therefore, the available information concerning these aspects will be discussed here.

Mitochondrial dysfunction and apoptosis

As discussed above, a critical step in the activation of the apoptotic cascade is the caspase activation at mitochondrial apoptosomes by release of proapoptotic factors from mitochondria (see Fig. 1). This brings the mitochondria and their disturbed function into play as an additional potential culprit for the induction of apoptosis in the failing heart. In the myocardium, these cytoplasmatic organelles in the μm^3 size range constitute up to 30 % of the cardiomyocyte volume and are composed of an outer and an inner membrane, which divide the organelle into the intermembrane space and the inner matrix, containing the enzymes of the respiratory chain for oxidative phosphorylation. Using the transmembrane proton gradient between the intermembrane space and matrix as driving force for ATP export, mitochondria produce the major part of ATP in most eukaryotic organisms (164). Until recently, disturbances in mitochondrial function have been seen mainly in the context of an insufficient cellular energy production. Disturbed mitochondrial function as a starting mechanism for the execution of cellular apoptosis is a mechanism which we expect to be identified very soon as a major factor for the induction of myocyte apoptosis in the failing heart.

For understanding mitochondrial disturbances, as might occur in the aging heart or in the overloaded myocardium with cytosolic calcium overload, it is necessary to remember that mitochondria in eukaryotic cells are assumed to stem from ancestral endosymbiosis between nucleated cells and bacteria capable of exploiting oxygen. As a consequence of that origin, mitochondria still own an autonomously replicating and expressing genome of about 16.6 kb, the mitochondrial DNA (mtDNA). Each mitochondrion has several copies of mtDNA. The mitochondrial genome has only a restricted set of genes coding for some proteins involved in oxidative phosphorylation, for mitochondrial ribosomal RNA, and for mitochondrial transfer RNA. However, the majority of genes required for mitochondrial biosynthesis and for proper mitochondrial function are encoded in the nucleus (for overview see (44, 52, 170)). Therefore, damage of mitochondrial DNA as a consequence of aging-associated mitochondrial dysfunction can primarily affect a certain fraction of the proteins of the mitochondrial respiratory chain, while nuclear encoded respiratory chain proteins remain primarily unaffected. We will summarize here the arguments indicating that this differential impairment of respiratory chain subunits can importantly contribute to the induction of programmed cell death in aging and/or calcium-overloaded cardiomyocytes.

The accumulating damage of cellular components, especially of the cellular DNA, through reactive oxygen species (ROS) is considered as one of the most important mechanisms contributing to the aging process (86). The mitochondrial respiratory chain is a major source of ROS in the cell (34, 178, 272). Because of its close proximity to the respiratory chain, the mitochondrial genome is especially exposed to oxidative free radicals and is, therefore, frequently damaged (75, 221, 249). This constellation in combination with an insufficiency of mitochondrial DNA repair mechanisms, with a lack of protection by histones, with a compact genome structure (mtDNA is mainly made up of exons and, therefore, mutations mostly affect coding areas), with an high error rate of the mitochondrial DNA-polymerase γ, and a high mitochondrial replication rate, results in the high mutation rate of coding sequences of the mitochondrial genome (244). Consequently, the spontaneous mtDNA mutation rate due to oxidative DNA damage is one to two magnitudes higher than in nuclear DNA (119). A hydroxyl-radical adduct of deoxyguanosine, 8-hydroxy-deoxyguanosine (8-OH-dG), is considered as a marker of oxidative DNA damage (75, 193). 8-OH-dG causes point mutations due to misreplication not only at its own position, but also at neighboring bases (128), and it increases in human hearts with aging (92). Furthermore, it has been shown that the frequency of a certain deletion of mitochondrial DNA in cardiac mitochondria as well as the overall number of deletions is increasing with age in human myocardium (92, 193). Interestingly, there is a clear correlation between the increase in 8-OH-dG and the total number of deletions (92). Altogether, these data indicate a clear rise in damaged mitochondrial DNA in the heart with aging.

These age-associated alterations in the myocardial mitochondrial genome of clinically asymptomatic cases should not be mixed up with the inherited mitochondrial myo- and neuropathies. These are characterized by deficiencies of proteins that function in the mitochondria and which demonstrate a variety of clinical manifestations, appearing in the central nervous system, skeletal muscle, and other organs at various ages in the patients (57, 280). The analysis of these diseases has helped to understand mitochondrial aging in individuals not affected by these syndromes (281).

As mentioned above, the mitochondrial DNA is coding for 13 protein subunits of the respiratory chain, whereas the other more than 60 subunits are encoded in the nucleus. The mitochondrially coded proteins are ND 1 – 6 (NADH dehydrogenase subunits) in complex I, cyt b (cytochrome b) in complex III, Cox I – III (cytochrome c oxidase subunits) in complex IV, and ATPase 6 and 8 in complex V of the respiratory chain. Only complex II is completely coded by nuclear DNA (44). Consequently, accumulation of damage to the mtDNA should lead to a defective synthesis of mt-genome-dependent proteins of the respiratory chain with subsequently impaired function of the complexes containing these proteins, but with no impairment in the function of complex II. In accordance with that expectation, it was reported that an increased 8-OH-dG contents in heart of old rats (100 weeks) is accompanied by a decreased activity of respiratory chain complexes I and IV, but not of complex II, in comparison with hearts of young rats of 7 weeks (92). Decreased rates of mitochondrial protein synthesis, which resulted in deficiencies of the respiratory chain in transmitochondrial cell lines containing cardiomyopathy-typical tRNA mutations in the mt-genome, also illustrate the possible impact of mt-genome alterations on several of the respiratory chain complexes (52). Respiratory chain enzyme defects due to mtDNA alterations are also observed in hearts from patients with idiopathic dilated cardiomyopathy (153).

There are three consequences resulting from a defective respiratory chain:
- ▶ the mitochondrial energy output can be diminished due to impaired proton pumping and possible defects in the FO/F1-ATPase;
- ▶ impaired pumping of protons from the matrix to the intermembrane space causes an increased generation of ROS in the mitochondrial matrix (202, 263);
- ▶ an enhanced mitochondrial radical formation causes an unstable or decreased mitochondrial transmembrane potential ($\Delta\Psi_m$), as discussed below.

Published data on myocardial energetics in the aging heart are controversial. Data favoring reduced mitochondrial energy output in old hearts (171) contrast with data indicating a maintained energy production (152). While part of these discrepancies might be due to the assessments of mitochondrial respiratory capacity under various *in vitro* conditions, there exists no convincing causal link between age-dependent mt-genome damage and impaired mitochondrial metabolic capacity. However, the enhanced formation of reactive oxygen species and the unstable transmembrane potential in hearts with a defective respiratory chain have a dual aspect: on the one hand, they are to be considered in the context of the mitochondrial defense against reactive oxygen species, and on the other hand, they can contribute to an enhanced susceptibility of cardiomyocytes to the initiation of the apoptotic program.

Even during normal respiratory conditions, a certain amount of the electron flux is continuously converted to free radicals at several specific sites of the respiratory chain (130, 272). A high cellular oxygen concentration, a reduced availability of reduced cofactors of the respiratory chain, and a high transmembrane potential of the inner mitochondrial membrane tend to enhance this mitochondrial radical formation, which is substantially enhanced in presence of defects or age-associated imbalances within the respiratory chain (84, 196, 272). Mitochondria apparently respond to this radical-induced oxidative stress with a defined antioxidant defense cascade, which includes membrane potential regulation at the inner mitochondrial membrane and which therefore affects the mitochondrial release of proapoptotic factors. Four steps can be discriminated in this mitochondrial defense cascade:

Step 1. Enzymatic radical scavenging is assumed to form the first protective barrier, consisting of mitochondrial superoxide-dismutase, the glutathione system, and the mitochondrial catalase (117, 163, 202, 253). Especially the glutathione system seems to play an important role, since the thiol redox status and the oxidation of mitochondrial sulfhydril groups seems to modify all the following steps of the defense cascade (46, 126).

Step 2. If the enzymatic scavenging mechanisms are exhausted, the oxidative stress is suggested to result in a so-called "mild uncoupling". This term means an increased proton conductance of the mitochondrial inner membrane, not coupled to the ATP synthesis, and resulting in a small dissipation of the mitochondrial transmembrane potential (252). A decrease of $\Delta\Psi_m$ as mitochondrial response to oxidative stress (235) without involving opening of permeability transition pores (see step 3) indicates the existence of not yet identified uncoupling mechanisms (30). Proteins of the recently identified UCP family (for "uncoupling proteins") could be candidates as mediators of this mild uncoupling. The activity of uncoupling proteins appears to depend on translocation of free fatty acids through the mitochondrial inner membrane (23, 123). Another candidate for mild uncoupling could be the F0/F1-ATPase itself, which contains essential thiol groups in the F0 sector. Modification of those groups through various agents can result in uncoupling (233, 292, 293).

Step 3. If under oxidative stress a certain $\Delta\Psi_m$ decline is reached due to mild uncoupling, a reversible opening of the so-called permeability transition pore is suggested to follow.

Since this process increases the permeability of the inner mitochondrial membrane for solutes up to 1500 Da (19), the consequence of the reversible permeability transition is a rapid and much stronger uncoupling than during step 2, resulting in a steep membrane potential decrease and in a stimulation of the respiratory rate with increased removal of cellular oxygen. Apart from activation by oxidative stress, this permeability transition is triggered by Ca^{2+} overload of the mitochondrial matrix (78, 151) by ADP, by the conversion of thiol groups to disulfide linkages, and by elevating the mitochondrial matrix pH (19, 300). Using patch clamp techniques at the inner mitochondrial membrane, a multiconductance ion channel, modified by Ca^{2+} and sensitive to cyclosporin A, has been described as likely candidate for the permeability transition pore (300). However, depolarization of the mitochondrial membrane potential is considered as the crucial inductor of the permeability transition, while other inductors are supposed merely to act by shifting the curve relating the open probability of the pore to the transmembrane potential (19, 241, 300). The proteins possibly contributing to the pore formation are not yet convincingly identified and the composition of the pore might vary (127). Recently, however, it has been demonstrated that the proapoptotic Bcl-2 protein Bax and the adenin nucleotide translocator (ANT) directly interact in contributing to the opening of the permeability transition pore in several cell types (157). A direct visualization of reversible permeability pore transition in response to oxidative stress has been obtained recently in isolated, single mitochondria from rat myocardium, directly illustrating step 3 of the defense cascade in cardiac mitochondria (100).

Step 4. Ongoing oxidative stress inspite of these described defense mechanisms is assumed to finally result in a so-called "irreversible" permeability transition (277), as has been shown *in vitro* in single cardiac mitochondria (100). This transition, if lasting long enough, results in a complete breakdown of the mitochondrial membrane potential, a cessation of ATP synthesis due to the uncoupling of the oxydative phosphorylation, and an hydrolysis of all available ATP (19). Furthermore, factors involved in the induction of programmed cell death, such as the intermembrane proteins cytochrome c and AIF (apoptosis inducing factor) are liberated from the mitochondria (47,127). As mentioned above, the cytochrome c released from the intermembrane space into the cellular cytosol promotes apoptosis by acting in concert with ATP and APAF-1 to activate procaspase-9. Activated caspase-9 then cleaves procaspase-3 to active caspase-3, which is responsible for many features of the apoptotic process. How the release of cytochrome c from the mitochondrion takes place is still a controversial matter and several mechanisms have been proposed (27, 200). The cell death following cytochrome c release apparently depends on the liberation of a sufficient amount of this protein, indicating that at least a certain number of mitochondria per cell has to undergo permeability transition before the cell is condemned to die (138). If only few damaged mitochondria in a given cell do release their cytochrome c in response to radical formation and Ca^{2+} loading, the apoptotic effector caspases activated around these mitochondria appear to contribute to the autophagy of these mitochondria without activating the process for the whole cell. This mitochondrial autophagy or "mitoptosis" is considered as important determinant of the limited half life of mitochondria in cardiomyocytes (for discussion, see (133)) and alterations of this process in aging hearts are not yet understood. Apoptotic removal of a cell with a majority of oxidatively damaged mitochondria can be considered as the ultimate step of the defense cascade prior to collapse of the entire organ function, as it occurs in terminal congestive heart failure. The final form of cell death following mitochondrial permeability transition and release of cytochrome c can occur as necrosis or apoptosis, and the equilibrium between these two forms of cell death probably depends on the availability of cellular ATP levels required for progredience of the caspase activation (127, 143).

Enhanced neuroendocrine activity as promoter of cardiomyocyte apoptosis?

β-Adrenoceptors

In rats, chronic β-adrenoceptor stimulation by isoproterenol caused myocyte apoptosis (251). This apoptosis is probably due to direct β-adrenergic stimulation of the cardiomyocytes and not secondary to the isoproterenol-associated moderate tachycardia, since it could not be mimicked by a similar pacing-induced tachycardia alone (251). Furthermore, norepinephrine-induced β-adrenoceptor stimulation of neonatal or adult rat cardioyocytes in culture also causes apoptosis (45, 158), which is prevented by β_1-selective blockade and which is attenuated by carbachol-mediated activation of G_i (45). Similarly, $G_{s\alpha}$ overexpression in transgenic mice causes apoptosis, which can be blocked by chronic β-blockade (8). Cardiac $G_{s\alpha}$ overexpression exacerbates in a β-blockade sensitive manner the apoptotic cardiomyopathy induced by an α-myosin heavy chain mutant (74).

The cellular mechanisms for the induction of cardiomyocyte apoptosis under prolonged activation of β-adrenergic signaling are not identified. However, it is an attractive hypothesis to assume an enhanced Ca^{2+} availability for cycling between cytosol and sarcoplasmic reticulum under β-adrenergic activation as the critical factor. In nonmyocyte cells, the Ca^{2+}-calmodulin activated phosphatase calcineurin has been shown to dephosphorylate the proapoptotic cytosolic Bcl-2 protein Bad. This dephosphorylation allows Bad to interact with the mitochondria-protecting, anti-apoptotic $Bcl-x_L$, thereby offsetting the protective potency of $Bcl-x_L$ (207, 216). Furthermore, temporarily enhanced cytosolic Ca^{2+} can enhance the Ca^{2+} burden for the mitochondrial matrix, rendering the mitochondria more sensitive to stimuli which induce the opening of the permeability transition pore (see previous section).

A similar elevation of the concentration-time integral of cytosolic Ca^{2+} is probably also the critical mechanism for the induction of heart failure and cardiomyocyte apoptosis, which can be induced by chronic tachypacing in larger mammals such as dog, sheep, swine or rabbit (89). In this model with activation of the tumor suppressor gene p53 and augmented expression of p53-dependent genes, apoptotic myocyte losses, hypertrophy of surviving myocytes, and nuclear mitotic divisions in myocytes are demonstrable (114, 135, 146).

The Ca^{2+}-calmodulin activated phosphatase calcineurin, however, is also involved in the hypertrophic response of the heart in response to various stimuli (166). In cardiomyocytes, the Ca^{2+}-activated calcineurin dephosphorylates not only the Bcl-2-protein Bad (see above), but also the transcription factor NF-AT3, a member of the multigene family of *nuclear factors of activated T cells,* which is expressed in the heart (97, 166). Dephosphorylated NF-AT3 is translocated to the nucleus and interacts with GATA4, a cardiac zink finger transcription factor involved in the cardiomyocyte hypertrophy in response to load or angiotensin II (88, 94, 166, 167). Transgenic mice with constitutively active mutated calcineurin or NF-AT3 under the control of the promoter of α-myosin heavy chain (which is active primarily after birth) demonstrated severe concentric cardiac hypertrophy, later progressing into dilatative cardiomegaly with signs of pulmonary congestion, cardiac interstitial fibrosis, cardiac fiber disarray, and premature death. Hearts of transgenic mice had elevated mRNA expression of β-myosin heavy chain, α-skeletal actin, and BNP, while α-myosin heavy chain, SERCA and phospholamban were downregulated (166). Although cardiomyocyte apoptosis was not specifically analyzed in these transgenics, its occurrence can be assumed for sure, since cardiomegalic myocardium of transgenic mice demonstrated histologic signs of myocyte degeneration (166). Similarly as in lymphocytes, the immunosuppressant drugs cyclosporin A or FK 506 abolished in neonatal rat cardiomyocytes under growth stimuli (angiotensin II or α_1-adrenoceptor agonist) the Ca^{2+} dependent dephosphorylation on NF-AT3, the cellular hypertrophy, and the induction of the fetal gene program. In transgenic mice with active calcineurin, the development of cardiac failure was prevented by the immunosuppressant cyclosporin A (166).

Thus, Ca^{2+} signaling in cardiomyocyte cytoplasma mediates not only contraction and hypertrophy, but appears also to be involved in the induction of apoptosis. Understanding the fine tuning of Ca^{2+} dependent, calcineurin-mediated processes, such as induction of hypertrophy via NF-AT3 dephosphorylation or induction of apoptosis via dephosphorylation of Bad, might be a core issue in discriminating adaptive or maladaptive responses of the heart to altered hemodynamic load and augmented neuroendocrine activation (see Survival factors section).

Angiotensin II

In neonatal rat cardiomyocytes in culture, angiotensin II acts as an autocrine mediator of stretch-induced trophic responses of these serum-deprived cardiomyocytes, grown on distensible membranes (232). Stretching of the myocytes by distension of the membranes caused a 100-fold increase in the angiotensin II concentration in the medium (without signs of cellular injury such as release of lactate or creatine kinase) and an activation of angiotensinogen expression (232). This distension-induced angiotensin II release was crucial for the trophic reactions triggered by the myocyte distension, such as immediate early gene expression and late hypertrophic responses (^{3}H-phenylalanine incorporation and expression of ANP and skeletal α-actin (232)). These early and late trophic reactions to stretch were suppressed by pretreatment of the myocyte cultures with angiotensin type I receptor (AT_1) blockade (232). A similar release of angiotensin II from secretory-like granules could also be demonstrated in cultured adult rat cardiomyocytes, stretched to a 9 % increase in sarcomere length and with membrane integrity documented by a membrane marker (136, 299). Stretching of these adult rat myocytes in culture resulted in a biphasic pattern of angiotensin II release: early release with immediate decline in cellular angiotensin II content, followed by enhanced angiotensinogen expression, augmented angiotensin II content, and activated angiotensin II release late after stretch, while ProANP mRNA expression was induced almost 100-fold by stretching (134). In those adult, resting cardiomyocytes, kept in serum-free medium, angiotensin II (threshold 10 pM) induces apoptosis of the myocytes, which is completely prevented by AT_1 blockade, but not affected by AT_2-receptor blockade, and which is associated with an increased cytosolic Ca^{2+} concentration due to protein kinase C activation with translocation of ϵ and δ isoforms (112). In contrast to neonatal cardiomyocytes, however, stretching of the adult cardiomyocytes is not associated with enhanced protein synthesis, but induces myocyte apoptosis, demonstrable by several techniques (134). For this stretch-apoptosis of the adult myocytes, the angiotensin II release is causal: pretreatment by AT_1 blockade prevents the stretch-induced apoptosis (134). The stretch-released angiotensin as well as exogenous angiotensin in nonstretched myocytes acts proapoptotic by inducing binding of the tumor suppressor gene product p53 to the promoters of angiotensinogen, AT_1 receptor, and bax (an apoptosis-promoting protein of the Bcl-2 family), resulting in augmented expression of these gene products (201) and AT_1 blockade attenuates this stretch-induced p53-binding (134).

Thus, the angiotensin II release from isolated, stretched cardiomyocytes *in vitro* can have a dual autocrine effect: induction of a hypertrophic growth response in neonatal cardiomyocytes (228, 231) and/or induction of apoptosis in adult cardiomyocytes (112, 134, 299). Both reactions are mediated by AT_1 receptor activation, and some kind of positive feedback is included in these stretch-induced reactions, since an upregulation of local angiotensin formation does occur later after stretching. The modulation of this autocrine angiotensin II action more toward growth or more toward apoptosis is not yet understood. In the neonatal cardiomyocytes, which still are able to proliferate and which have a high basal apoptotic rate, the trophic pattern seems to prevail, but some angiotensin-induced apoptosis has also been observed in this preparation (40). In the terminally differentiated adult cardiomyocytes, which have a very limited capacity to survive in an differentiated state in culture and which have nearly lost their capacity to reenter the cell cycle, the same autocrine stimulus induces only apoptosis. Presently we do not understand the antonymy of the adult myocardium *in vivo*, when it is exposed to enhanced hemodynamic load and local or systemic growth factors (98). Antonymy is a state with incompatible growth signals in the presence of a constitutive proliferation block, which results in the induction of apoptosis (95). Whether antonymy-induced apoptosis is the response of myocytes in the intact myocardium under overload and angiotensin II stimulation cannot be deduced from analyses of isolated myocytes in culture: disconnection of intercellular contacts via cell adhesion molecules for the isolation of cells can act as a strong stimulus for apoptosis in some tissues, and this isolation-induced apoptosis has been called anoikis (70, 161). It is well conceivable that anoikis in isolated cardiomyocytes completely alters the response to a trophic signal with a proapoptotic potential such as angiotensin II.

Atrial natriuretic peptide

Similar problems appear for understanding the autocrine effects of atrial natriuretic peptide (ANP) on the intact myocardium *in vivo*: natriuretic peptide receptors type A (NPR-A) are present in the heart and induce cGMP formation upon activation by ANP (48, 172, 179). This ANP-induced NPR-A activation causes some negative inotropic action *in vitro* and *in vivo* (162, 211, 258). Recently, it was shown that ANP induces apoptosis of cultured neonatal rat cardiomyocytes within 24 h in culture via NPR-A-mediated cGMP formation, and this effect had a threshold in the subnanomolar range of ANP concentrations (291). Enhanced formation and release of ANP from ventricular myocardium is a hallmark of overload-induced cardiac hypertrophy and heart failure (53), and an autocrine apoptotic action of this overload-induced cardiac ANP release could be considered as a straight forward hypothesis explaining myocyte apoptosis and progressive myocardial failure. However, chronic elevation of circulating ANP in intact rats did not enhance cardiomyocyte apoptosis, neither in normotensive rats nor in spontaneously hypertensive rats with cardiac hypertrophy and ongoing myocyte apoptosis (Heinrich et al., unpublished observation).

Presently, the pathophysiological role of the potentially proapoptotic action of activated β-adrenoceptors, AT_1 receptors or natriuretic peptide type A receptors on cardiomyocytes in culture (45, 112, 134, 158, 291, 299) for the failing heart *in vivo* remains open. Isolated myocytes in culture with their high basal apoptotic rate and their susceptibility to anoikis cannot predict the reactions of the intact organ, as is true for models with transgenic overexpression of receptor signal transduction elements (8, 74). Some contributory role of enhanced neuroendocrine activity for myocardial apoptosis in heart failure remains a plausible, but unproven hypothesis.

Survival factors

Gp130 signaling

The relevance of this membrane glycoprotein receptor for cardiac myocyte survival during cardiac growth processes became clear with the identification and expression cloning of the cytokine *cardiotrophin-1* from embryonic stem cells during genesis of cardiogenic progenitor cells in embryoid bodies (197). Cardiotrophin-1 is a member of the IL-6-like family of cytokines, which use gp130 as a part of their transmembrane signal transduction complexes (197). For cardiotrophin-1, this membrane receptor complex consists of gp130, gp190 or LIF-Rβ (for leukemia inhibitory factor receptor β) and a third 80 kDa element (198, 223). During embryonic development, cardiotrophin-1 is highly expressed in the myocardial cells of the early embryonic heart tube and augments survival and proliferation of cultured neonatal cardiac myocytes (246), while knockout of gp130 in mice resulted in prenatal mortality of the pups with hypoplastic ventricular myocardium (295), suggesting an autocrine role of cardiotrophin-1 during cardiac embryonic organogenesis. In the adult rat, cardiotrophin-1 is expressed (among several other organs) in ventricular myocytes, and this expression is substantially enhanced in hearts of spontaneously hypertensive rats with established cardiac hypertrophy (103). Chronic treatment of mice with exogenous cardiotrophin-1 (0.5 – 2.0 μg twice daily for 2 weeks) induced a dose-dependent ventricular hypertrophy (and some enlargement of liver, kidney, and spleen) (109). In cultured cardiac myocytes, gp130 is activated by stretching and this activation contributes to stretch-induced activation of MAP kinase (for mitogen activated protein kinase) independently from angiotensin II (183).

The cardiotrophin-1-induced enlargement of cardiomyocytes in culture (197) differs from the enlargement induced by other hypertrophic stimuli: under cardiotrophin-1, myocyte enlargement occurs preferentially by an assembly of new sarcomeric units in series and by an increase in cell length, not in cell width, while enlargement under another cardiotrophic signal occurs by assembly in parallel and augmentation in cell width (289). This cardiotrophin-1-mediated myocyte elongation involves gp130 and LIF-receptor-β, which are tyrosine phosphorylated (289). This reaction induces activation of phosphatidylinositol 3-kinase (PI 3-kinase), activation of JAK-STAT (Janus kinase – signal transducer and activator of transcription), and association of PI 3-kinase with JAK1 in cultured cardiomyocytes; this PI 3-kinase activation is crucial for the downstream activation of PKB (protein kinase B) in these myocytes (185). Analyses in myocytes with adenovirus transfection demonstrated that JAK3 within the JAK-STAT is critically involved in these cardiotrophin-1-induced, gp130-mediated trophic reactions of myocytes with enhanced protein synthesis and ANP expression (129). A similar activation of the JAK-STAT pathway is also demonstrated during gp130-mediated growth stimulation of cardiomyocytes in response to the cardiotrophin-related cytokine LIF (122).

Besides causing myocyte enlargement, cardiotrophin also enhances survival of cardiomyocytes in culture by attenuating cytokine-activated apoptosis (206, 246). In cardiomyocytes under serum-deprived culture, the signal transduction of the antiapoptotic protective effect of cardiotrophin-1 is less dependent on JAK3 than the trophic reactions (245). In contrast, the critical element for the antiapoptotic effect of gp130-activating cytokines in cardiomyocytes is the PI 3-kinase/Akt-kinase pathway, as is demonstrable in cultured cardiomyocytes with activation of apoptosis by doxorubicin or serum deprivation (186, 187). Protein kinase B (PKB or RAC-protein kinase) is a serine/threonine kinase, and the activation of the PKB/Akt-kinase axis by PI 3-kinase is involved in protective, antiapoptotic actions of gp130 pathways in cardiomyocytes (186) and in the protective pathways of angiopoietin, VEGF, FGF and angiotensin II in endothelial and vascular smooth muscle cells (71, 124, 165, 260). Akt kinase can phosphorylate proteins of the Bcl-2 family, and we expect that ongoing research will demonstrate that gp130/PI 3-kinase/Akt kinase-mediated phosphorylation of cytosolic proapoptotic Bcl-proteins, e.g., Bad, is the critical antiapoptotic mechanism of this protective signal cascade in cardiomyocytes, as is indicated in Fig. 1. Phosphorylation of Bad prevents complexation with the protective Bcl-proteins Bcl-x$_L$ and Bcl-2, while growth factor- and Ca^{2+}-regulated activation of the phosphatase calcineurin dephosphorylates Bad (see previous section: β-adrenoceptors, and part this section: IGFs), allowing inactivation of the protective Bcl-x$_L$/Bcl-2 function by complex formation (Fig. 1).

The gp130-dependent survival signaling via activation of Akt kinase not only affects the interaction between Bad and Bcl-x$_L$/Bcl-2 by counteracting the proapoptotic Ca^{2+}-activated phosphatase calcineurin (Fig. 1), but also includes further protective actions in cardiomyocytes: upregulation of antiapoptotic Bcl-x$_L$ expression (72) and strong induction of the protective heat shock proteins Hsp-70 and Hsp-90 (256). Furthermore, cardiotrophin-1 inhibits the endotoxin-stimulated cardiac TNF production *in vivo* (18), similarly as it acts immunomodulating by IL-6 induction in other cells (222).

From these data on the protective role of the cardiotrophin-1/gp130 axis in cardiomyocytes, it is reasonable to assume that the upregulation of cardiotrophin in hypertension-associated cardiac hypertrophy (103) and in experimental Chagasic cardiomyopathy (35) is a protective adaptation, which attenuates the apoptotic program activated by cardiac overload.

Insulin-like growth factors (IGFs)

There are several reasons for assuming an involvement of IGF-I in the regulation of overload-induced trophic reactions of the myocardium and for considering the IGF-I/IGF receptor type I (IGF-IR) axis as a potential target for antiapoptotic therapy in overload induced heart failure:

▶ IGF-I, classically considered as an autocrine/paracrine growth factor, involved in the regulation of cellular proliferation and differentiation, recently triggered substantial interest because of its antiapoptotic efficacy, mediated by activation of IGF-IR, and because of the permissive role of IGF-IR-mediated antiapoptotic protection for tumorigenesis (13, 15, 131, 302).

▶ In ischemic heart disease, IGF-I-mediated activation of IGF-IR prevents necrotic, ischemia/reperfusion-induced cardiomyocyte losses (31), consistent with the concept that important apoptotic steps contribute to ischemic cell losses (11).

▶ Myocardial IGF-I expression is upregulated in overload-induced cardiac hypertrophy in patients and in most experimental models (69), while in overload models without enhanced IGF-I expression and without augmented ventricular mass, myocyte enlargement with reduced myocyte numbers is observed (261), suggestive of apoptotic myocyte losses.

▶ Growth hormone and IGF-I may improve cardiac function in severe heart failure (42, 148), a condition in which apoptosis of cardiomyocytes contributes to the progression of cardiac dysfunction.

The IFG-IR belongs to the family of tyrosine kinase receptors and is a heterodimeric receptor, consisting of two extracellular, ligand binding α-subunits and 2 transmembrane β-subunits with an intracellular tyrosine kinase domain and binding sites for IGF-IR tyrosine kinase (132, 238). These 4 subunits are linked by disulfide bonds, similarly as in the insulin receptor, to which the IGF-IR is closely related in its protein and gene structure. The IGR-IR is activated by IGF-I, by IGF-II, and by supraphysiological concentrations of insulin (248). The availability of IGFs at the IGF-IR is substantially modified by ten different IGF-binding proteins (IGFBPs, see below) and by the IGF receptor type II. This single peptide chain receptor is a multifunctional transmembrane glycoprotein with a large extracellular domain, binding at distinct sites IGFs (which are internalized and degraded by lysosomal enzymes after binding to this receptor), mannose-6-phosphate (M6P) and M6P-bearing glyoproteins, and retinoic acid (115). Thus, activation of this receptor may counteract the antiapoptotic IGF-IR actions by sequestering IGFs and by transmitting a proapoptotic signal upon retinoic acid binding (285).

The protective, antiapoptotic effect of an activated IGF-IR has been detected in cells of the central nervous system (132, 257) and in pancreas islets (87). Later it was shown that activated IGF-IR also inhibited apoptosis induced *in vitro* by growth factor withdrawal or overexpression, by tumor promoters, by toxin, and by ligands of death domain receptors. Furthermore, a permissive role of activated IGF-IR for tumor growth could be demonstrated *in vivo*: experimental lowering of IGF-IR levels or the use of a dominant negative mutant of the IGF-IR caused massive apoptosis of tumors *in vivo* (for recent reviews see (14, 15, 131, 302)). The upregulation of an IGF-I antagonsist (IGFBP3, see below) appears to be one of the mechanisms by which the tumor suppressor p53 fosters tumor cell apoptosis (176). Mutational analyses of the IGF-IR demonstrated that the mitogenic and transforming domains of the receptor can be separated from the receptor domain transmitting the antiapoptotic signal, which is not present in the closely related insulin receptor (73, 184). The antiapoptotic signal transduction of activated IGF-IR is largely unknown and appears to include various kinase pathways and 14-3-3-proteins, a group of phosphoserine-binding proteins, which are involved in several apoptotic pathways (73, 131).

In neonatal rat cardiomyocytes *in vitro* and *in vivo*, IGF-I induces a trophic response with increased expression of muscle-specific genes (63, 79, 104), which is mediated by IGF-IR and which includes the activation of several phosphorylation cascades (68). Furthermore, stimulation of IGF-IR in cultured neonatal cardiomyocytes suppresses doxorubicin-induced apoptosis (283). The first demonstration of an antiapoptotic protection of cardiomyocytes in the intact heart, however, was obtained earlier: IGF-I application in intact rats one hour prior to coronary occlusion significantly attenuated myocardial injury and myocyte apoptosis induced by 20 min coronary occlusion, followed by 24 h reperfusion (31). Similarly, transgenic overexpression of IGF-I in mice reduced infarct size and cardiomyocyte losses resulting from permanent coronary occlusion and attenuated the subsequent postinfarction dilatory ventricular remodeling (140). Myocyte death in myocardial infarction is a mixed form of cell death, including steps of the apoptotic program (for review see (11, 108)), which means that infarct-induced myocyte losses can be diminished by antiapoptotic interventions such as IGF-IR activation.

The efficacy of IGF-I as a protective intervention in experimental myocardial infarction must not mean that IGF-IR activation is an effective antiapoptotic treatment in severe heart failure with overload-induced cardiomyocyte apoptosis. In experimental heart failure models such as postinfarction overload or doxorubicin-induced myocardial injury, short-term treatment with IGF-I or growth hormone improved cardiac function (4, 41, 61, 110). Similarly, in patients with dilated cardiomyopathy, treatment for three months with growth hormone increased myocardial mass and improved cardiac function (66) (but not always clinical status (192)), probably by an IGF-I-mediated effect. However, these experimental and clinical studies analyzed the growth hormone/ IGF-I effects under the aspect of augmented cardiac growth and altered cardiac function (147), while effects on myocardial apoptosis were not analyzed. Similarly, the enhanced IGF-I expression in models of cardiac pressure or volume overload (58, 59, 69, 80, 85, 102, 218, 219, 227, 279) or in patients with hypertrophic cardiomyopathy (141) were considered under the aspect of IGF-I acting as an endogenous growth factor, contributing to the load-induced myocyte hypertrophy. However, transfection-induced cardiac overexpression of IGF-I in mice did not induce cardiomyocyte hypertrophy, but cardiomegaly due to myocyte proliferation (217). This is consistent with an antiapoptotic effect of the excess IGF-I during cardiac development, since myocyte apoptosis substantially contributes to normal perinatal cardiac development (107). Another preliminary hint for an antiapoptotic effect of IGF-I in the overloaded heart came from experiments on hypertension, induced by chronic inhibition of NO synthases. Surprisingly, chronic pressure overload in this model does not induce cardiac hypertrophy (6, 7, 261, 262) and the overload-typical enhanced cardiac expression of IGF-I or its receptor does not take place (288). Histological analysis of the left ventricular myocardium in rats under chronic inhibition of NO synthase, however, revealed enhanced size of the cardiomyocytes, although the ventricular weight was not augmented (262). This can be explained only by a loss of cardiomyocytes under chronic NO synthase inhibition (262). Although cardioyocyte apoptosis was not analyzed, overload-induced cardiomyocyte apoptosis in the absence of enhanced expression of the antiapoptotic IGF-I is the plausible explanation for these data.

Taken together, these data strongly suggest that IGF-I, either by therapeutic application or by enhanced expression in the myocardium, can suppress the overload-induced apoptosis of cardiomyocytes in the failing heart, although definitive experimental or clinical proof is still lacking. The favorable cardiac effects of growth hormone therapy for dilated cardiomyopathy in a small, preliminary clinical study resulting in a doubling of plasma IGF-I (66) are assumed to result from this enhanced IGF-I formation (42, 147, 148). However, this exciting study is far from yielding conclusive arguments: the study was not placebo-controlled, randomized or blinded and could not delineate the beneficial cardiac effects of short-term growth hormone treatment. Furthermore, the striking clinical improvement in this study could not be confirmed in a larger, randomized study in somewhat elder patients with dilated cardiomyopathy, although an elevation in plasma IGF-I, significantly related to the increase in left ventricular mass, was observed (192). This suggests that a positive cardiac response to growth hormone therapy is not a general finding in heart failure and that we do not yet know the exact type of patient which experiences a clinical benefit from this therapy.

Growth hormone exerts a broad spectrum of endocrine effects, including actions with a potential anti-IGF-I efficacy (42, 148). Such potentially IGF-I antagonistic effects may result from growth hormone-induced expression of IGF-II (see above) and from IGF-I binding proteins (IGFBPs) (210, 215). Basically, IGFBPs counteract IGF-I in two ways: by complexing IGFs and thereby preventing their access to the IGF receptors, and by IGF independent actions mediated via activation of not yet identified IGFBP receptors. Several different IGFBPs (IGFBP-1 – IGFBP-6) with high affinity for IGFs are known to occur in human serum and contribute to the complexing of circulating IGFs. IGFBP-7 – IGFBP-10 have lower affinities for IGFs, but may be more involved in IGF independent signaling of IGFBPs (188, 215).

In human serum, IGFs occur in a large 150 kDa complex (consisting of an IGF, IGFBP-3, and a large glycoprotein, the acid-labile subunit = ALS), in a medium-sized 50 kDa complex (IGF and IGFBP-1, -2, -4, -5, or -6), and in less than 1 % of serum IGF concentration as free proteins. The 150 kDa complex does not cross the vascular barrier and serves as circulating reservoir of IGF-I, determining its bioavailability and circulating half-life of 15 h. Formation of the 150 kDa complex is determined by growth hormone-induced synthesis of ALS and IGFBP-3; an endothelium-derived IGFBP-3 protease disrupts the complex and releases the IGF, which is transported into the tissue extracellular space in the 50 kDa complex, protecting the IGF-I from degradation. At the target tissues, proteases for the IGFBPs of the 50 kDa complex regulate liberation of IGF-I and its bioavailability at the target organ receptor (210). IGF independent actions of IGFBPs are best known for IGFBP-3 and include inhibition of cellular proliferation without binding of IGF-I, binding to cell membrane-associated proteins and incorporation into the cell nucleus, and induction of apoptosis (116, 177, 209). Furthermore, induced expression of IGFBP-3 at least partially mediates the antiproliferative effects of TGF-ß, retinoic acid, antiestrogens and of the tumor suppressor p53 (for review see (215)). Similarly, the other IGFBPs also may have actions independent from binding and inactivation of IGF-I, but these are less well studied. Presently, it is not clear to what extent the expression of IGFBP-3 or other IGFBPs, and of IGF-II, induced by therapeutic application of growth hormone, modify the desired IGF-I-mediated cardiac effects of this therapeutic approach. In the randomized, placebo-controlled growth hormone trial in patients with dilated cardiomyopathy, the hormonal treatment significantly enhanced serum IGFBP-3 levels (192). Circulating growth hormone-binding proteins, age-dependent differences in the activity of the growth hormone/ IGF-I axis and other variable determinants of growth hormone responsivenes (111) may contribute to modify the clinical outcome of growth hormone therapy in chronic heart failure.

Probably, the application of IGF-I or a synthetic IGF-IR activating agonist in overload-induced heart failure is a more effective antiapoptotic approach than the therapy with growth hormone. Although clinical evidence is lacking, the available experimental data suggest that IGF-IR activation should be investigated as a promising approach for the suppression of overload-induced myocyte apoptosis in terminal heart failure.

"Polarity"-regulating signal pathways

Polarity-regulating genes and their functions have been detected in insects, very often in *Drosophila*, and their highly conserved homologs in mammals appear to have important roles in embryonic development and tissue differentiation (2, 191, 156). Speculations on a role of polarity-regulating genes in the myocardial phenotype changes induced by hemo-dynamic overload arouse from the impression that overload-induced cardiac growth processes should follow a spatial pattern strictly determined by the direction of the mechanical forces operating in an overloaded heart, and those speculations triggered the identification of *fz-2* (a rat homolog of the *Drosophila* gene *frizzled*) as the first known polarity-regulating gene in the myocardium, which is upregulated in response to cardiac pressure or volume overload (25). In *Drosophila, frizzled* transcripts appear to transduce polarity signals for hair and bristle development on the epidermal cells of developing wings, probably through an interaction with the cytoskeleton (290).

The *frizzled* gene, the prototype of a whole gene family, encodes a serpentine (i.e., a seven transmembrane domain containing) receptor protein (33, 279, 286). Unlike serpentine receptors for catecholamines and other mediators, however, no G-protein coupling of receptors from the *frizzled* family in the transmission of agonist-induced activation has yet been demonstrated (278). These receptors from the *frizzled* family were recently shown to be the receptors for *wingless* and its homologs, which mediate decisive cell-cell interactions during the development of insects and vertebrates (21, 191, 199, 294). The *wnt* genes and their *Drosophila* ortholog *wingless* form a very large gene family, highly conserved over several phyla including vertebrates and insects, and encode cysteine-rich, N-glycosylated secreted proteins, which bind to the extracellular matrix and which act as short-rang-

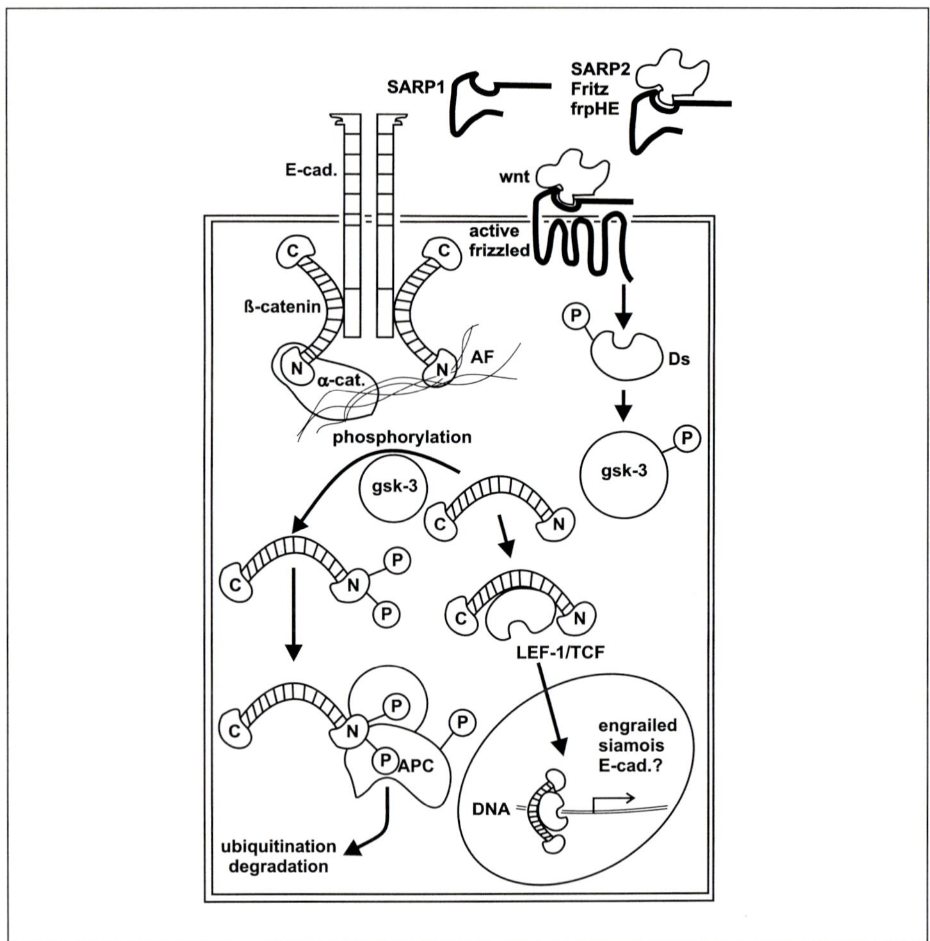

Fig. 2. Dual cellular function of β-catenin.
Complexation of β-catenin with α-catenin contributes to anchoring of cell adhesion molecule E-cadherin (E-cad) to actin filaments (AF). Soluble β-catenin is an element of the signal transduction of the membrane receptor *frizzled*: activated *frizzled* causes an inactivating phosphorylation of the glycogen synthase kinase-3 (gsk-3) via the homolog of the phosphoprotein *dishevelled* (Ds).
When gsk-3 is inactive due to phosphorylation, free β-catenin in high cytosolic concentration is available for association with the transcription factor LEF-1/TCF (T cell factor/lymphoid enhancer binding factor-1). After association with LEF-1/TCF, β-catenin is translocated into the nucleus, inducing alterations in gene transcription. When *frizzled* is blocked, gsk-3 is active and lowers free β-catenin by phosphorylation and ubiquitin-dependent degradation via complexation of phosphorylated β-catenin with tumor suppressor APC proteins.
Proteins of the *wnt* family stimulate the *frizzled* receptor. SARPs (secreted apoptosis regulating proteins) lower cytosolic free β-catenin by blocking *frizzled* activation (SARP$_2$) and enhance apoptosis, or enhance free β-catenin by activating *frizzled* (SARP$_1$) and attenuate apoptotic susceptibility. Myocardial SARP expression is altered in cardiac overload or myocardial damage.
Note that many homologs and isoforms of β-catenin regulating proteins exist, which are not listed here. For details see (90).

ing signaling molecules, involved in developmental pattern formation and tissue polarity, in experimental carcinogenesis and in cellular differentiation (181). The first cloned gene of the *wnt* family, the mouse gene *int-1* (for mammary tumor virus *int*egration site *1*), was identified in the context of oncogene research (180), and the name *wnt* is an amalgam of *int* and *wingless*, which is one of roughly a dozen segment polarity genes identified and classified according to the region of the cuticle deleted in *Drosophila* mutants (182).

The identification of *frizzled* proteins as membrane receptors for the *wnt* family substantially helped to unravel the *wnt*-activated signal transduction toward polarity forming gene expression, and this transduction turned out to include elements of the cytoskeleton in the form of certain proteins of the *armadillo* family (90). Proteins of this family, such as the vertebrate β-catenin or plakoglobin, are involved in two different functions: they are cytoskeleton components of the junctional plaques in desmosomes and in similar junctional structures (where they are required for stable cytoskeletal interactions and cluster formation with adhesion molecules) and on the other hand, they participate in the *wnt/frizzled* signal transduction for pattern formation during embryogenesis (90). This signal transduction is schematically depicted in Fig. 2. In the absence of *frizzled*-receptor activation by *wnt*-proteins, free cytosolic β-catenin is phosphorylated in its N-terminal region by glycogen synthase kinase-3 (GSK-3) (296), and phosphorylated β-catenin is degraded by the ubiquitin/proteasome pathway after complex formation with the tumor suppressor APC (168, 226). Thus, the cytosolic level of free β-catenin is kept low without *wnt*-signaling. *Wnt*-mediated activation of a *frizzled*-receptor, however, inactivates GSK-3 by phosphorylation via activation of the phosphoprotein *dishevelled* (or its vertebrate homolog, (205, 271)), resulting in cytosolic accumulation of free β-catenin (51), which directly binds to a family of transcription factors called TCF/LEF-1 (T cell factor/ lymphoid enhancer binding factor-1; (16)). This binding of β-catenin to the TCFs causes the translocation of this complex into the nucleus and enhances the transcriptional activity of TCFs, resulting in ectopic axis induction and in expression of cell adhesion elements (for review see (90)). Thus, β-catenin and other *armadillo*-proteins appear to be involved in cell adhesion as well as in *Wnt*-mediated polarity signaling: *wnt*-signals may stabilize cell adhesion, and elements of cell adhesion may regulate the response to *wnt*-signals by modifying the free β-catenin pool available for signaling (90).

The involvement of β-catenin-mediated *wnt*-signaling in the regulation of apoptosis became apparent, when an antiapoptotic activity was detected in culture media conditioned by quiescent (but not by proliferating) CH3/T10 fibroblasts, and a group of SARPs (= secreted apoptosis regulating proteins) with structural relations to *frizzled*-like proteins was cloned from these cells (160). SARP$_1$ causes an elevation in cytosolic free β-catenin content, induces resistance to apoptotic stimuli and acts like an agonist activating *frizzled*-like receptors while SARP$_2$ lowers free β-catenin, causes increased apoptotic sensitivity, and inactivates *wnt*-mediated signaling (either by inactivating a *wnt*-protein or by blocking a *frizzled*-receptor (see Fig. 2). Presently, it is not known whether the modulation of cytosolic free β-catenin is the critical signal for the modulation of the apoptotic susceptibility, but β-catenin is accumulating in certain apoptosis-resistant tumor cells with mutations in the tumor suppressor APC (125, 168, 226).

SARP$_1$ and SARP$_2$ mRNAs are expressed in the human heart (160); in ventricular myocardium from hearts with endstage heart failure, removed for transplantation, the antiapoptotic SARP$_1$ appears downregulated in contrast to the pro-apoptotic SARP$_2$ (Hatzfeld unpublished observation), consistent with an enhanced apoptotic susceptibility of failing human hearts, in which myocyte apoptosis is demonstrable (24, 174, 189). It appears fascinating that short range signaling molecules, known from developmental biology, may be involved in organizing the architecture of the adult heart after changes of its working conditions and that those short range signaling molecules are involved in apoptosis regulation. Strongly altered architecture of the heart occurs following myocardial infarction, and a *frizzled* related gene, *fz2*, appears to be involved in the spatial control of cardiac wound repair after infarction (26). Meanwhile, further homologs of the SARPs, also called sFRPs (for secreted *frizzled*-related proteins), modulating *wnt*-signaling in various organisms, have been identified (67, 96, 137, 213, 250, 284). Their role in myocardial *wnt*-signaling and the contribution of *wnt*-signaling to the myocardial plasticity in response to cardiac overload remains to be fully delineated, but speculations on *wnt*-signaling as target for therapeutic, antiapoptotic interventions in overload cardiomyopathy appear justified.

Summary and perspectives

Enhanced myocyte apoptosis is demonstrable in several models of acute myocyte distension *in vitro*, in many experimental models with volume and/or pressure overload, and in the dilated myocardium of patients with terminally failing hearts. Although distension-induced myocyte apoptosis is proposed as an attractive mechanism for the transition from compensated overload to ouvert failure and for the progression of failure, neither a causal role of apoptosis in failure nor its quantitative relevance can be assessed at present. Furthermore, the signal mechanism triggering myocyte apoptosis in response to myocardial overload and/or myocyte distension is unknown.

In cardiomyocytes as in any other eukaryotic cell, apoptosis is mediated by an activated cascade of caspases. Activation of this cascade originates from autoactivation by oligomerization of low activity initiator caspases, occuring at mitochondrial "apoptosome" and/or at "death-inducing signal complexes" (disc) of death domain-containing receptors from the TNF receptor family. Although most known receptors of this family are expressed in the myocardium, a contribution of their activation to overload-induced cardiac apoptosis appears at best marginal. On the other hand, caspase autoactivation at myocardial apoptosomes is triggered by release of proapoptotic mitochondrial signals such as cytochrome c, AIF (apoptosis inducing factor), ATP, and others. This release is associated with depolarization of the mitochondrial (inner) membrane potential and is elicited by disturbances of mitochondrial function due to oxidative stress, Ca^{2+} overload, advanced age, and signals arising from activated discs. A further potentiation of this proapoptotic release in a kind of positive feedback is obtained by activated caspases, which mediate cleavage and inactivation of antiapoptotic mitochondrial proteins of the Bcl-2 family. These antiapoptotic Bcl-2 proteins protect the mitochondria against depolarizing stimuli and they attenuate the release of caspase activating signals; their protective function is blocked by complexation with proapoptotic proteins such as Bad and/or Bax, and their protective function is supported by survival signals from gp130-containing receptor complexes for the interleukin-6 family, by IGF-receptor I activation and probably by polarity signals, which regulate cytosolic β-catenin. Survival signals phosphorylate proapoptotic Bad and prevent its inhibitory complexation with antiapoptotic Bcl-2 proteins. Proapoptotic growth factor signals dephosphorylate Bad by activation of calcineurin, allowing this complexation.

In isolated cardiomyocytes, receptors of the neuroendocrine activity (AT_1 receptor, β-adrenoceptors, ANP receptor Type A) can induce apoptosis upon activation. However, analysis from apoptotic signaling in isolated myocytes in culture cannot predict the relevance of this signaling in the intact tissue, since the process of cellular isolation strongly alters the control of apoptotic thresholds by elements of the cytoskeleton. Nevertheless, a preliminary working hypothesis for the induction of apoptosis in overloaded myocardium is possible, postulating a combined action of impaired mitochondrial function, enhanced neuroendocrine activity, cytosolic calcium overload, and altered survival signaling as mechanism.

Acknowledgment Our own research on apoptosis in the overloaded myocardium is generously supported by grants from the Bundesministerium für Bildung, Wissenschaft, Forschung und Technologie (BMBF 01 ZZ 9512/0) and by a stipendium from the Deutsche Herzstiftung for H. H.

References

1. Adams JM, Cory S (1998) The Bcl-2 protein family: arbiters of cell survival. Science 281: 1322–1325
2. Adler PN (1992) The genetic control of tissue polarity in Drosophila. BioEssays 4: 735–741
3. Alnemri ES, Livingston DJ, Nicholson DW, Salvesen G, Thornberry ND, Wong WW, Yuan J (1996) Human ICE/CED-3 protease nomenclature. Cell 87: 171
4. Ambler GR, Johnston BM, Maxwell B, Gavin JB, Gluckman PD (1993) Improvement of doxorubicin induced cardiomyopathy in rats treated with insulin-like growth factor I. Cardiovasc Res 27: 1368–1373
5. Ambrosini G, Adida C, Altieri DC (1997) A novel anti-apoptosis gene, survivin, expressed in cancer and lymphoma. Nature Med 3: 917–921
6. Arnal JF, El Amrani AI, Chatellier G, Mé J, Michel JB (1993) Cardiac weight in hypertension induced by nitric oxide synthase blockade. Hypertension 22: 380–387
7. Arnal JF, Warin L, Michel JB (1992) Determinants of aortic cyclic guanosine monophosphate in hypertension induced by chronic inhibition of nitric oxide synthase. J Clin Invest 90: 647–652
8. Asai K, Meguro T, Coast DA, Smith AB, Ishikawa Y, Homcy CJ, Vatner DE, Vatner SF (1998) Chronic β-adrenergic receptor blockade prevents the depression in cardiac function in older mice with cardiac $G_{s\alpha}$ overexpression (abstr). Circulation 98: I-69
9. Ashkenazi A, Dixit VM (1998) Death receptors: signaling and modulation. Science 281: 1305–1308
10. Au JLS, Panchal N, Li D, Gan Y (1997) Apoptosis: a new pharmacodynamic endpoint. Pharmaceutical Res 14: 1659-1671
11. Bartling B, Holtz J, Darmer D (1998) Contribution of myocyte apoptosis to myocardial infarction? Basic Res Cardiol 93: 71–84
12. Bartling B, Milting H, Schumann H, El-Banayosy A, Koerner M, Koerfer R, Darmer D, Holtz J, Zerkowski HR (1998) Improved myocardial expression of anti-apoptotic genes under support by ventricular assist devices (VAD) in terminal heart failure (abstr). Circulation 98 (suppl): I-200
13. Baserga R (1995) The insulin-like growth factor I receptor: a key to tumor growth? Cancer Res 55: 249–252
14. Baserga R, Hongo A, Rubini M, Prisco M, Valentinis B (1997) The IGF-I receptor in cell growth, transformation and apoptosis. Biochim Biophys Acta 1332: F105–F126
15. Baserga R, Resnicoff M, Dews M (1997) The IGF-I receptor and cancer. Endocrine 7: 99–102
16. Behrens J, Von Kries JP, Kuhl M, Bruhn L, Wedlich D, Grosschedl R, Birchmeier W (1996) Functional interaction of β-catenin with the transcription factor LEF-1. Nature 382: 638–642
17. Beidler DR, Tewari M, Friesen PD, Poirier G, Dixit VM (1995) The baculovirus p35 protein inhibits Fas- and tumor necrosis factor-induced apoptosis. J Biol Chem 270: 16526–16528
18. Benigni F, Sacco S, Pennica D, Ghezzi P (1996) Cardiotrophin-1 inhibits tumor necrosis factor production in the heart and serum of lipopolysaccharide-treated mice and in vitro in mouse blood cells. Am J Pathol 149: 1847–1850
19. Bernardi P (1996) The permeability transition pore: control point of a cyclosporin-A-sensitive mitochondrial channel involved in cell death. Biochim Biophys Acta 1275: 5–9
20. Bertin J, Armstrong RC, Ottilie S, Martin DA, Wang Y, Banks S, Wang G-H, Senkewich TG, Alnemri ES, Moss B, Lenardo MJ, Tomaselli KJ, Cohen JI (1997) Death effector domain-containing herpesvirus and poxvirus proteins inhibit both Fas- and TNFR1-induced apoptosis. Proc Natl Acad Sci USA 94: 1172–1176
21. Bhanot P, Brink M, Samos CH, Hsieh JC, Wang Y, Macke JP, Andrew D, Nathans J, Nuse R (1996) A new member of the frizzled family from Drosophila functions as a Wingless receptor. Nature 382: 255–230
22. Bialik S, Cryns V, Drincic A, Srinivasan A, Kitsis RN (1998) Cytochrome c release from the mitochondria precedes caspase activation in apoptotic myocytes during ischemia. Circulation 98: I-462
23. Bienengraeber M, Echtay KS, Klingenberg M (1998) H+ transport by uncoupling protein (UCP-1) is dependent on a histidine pair, absent in UCP-2 and UCP-3. Biochemistry 37: 3–8
24. Bing OHL (1994) Hypothesis: apoptosis may be a mechanism for the transition to heart failure with chronic pressure overload. J Mol Cell Cardiol 26: 943–948

25. Blankesteijn WM, Essers-Janssen YPG, Ulrich MMW, Smits JFM (1996) Increased expression of a homologue of Drosophila tissue polarity gene "frizzled" in left ventricular hypertrophy in the rat, as identified by subtractive hybridization. J Mol Cell Cardiol 28: 1187–1191

26. Blankesteijn WM, Essers-Janssen YPG, Verluyten MJA, Daemen MJAP, Smits JFM (1997) A homologue of Drosophila tissue polarity gene frizzled is expressed in migrating myofibroblasts in the infarcted rat heart. Nature Med 5: 541–544

27. Bossy-Wetzel E, Newmeyer DD, Green DR (1998) Mitochondrial cytochrome c release in apoptosis occurs upstream of DEVD-specific caspase activation and independently of mitochondrial transmembrane depolarization. Embo J 17: 37–49

28. Bozkurt B, Kribbs SB, Clubb FJ, Michael LH, Didenko VV, Hornsby PJ, Seta Y, Oral H, Spinale FG, Mann DL (1998) Pathophysiologically relevant concentrations of tumor necrosis factor-α promote progressive left ventricular dysfunction and remodeling in rats. Circulation 97: 1382–1391

29. Brömme HJ, Holtz J (1996) Apoptosis in the heart: when and why? Molecular and Cellular Biochemistry 163/164: 261–275

30. Brooke PS, Land JM, Clark JB, Heales SJ (1998) Peroxynitrite and brain mitochondria: evidence for increased proton leak. J Neurochem 70: 2195–2202

31. Buerke M, Murohara T, Skurk C, Nuss C, Tomaselli K, Lefer AM (1995) Cardioprotective effect of insulin-like growth factor I in myocardial ischemia followed by reperfusion. Proc Natl Acad Sci 92: 8031–8035

32. Buja LM, Entman ML (1998) Modes of myocardial cell injury and cell death in ischemic heart disease. Circulation 98: 1355–1357

33. Chan SDH, Karpf DB, Fowlkes ME, Hooks M, Bradley MS, Vuong V, Bambino T, Liu MY, Arnaud CD, Strewler GJ, Nissenson RA (1992) Two homologs of the Drosophila polarity gene frizzled (fz) are widely expressed in mammalian tissues. J Biol Chem 267: 25202–25207

34. Chance B, Sies H, Boveris A (1979) Hydroperoxide metabolism in mammalian organs. Physiol Rev 59: 527–603

35. Chandrasekar B, Melby PC, Pennica D, Freeman GL (1998) Overexpression of cardiotrophin-1 and gp130 during experimental acute Chagasic cardiomyopathy. Immunol Lett 61: 89–95

36. Cheng W, Kajstura J, Nitahara JA, Li B, Reiss K, Liu Y, Clark WA, Krajewski S, Reed JC, Olivetti G, Anversa P (1996) Programmed myocyte cell death affects viable myocardium after infarction in rats. Exp Cell Res 226: 316–327

37. Cheng W, Li B, Kajstura J, Li P, Wolin MS, Sonnenblick EH, Hintze TH, Olivetti G, Anversa P (1995) Stretch induced programmed myocyte cell death. J Clin Invest 96: 2247–2259

38. Chicheportiche Y, Bourdon PR, Xu H, Hsu YM, Scott H, Hession C, Garcia I, Browning JL (1997) TWEAK, a new secreted ligand in the tumor necrosis factor family that weakly induces apoptosis. J Biol Chem 272: 32401–32410

39. Chu ZL, McKinsey TA, Liu L, Gentry JJ, Malim MH, Ballard DW (1997) Suppression of tumor necrosis factor-induced cell death by inhibitor of apoptosis c-IAP2 is under NF-$_{\kappa B}$ control. Proc Natl Acad Sci 94: 10057–10062

40. Cigola E, Kajstura J, Li B, Meggs LG, Anversa P (1997) Angiotensin II activates programmed myocyte cell death in vitro. Exp Cell Res 231: 363–371

41. Cittadini A, Grossmen JD, Napoli R, Katz SE, Stromer H, Smith RJ, Clark R, Morgan JP, Douglas PS (1997) Growth hormone attenuates early left ventricular remodeling and improves cardiac function in rats with large myocardial infarction. J Am Coll Cardiol 29: 1109–1116

42. Clark R (1997) Growth hormone and insulin-like growth factor 1: new endocrine therapies in cardiology. Trends Cardiovasc Med 7: 264–268

43. Clem RJ, Miller LK (1994) Control of programmed cell death by the baculovirus genes p35 and iap. Mol. Cell Biol. 14: 5212–5222

44. Collombet JM, Coutelle C (1998) Towards gene therapy of mitochondrial disorders. Mol Med Today 4: 31–38

45. Communal K, Singh K, Colucci WS (1998) Gi protein protects adult rat ventricular myocytes from ß-adrenergic receptor-stimulated apoptosis in vitro (abstr). Circulation 98: I-742

46. Constantini P, Chernyak BV, Petronilli V, Bernardi P (1996) Modulation of the mitochondrial permeability transition pore by pyridine nucleotides and dithiol oxidation at two separate sites. J Biol Chem 271: 6746–6751

47. Cory S, Adams JM (1998) Matters of live and death: programmed cell death at cold spring harbor. Biochim Biophys Acta 1377: R25–R44

48. Cramb G, Banks R, Rugg EL, Aiton JF (1987) Actions of atrial natriuretic peptide (ANP) on cyclic nucleotide concentrations and phosphatidylinositol turnover in ventricular myocytes. Biochem Biophys Res Comm 148: 962–970

49. Crook NE, Clem RJ, Miller LK (1993) An apoptosis-inhibiting baculovirus gene with a zinc finger-like motif. J Virol 67: 2168–2174

50. Cryns V, Yuan J (1998) Proteases to die for. Genes Dev 12: 1551–1556

51. Dale TC (1998) Signal transduction by the Wnt family of ligands. Biochem J 329: 209–223
52. Davidson E, King MP (1997) Advances in human mitochondrial diseases: molecular genetic analysis of pathogenic mtDNA mutations. Trends Cardiovasc Med 7: 16–24
53. DeBold AJ, Bruneau BG, DeBold MLK (1996) Mechanical and neuroendocrine regulation of the endocrine heart. Cardiovasc Res 31: 7–18
54. Devaux PF (1991) Static and dynamic lipid asymmetry in cell membranes. Biochemistry 30: 1163–1173
55. Deveraux QL, Takahashi R, Salvesen GS, Reed JC (1997) X-linked IAP is a direct inhibitor of cell-death proteases. Nature 388: 300–304
56. Díez J, Panizo A, Hernández M, Vega F, Sola I, Fortuno MA, Pardo J (1997) Cardiomyocyte apoptosis and cardiac angiotensin-converting enzyme in spontaneously hypertensive rats. Hypertension 30: 1029–1034
57. DiMauro S, Hirano M (1998) Mitochondria and heart disease. Curr Opin Cardiol 13: 190–197
58. Donohue TJ, Dworkin LD, Lango MN, Fliegner K, Lango RP, Bernstein JA, Slater WR, Catanese VM (1994) Induction of myocardial insulin-like growth factor-I gene expression in left ventricular hypertrophy. Circulation 89: 799–809
59. Donohue TJ, Dworkin LD, Ma J, Lango MN, Catanese VM (1997) Antihypertensive agents that limit ventricular hypertrophy inhibit cardiac expression of insulin-like growth factor-I. J Investig Med 45: 584–591
60. Ducket CS, Li F, Wang Y, Tomaselli KJ, Thompson CB, Armstrong RC (1998) Human IAP-like protein regulates programmed cell death downstream of Bcl-xL and cytochrome c. Mol Cell Biol 18: 608–615
61. Duerr RL, Huang S, Miraliakbar HR, Clark R, Chien KR, Ross J (1995) Insulin-like growth factor-1 enhances ventricular hypertrophy and function during the onset of experimental cardiac failure. J Clin Invest 95: 619–627
62. Enari M, Sakahira H, Yokoyama H, Okawa K, Iwamatsu A, Nagata S (1998) A caspase-activated DNase that degrades DNA during apoptosis, and its inhibitor ICAD. Nature 391: 43–50
63. Engelmann GL, Boehm KD, Haskell JF, Khairallah PA, Ilan J (1989) Insulin-like growth factors and neonatal cardiomyocyte development: ventricular gene expression and membrane receptor variations in normotensive and hypertensive rats. Mol Cell Endocrinol 63: 1–14
64. Eriksson PS, Perfilieva E, Björk-Eriksson T, Alborn AM, Nordborg C, Peterson DA, Gage FH (1998) Neurogenesis in the adult human hippocampus. Nature Med 4: 1313–1317
65. Evan G, Littlewood T (1998) A matter of life and death. Science 281: 1317–1321
66. Fazio S, Cittadini A, Sabatini D, Merola B, Colao A, Biondi B, Lombardi G, Saccà L (1996) A preliminary study of growth hormone in the treatment of dilated cardiomyopathy. N Engl J Med 334: 811–814
67. Finch PW, He X, Kelley MJ, Uren A, Schaudies RP, Popescu NC, Rudikoff S, Aaronson SA, Varmus HE, Rubin JS (1997) Purification and molecular cloning of a secreted, Frizzled-related antagonist of Wnt action. Proc Natl Acad Sci 94: 6770–6775
68. Foncea R, Andersson M, Ketterman A, Blakesley V, Sapag-Hagar M, Sugden PH, LeRoith D, Lavandero S (1997) Insulin-like growth factor-I rapidly activates multiple signal transduction pathways in cultured rat cardiac myocytes. J Biol Chem 272: 19115–19124
69. Friberg P, Isgaard J, Wahlander H, Wickman A, Guron G, Adams MA (1995) Cardiac hypertrophy and related growth processes: the role of insulin-like growth factor-I. Blood Pressure 4 (suppl 2): 22–29
70. Frisch SM, Ruoslahti E (1997) Integrins and anoikis. Curr Opin Cell Biol 9: 701–706
71. Fujio K, Mano T, Takahashi T, Walsh K (1998) Akt mediates the cell survival effects of vascular endothelial growth factor (abstr). Circulation 98 (suppl-I): I-463
72. Fujio Y, Kunisada K, Hirota H, Matsui H, Yamauchi-Takihara K, Kishimoto T (1997) Signals through gp130 upregulate bcl-x gene expression via STAT1-binding cis-element in cardiac myocytes. J Clin Invest 99: 2898–2905
73. Furlanetto RW, Dey BR, Lopaczynski W, Nissley SP (1997) 14-3-3 proteins interact with the insulin-like growth factor receptor but not the insulin receptor. Biochem J 327: 765–771
74. Geng YJ, Bishop SS, Wagner TE, Yang G, Mathier MA, Yun JS, Vatner DE, Shannon RP, Homcy CJ, Seidman CE, Seidman JG, Vatner SF (1998) Exacerbated cardiomyopathy in mice with both cardiac overexpression of $G_{s\alpha}$ and missense mutation of α-myosin heavy chain (abstr). Circulation 98: I467
75. Giulivi C, Boveris A, Cadenas E (1995) Hydroxyl radical generation during mitochondrial electron transfer and the formation of 8-hydroxydesoxyguanosine in mitochondrial DNA. Arch Biochem Biophys 316: 909–916
76. Glinsky GV (1997) Apoptosis in metastatic cancer cells. Crit Rev Oncol Hematol 25: 175–186
77. Gross A, Yin XM, Wang K, Wei MC, Jockel J, Milliman C, Erdjument-Bromage H, Tempst P, Korsmeyer SJ (1999) Caspase cleaved BID targets mitochondria and is required for cytochrome c release, while BCL-XL prevents this release but not tumor necrosis-R1/Fas death. J Biol Chem 274: 1156–1163
78. Gunter TE, Pfeiffer DR (1990) Mechanisms by which mitochondria transport calcium. Am J Physiol 258: C755–C786
79. Guo W, Kada K, Kamiya K, Toyama J (1997) IGF-I regulates K^+-channel expression of cultured neonatal rat ventricular myocytes. Am J Physiol 272: H2599–H2606

80. Guron G, Friberg P, Wickman A, Brantsing C, Gabrielsson B, Isgaard J (1996) Cardiac insulin-like growth factor I and growth hormone receptor expression in renal hypertension. Hypertension 27: 636–642
81. Hamet P, Richard L, Dam TV, Teiger E, Orlov SN, Gaboury L, Gossard F, Tremblay J (1995) Apoptosis in target organs of hypertension. Hypertension 26: 642–648
82. Han Z, Bhalla K, Pantazis P, Hendrickson EA, Wyche JH (1999) Cif (Cytochrome c efflux-inducing factor) activity is regulated by bcl-2 and caspase and correlates with the activation of Bid. Mol Cell Biol 19: 1381–1389
83. Han Z, Li G, Bremner TA, Lange TS, Zhang G, Jemmerson R, Wyche JH, Hendrickson EA (1998) A cytosolic factor is required for mitochondrial cytochrome c efflux during apoptosis. Cell Death Diff 5: 469–479
84. Hansford RG, Hogue BA, Mildaziene V (1997) Dependence of H_2O_2 formation by rat heart mitochondria on substrate availability and donor age. J Bioenerg Biomembr 29: 89–95
85. Hanson MC, Fath KA, Alexander RW, DeLafontaine P (1993) Induction of cardiac insulin-like growth factor I gene expression in pressure overload hypertrophy. Am J Med Sci 306: 69–74
86. Harman D (1991) The aging process: major risk factor for the disease and death. Proc Natl Acad Sci 88: 5360–5364
87. Harrington EA, Bennett MR, Fanidi A, Evan GI (1994) C-myc-induced apoptosis in fibroblasts is inhibited by specific cytokines. Embo J 13: 3286–3295
88. Hasegawa K, Lee SJ, Jobe SM, Markham BE, Kitsis RN (1997) Cis-acting sequences that mediate induction of β-myosin heavy chain gene expression during left ventricular hypertrophy due to aortic constriction. Circulation 96: 3943–3953
89. Hasenfuss G (1998) Animal models of human cardiovascular disease, heart failure and hypertrophy. Cardiovasc Res 39: 60–76
90. Hatzfeld M (1998) The armadillo family of structural proteins. Int Rev Cytol 186: 179–224
91. Haunstetter A, Izumo S (1998) Apoptosis: basic mechanisms and implications for cardiovascular disease. Circ Res 82: 1111–1129
92. Hayakawa M, Sugiyama S, Hattori K, Takasawa M, Ozawa T (1993) Age-associated damage in mitochondrial DNA in human hearts. Mol Cell Biochem 119: 95–103
93. Hengartner MO (1997) CED-4 is a stranger no more. Nature 388: 714–715
94. Herzig TC, Jobe SM, Aoki H, Molketin JD, Cowley AW, Izumo S, Markham BE (1997) Angiotensin II type 1a receptor gene expression in the heart: AP-1 and GATA-4 participate in the response to pressure overload. Proc Natl Acad Sci 94: 7543–7548
95. Hibner U, Coutinho A (1994) Signal antonymy: a mechanism for apoptosis induction. Cell Death Diff 1: 33–37
96. Hoang B, Moos M, Vukicevic S, Luyten FP (1996) Primary structure and tissue distribution of FRZB, a novel protein related to Drosophila frizzled, suggest a role in skeletal morphogenesis. J Biol Chem 271: 26131–26137
97. Hoey T, Sun YL, Williamson K, Xu X (1995) Isolation of two new members of the NF-AT gene family and functional characterization of the NF-AT proteins. Immunity 2: 461–472
98. Holtz J (1998) Role of ACE-inhibition or AT_1-blockade in the remodeling following myocardial infarction. Basic Res Cardiol 93 (suppl 2): 92–100
99. Hu S, Vincenz C, Bullers M, Dixit VM (1997) A novel family of viral death effector domain-containing molecules that inhibit both CD-95- and tumor necrosis factor receptor-1-induced apoptosis. J Biol Chem 272: 9621–9624
100. Hüser J, Rechenmacher CE, Blatter LA (1998) Imaging the permeability pore transition in single mitochondria. Biophys J 74: 2129–2137
101. Irmler M, Thome M, Hahne M, Schneider P, Hofmann K, Steiner V, Bodmer JL, Schroeter M, Burns K, Mattmann C, Rimoldi D, French LE, Tschopp J (1997) Inhibition of death receptor signals by cellular FLIP. Nature 388: 190–195
102. Isgaard J, Wahlander H, Adams MA, Friberg P (1994) Increased expression of growth hormone receptor mRNA and insulin-like growth factor-I mRNA in volume-overloaded hearts. Hypertension 23: 884–888
103. Ishikawa M, Saito Y, Miyamoto Y, Kuwahara K, Ogawa E, Nakagawa O, Harada M, Masuda I, Nakao K (1996) cDNA cloning of rat Cardiotrophin-1 (CT-1): augmented expression of CT-1 gene in ventricle of genetically hypertensive rats. Biochem Biophys Res Comm 219: 377–381
104. Ito H, Hiroe M, Hirata Y, Tsujino M, Adachi S, Shichiri M, Koike A, Nogami A, Marumo F (1993) Insulin-like growth factor-I induces hypertrophy with enhanced expression of muscle specific genes in cultured rat cardiomyocytes. Circulation 87: 1715–1721
105. Jacobson MD, Weil M, Raff MC (1997) Programmed cell death in animal development. Cell 88: 347–354
106. James TN (1994) Normal and abnormal consequences of apoptosis in the human heart from postnatal morphogenesis to paroxysmal arrhythmias. Circulation 90: 556–573
107. James TN (1997) Apoptosis in congenital heart disease. Coronary Art Dis 8: 599–616
108. James TN (1997) Complex causes of fatal myocardial infarction. Circulation 96: 1696–1700

109. Jin H, Yang R, Keller GA, Ryan A, Finkle D, Swanson TA, Li W, Pennica D, Wood WI, Paoni NF (1996) In vivo effects of cardiotrophin-1. Cytokine 8: 920–926

110. Jin H, Yang RNG, Clark RG, Ko A, Paoni NF (1995) Beneficial effects of growth hormone and insulin-like growth factor I in experimental heart failure in rats treated with chronic ACE inhibition. J Cardiovasc Pharmacol 26: 420–425

111. Johannson G, Bjarnason G, Brammert M, Carlsson LM, Degerblad M, Manhem P, Rosen T, Thoren U, Bengtsson BA (1996) The individual responsiveness to growth hormone (GH) treatment in GH-deficient adults is dependent on the level of GH-binding protein, body mass index, age, and gender. J Clin Endocrinol Metab 81: 1575–1581

112. Kajstura J, Cigola E, Malhotra A, Li P, Cheng W, Meggs LG, Anversa P (1997) Angiotensin II induces apoptosis of adult ventricular myocytes in vitro. J Mol Cell Cardiol 29: 859–870

113. Kajstura J, Leri A, Finato N, Di Loreto C, Beltrami CA, Anversa P (1998) Myocyte proliferation in end-stage cardiac failure in humans. Proc Natl Acad Sci 95: 8801–8805

114. Kajstura J, Zhang X, Liu Y, Szoke E, Cheng W, Olivetti G, Hintze TH, Anversa P (1995) The cellular basis of pacing-induced dilated cardiomyopathy: myocyte cell loss and myocyte cellular reactive hypertrophy. Circulation 92: 2306–2317

115. Kang JX, Li Y, Leaf A (1997) Mannose-6-phosphate/insulin-like growth factor-II receptor is a receptor for retinoic acid. Proc Natl Acad Sci 95: 13671–13676

116. Karas M, Danilenko M, Fishman D, LeRoith D, Levy J, Sharoni Y (1997) Membrane-associated insulin-like growth factor-binding protein-3 inhibits insulin-like growth factor-I-induced insulin-like growth factor-I receptor signaling in ishikawa endometrial cancer cells. J Biol Chem 272: 16514–16520

117. Keller JN, Kindy MS, Holtsberg FW, Clair DKS, Yen HC, Germeyer A, Steiner SM, Bruce-Keller AJ, Hutchins JB, Mattson MP (1998) Mitochondrial manganese superoxide dismutase prevents neural apoptosis and reduces ischemic brain injury: suppression of peroxynitrite production, lipid peroxidation, and mitochondrial dysfunction. J Neurosci 18: 687–697

118. Kharbanda S, Pandey P, Saxena SP, Haider N, Iskandrian A, Narula J (1998) Translocation of stress-induced JNK to mitochondria and release of cytochrome-c during apoptosis (abstr). Circulation 98: I-683

119. Khrapko K, Coller HA, André PC, Li XC, Hanekamp JS (1997) Mitochondrial mutational spectra in human cells and tissues. Proc Natl Acad Sci 94: 13798–13803

120. Kluck RM, Bossy-Wetzel E, Green DR, Newmeyer DD (1997) The release of cytochrome c from mitochondria: a primary site for bcl-2 regulation of apoptosis. Science 275: 1132–1136

121. Kluck RM, Martin SJ, Hoffman BM, Zhou JS, Green DR, Newmeyer DD (1997) Cytochrome c activation of CPP32-like proteolysis plays a critical role in a Xenopus cell-free apoptosis system. Embo J 16: 4639–4649

122. Kodama H, Fukuda K, Pan J, Makino S, Baba A, Hori S, Ogawa S (1997) Leukemia inhibitory factor, a potent cardiac hypertrophic cytokine, activates the JAK/STAT pathway in rat cardiomyocytes. Circ Res 81: 656–663

123. Kohnke D, Ludwig B, Kadenbach B (1993) A threshold membrane potential accounts for controversial effects of fatty acids on mitochondrial oxydative phosphorylation. FEBS Letters 336: 90–94

124. Kontos CD, Sankar S, Stauffer TP, York JD, Meyer T, Peters KG (1998) The endothelial receptor kinase Tie2 activates phosphatidylinositol 3-kinase and Akt and mediates endothelial cell survival (abstr). Circulation 98 (suppl-I): I-463

125. Korinek V, Barker N, Morin PJ, Van Wichen D, De Weger R, Kinzler KW, Vogelstein B, Clevers H (1997) Constitutive transcriptional activation by a β-catenin-Tcf-complex in APC-/-colon carcinoma. Science 275: 1784–1787

126. Kowaltowski AJ, Netto LE, Vercesi AE (1998) The thiol-specific antioxidant enzyme prevents mitochondrial permeability transition. Evidence for the participation of reactive oxygen species in this mechanism. J Biol Chem 273: 12766–12769

127. Kroemer G, Dallaporta B, Resche-Rigon M (1998) The mitochondrial death/life regulator in apoptosis and necrosis. Ann Rev Physiol 60: 619–642

128. Kuchino Y, Mori F, Kasai H, Inoue H, Iwai S, Miura K, Ohtsuka E, Nishimura S (1987) Misreading of DNA templates containing 8-hydroxydeoxyguanosine at the modified base and at adjacent residues. Nature 327: 77–79

129. Kunisada K, Tone E, Fujio Y, Matsui H, Yamauchi-Takihara K, Kishimoto T (1998) Activation of gp130 transduces hypertrophic signals via STAT3 in cardiac myocytes. Circulation 98: 346–352

130. Kwong LK, Sohal RS (1998) Substrate and site specificity of hydrogen peroxide generation in mouse mitochondria. Arch Biochem Biophys 350: 118–126

131. Le Roith D, Parrizas M, Blakesley VA (1997) The insulin-like growth factor-I receptor and apoptosis: implications for the aging process. Endocrine 7: 103–105

132. Le Roith D, Werner H, Faria TN, Kato H, Adamo M, Roberts CT (1993) Insulin-like growth factor receptors: implications for nervous system function. Ann N Y Acad Sci 692: 22–32

133. Lemasters JJ, Nieminen AL, Qian T, Trost LC, Elmore SP, Nishimura Y, Crowe RA, Cascio WE, Bradham CA, Brenner DA, Herman B (1998) The mitochondrial permeability transition in cell death: a common mechanism in necrosis, apoptosis and autophagy. Biochim Biophys Acta 1366: 177–196

134. Leri A, Claudio PP, Li Q, Wang X, Reiss K, Wang S, Malhotra A, Kajstura J, Anversa P (1998) Stretch-mediated release of angiotensin II induces myocyte apoptosis by activating p53 that enhances the local renin-angiotensin system and decreases the bcl-2-to-bax ratio in the cell. J Clin Invest 101: 1326–1342

135. Leri A, Liu Y, Malhotra A, Li Q, Stiegler P, Claudio PP, Giordano A, Kajstura J, Hintze TH, Anversa P (1998) Pacing-induced heart failure in dogs enhances the expression of p53 and p53-dependent genes in ventricular myocytes. Circulation 97: 194–203

136. Leto TL, Lomax KJ, Volpp BD, Nunoi H, Sechler JM, Nauseef WM, Clark RA, Gallin JI, Malech HL (1990) Cloning of a 67-kD neutrophil oxidase factor with similarity to a noncatalytic region of $p60^{c-src}$. Science 248: 727–730

137. Leyns L, Bouwmeester T, Kim SH, Piccolo S, De Robertis EM (1997) Frzb-1 is a secreted antagonist of Wnt signaling expressed in the Spemann organizer. Cell 88: 747–756

138. Li F, Srinivasan A, Wang Y, Armstrong RC, Tomaselli KJ, Fritz LC (1997) Cell-specific induction of apoptosis by microinjection of cytochrome c. J Biol Chem 272: 30299–30305

139. Li P, Nijhawan D, Budihardjo I, Srinivasula SM, Ahmad M, Alnemri ES, Wang X (1997) Cytochrome c and dATP-dependent formation of Apaf-1/caspase-9 complex initiates an apoptotic protease cascade. Cell 91: 479–489

140. Li Q, Li B, Wang X, Levi A, Jana KP, Liu X, Kajstura J, Baserga R, Anversa P (1997) Overexpression of insulin growth factor-1 in mice protects from myocyte death after infarction, attenuating ventricular dilation, wall stress and cardiac hypertrophy. J Clin Invest 100: 1991–1999

141. Li RK, Li G, Mickle DAG, Weisel RD, Merante F, Luss H, Rao V, Christakis GT, Williams WG (1997) Overexpression of transforming growth factor-β1 and insulin-like growth factor-I in patients with idiopathic hypertrophic cardiomyopathy. Circulation 96: 874–881

142. Li ZH, Bing OHL, Long XL, Robinson KG, Lakatta EG (1997) Increased cardiocyte apoptosis during the transition to heart failure in the spontaneously hypertensive rat. Am J Heart 272: H2313–H2319

143. Lipton SA, Nicotera P (1998) Calcium, free radicals and excitotoxins in neuronal apoptosis. Cell Calcium 23: 165–171

144. Liston P, Roy N, Tamai K, Lefebvre C, Baird S, Cherton-Horvat G, Farahani R, McLean M, Ikeda JE, Mackenzie A, Korneluk RG (1996) Suppression of apoptosis in mammalian cells by NIAP and a related family of IAP genes. Nature 379: 349–353

145. Liu X, Kim CN, Yang J, Jemmerson R, Wang X (1996) Induction of apoptotic program in cell-free extracts: requirement for dATP and cytochrome c. Cell 86: 147–157

146. Liu Y, Cigola E, Cheng W, Kajastura J, Olivetti G, Hintze TH, Anversa P (1995) Myocyte nuclear mitotic division and programmed myocyte cell death characterize the cardiac myopathy induced by rapid ventricular pacing in dogs. Lab Invest 73: 771–787

147. Loh E, Swain JL (1996) Growth hormone for heart failure – cause for cautious optimism. N Engl J Med 334: 836–837

148. Lombardi G, Colao A, Ferone D, Marzullo P, Orio F, Longobardi S, Merola B (1997) Effect of growth hormone on cardiac function. Hormone Res 48 (suppl 4): 38–42

149. Long X, Boluyt MO, De Lourdes Hipolito M, Lundberg MS, Zheng JS, L ON, Cirielli C, Lakatta EG, Crow MT (1997) P53 and the hypoxia-induced apoptosis of cultured neonatal rat cardiac myocytes. J Clin Invest 99: 2635–2643

150. MacLellan WR, Schneider MD (1997) Death by design: programmed cell death in cardiovascular biology and disease. Circ Res 81: 137–144

151. Magnus G, Keizer J (1998) Model of β-cell mitochondrial calcium handling and electrical activity. II. Mitochondrial variables. Am J Physiol 274: C1174–C1184

152. Manzelmann MS, Harmon HJ (1987) Lack of age-dependent changes in rat heart mitochondria. Mech Ageing Dev 39: 281–288

153. Maria-Garcia J, Goldenthal MJ, Pierpont ME, Ananthakrishnan R (1995) Impaired mitochondrial function in idiopathic dilated cardiomyopathy: biochemical and molecular analysis. J Card Fail 1: 285–291

154. Marsters SA, Sheridan JP, Donahue CJ, Pitti RM, Gray CL, Goddard AD, Bauer KD, Ashkenazi A (1996) Apo-3, a new member of the tumor necrosis factor receptor family, contains a death domain and activates apoptosis and NF-κB. Current Biol 6: 1669–1676

155. Marsters SA, Sheridan JP, Pitti RM, Brush J, Goddard A, Ashkenazi A (1998) Identification of a ligand for the death domain-containing receptor apo3. Curr Biol 8: 525–528

156. Martinez-Arias A, Baker NE, Ingham PW (1988) Role of segment polarity genes in the definition and maintenance of cell states in the Drosophila embryo. Development 103: 157–170

157. Marzo I, Brenner C, Zamzami N, Jürgensmeier JM, Susin SA, Vieira HLA, Prévost MC, Xie Z, Matsuyama S, Reed JC, Kroemer G (1998) Bax and adenin nucleotide translocator cooperate in the mitochondrial control of apoptosis. Science 281: 2027–2031

158. Matsui T, Hajjar RJ, Kang JX, Rosenzweig A (1997) Norepinephrine directly induces apoptosis in neonatal rat myocytes (abstr.). J Am Coll Cardiol 29: A-230
159. Meldrum DR (1998) Tumor necrosis factor in the heart. Am J Physiol 274: R577–R595
160. Melkonyan HS, Chang WC, Shapiro JP, Mahadevappa M, Fitzpatrick PA, Kiefer MC, Tomei LD, Umansky SR (1997) SARPs: a family of secreted apoptosis-related proteins. Proc Natl Acad Sci 94: 13636–13641
161. Meredith JE, Schwartz MA (1997) Integrins, adhesion and apoptosis. Trends Cell Biol 7: 146–150
162. Meulemans AL, Sipido KR, Sys SU, Brutsaert DL (1988) Atriopeptin III induces early relaxation of isolated mammalian papillary muscle. Circ Res 62: 1171–1174
163. Mignotte B, Vayssiere JL (1998) Mitochondria and apoptosis. Eur J Biochem 252: 1–15
164. Mitchell P (1966) Chemiosmotic coupling in oxidative and photosynthetic phosphorylation. Biol Rev 41: 445–502
165. Miyamoto T, Fox JC (1998) Ras regulates apoptosis through both MAPK and PI-3/Akt in vascular smooth muscle cells (abstr). Circulation 98 (suppl-I): I-463
166. Molketin JD, Lu JR, Antos CL, Markham B, Richardson J, Robbins J, Grant SR, Olson EN (1998) A calcineurin-dependent transcriptional pathway for cardiac hypertrophy. Cell 93: 215–228
167. Molketin JD, Olson EN (1997) GATA-4: a novel transcriptional regulator of cardiac hypertrophy? Circulation 96: 3833–3835
168. Morin PJ, Sparks AB, Korinek V, Barker N, Clevers H, Vogelstein B, Kinzler KW (1997) Activation of β-catenin-Tcf signaling in colon cancer by mutations in β-catenin or APC. Science 275: 1787–1790
169. Möröy T, Zoernig M (1996) Regulators of life and death: the bcl-2 gene family. Cell Physiol Biochem 6: 312–336
170. Moyes CD, Battersby BJ, Leary SC (1998) Regulation of muscle mitochondrial design. J Exp Biol 201: 299–307
171. Muscari C, Giaccari A, Giordano E, Clo C, Guarneri C, Caldarera CM (1996) Role of reactive oxygen species in cardiovascular aging. Mol Cell Biochem 160/161: 159–166
172. Nachshon S, Zamir O, Matsuda Y, Zamir N (1995) Effect of ANP receptor antagonists on ANP secretion from adult cultured atrial myocytes. Am J Physiol 268: E428–E432
173. Nagata S (1997) Apoptosis by death factor. Cell 88: 355–365
174. Narula J, Haider N, Virmani R, DiSalvo T, Kolodgie FD, Hajjar RJ, Schmidt U, Semigran MJ, Dec W, Khaw BA (1996) Apoptosis in myocytes in end-stage heart failure. N Engl J Med 335: 1182–1189
175. Narula J, Kharbanda S, Khaw BA (1997) Apoptosis and the heart. Chest 112: 1358–1362
176. Neuberg M, Buckbinder L, Seizinger B, Kley N (1997) The p53/IFF-1 receptor axis in the regulation of programmed cell death. Endocrine 7: 107–109
177. Nickerson T, Huynh H, Pollak M (1997) Insulin-like growth factor binding protein-3 induces apoptosis in MCF7 breast cancer cells. Biochem Biophys Res Comm 237: 690–693
178. Nohl H, Hegner D (1978) Do mitochondria produce oxygen radicals in vivo? Eur J Biochem 82: 563–567
179. Nunez DJR, Dickson MC, Brown MJ (1992) Natriuretic peptide receptor mRNAs in the rat and human heart. J Clin Invest 90: 1966–1971
180. Nusse R, Varmus HE (1982) Many tumors induced by the mouse mammary tumor virous contain a provirus integrated in the same region of the host genome. Cell 31: 99–109
181. Nusse R, Varmus HE (1992) Wnt genes. Cell 69: 1073–1087
182. Nüsslein-Volhard C, Wieschaus E (1980) Mutations affecting segment number and polarity in Drosophila. Nature 287: 792–801
183. Nyui N, Tamura K, Mizuno K, Ishigami T, Kihara M, Ochiai H, Kimura K, Umemura S, Ohno S, Taga T, Ishii M (1998) Gp130 is involved in stretch-induced MAP kinase activation in cardiac myocytes. Biochem Biophys Res Comm 245: 928–932
184. O'Connor R, Kauffmann-Zeh A, Liu Y, Lehar S, Evan GI, Baserga R, Blattler WA (1997) Identification of domains of the insulin-like growth factor I receptor that are required for protection from apoptosis. Mol Cell Biol 17: 427–435
185. Oh H, Fujio Y, Kunisada K, Hirota H, Matsui H, Kishimoto T, Yamauchi-Takihara K (1998) Activation of phosphatidylinositol 3-kinase through glycoprotein 130 induces protein kinase B and p70S6 kinase phosphorylation in cardiac myocytes. J Biol Chem 273: 9703–9710
186. Oh H, Kunasada K, Matsui H, Yamauchi-Takihara K (1998) Phosphatidylinositol 3-kinase transduces survival and hypertrophic signals via Akt/MAP kinase and p70 S6 kinase pathways in cardiac myocytes. Circulation 98: I-462
187. Oh H, Kunisada K, Funamoto M, Yamauchi-Takihara K (1998) Activation of gp 130 inhibits doxorubicin induced cell death by Bcl-x$_L$/caspase 3 interaction and PI 3-kinase/Akt pathway in cardiac myocytes. Circulation 98: I-462
188. Oh Y, Mueller HL, Lamson G, Rosenfeld RG (1993) Insulin-like growth factor (IGF)-independent action to IGF-binding protein-3 in Hs578T human breast cancer cells. J Biol Chem 268: 14964–14971
189. Olivetti G, Abbi R, Quaini F, Kajstura J, Cheng W, Nitahara JA, Quaini E, DiLoreto C, Beltrami CA, Krajewski S, Reed JC, Anversa P (1997) Apoptosis in the failing human heart. N Engl J Med 336: 1131–1141

190. Olivetti G, Quiani F, Sala R, Lagrasta C, Corradi D, Bonancia E, Gambert SR, Cigola E, Anversa P (1996) Acute myocardial infarction in humans is associated with activation of programmed myocyte cell death in the surviving portion of the heart. J Moll Cardiol 28: 2005–2016
191. Orsulic S, Pfeifer M (1996) Cell-cell signaling: wingless lands at last. Curr Biol 6: 1363–1367
192. Osterziel KJ, Strohm O, Schuler J, Friedrich M, Hänlein D, Willenbrock R, Anker SD, Poole-Wilson PA, Ranke MB, Dietz R (1998) Randomised, double-blind, placebo-controlled trial of human recombinant growth hormone in patients with chronic heart failure due to dilated cardiomyopathy. Lancet 351: 1233–1237
193. Ozawa T (1997) Genetic and functional changes in mitochondria associated with aging. Physiol Rev 77: 425–464
194. Pan G, Bauer JH, Haridas V, Wang S, Liu D, Yu G, Vincenz C, Aggarwal BB, Ni J, Dixit VM (1998) Identification and functional characterization of DR6, a novel death domain-containing TNF receptor. FEBS Lett 431: 351–356
195. Pan G, Ni J, Wei YF, Yu QL, Gentz R, Dixit VM (1997) An antagonist decoy receptor and a death domain-containing receptor for TRAIL. Science 277: 815–818
196. Papa S, Skulachev VP (1997) Reactive oxygen species, mitochodria, apoptosis and aging. Mol Cell Biochem 174: 305–319
197. Pennica D, King KL, Shaw KJ, Luis E, Rullamas J, Luoh SM, Darbonne WC, Knutzon DS, Yen R, Chien KR, Et AL (1995) Expression cloning of cardiotrophin 1, a cytokine that induces cardiac myocyte hypertrophy. Proc Natl Acad Sci 92: 1142–1146
198. Pennica D, Shaw KJ, Swanson TA, Moore MW, Shelton DL, Zioncheck KA, Rosenthal A, Taga T, Paoni NF, Wood WI (1995) Cardiotrophin-1: biological activities and binding to the leukemia inhibitory factor/gp130 signaling complex. J Biol Chem 270: 10915–10922
199. Perrimon N (1996) Serpentine receptors slither into the wingless and hedgehog fields. Cell 86: 513–516
200. Petit PX, Goubern M, Diolez P, Susin A, Zamzani N, Kroemer G (1998) Disruption of the outer mitochondrial membrane as a result of large amplitude swelling: the impact of irreversible permeability transition. FEBS Letters 426: 111–116
201. Pierzchalski P, Reiss K, Cheng W, Cirielli C, Kajstura J, Nitahara JA, Rizk M, Capogrossi MC, Anversa P (1997) P53 induces myocyte apoptosis via the activation of the renin-angiotensin system. Exp Cell Res 234: 57–65
202. Pitkaenen S, Robinson BH (1996) Mitochondrial complex I deficiency leads to increased production of superoxide radicals and induction of superoxide dismutase. J Clin Invest 98: 345–351
203. Pitti RM, Marsters SA, Lawrence DA, Roy M, Kischkel FC, Dowd P, Huang A, Donahue CJ, Sherwood SW, Gurney AL, Hillan KJ, Cohen RL, Goddard AD, Botstein D, Ashkenazi A (1998) Genomic amplification of a decoy receptor for Fas ligand in lung and colon cancer. Nature 396: 699–703
204. Pitti RM, Marsters SA, Ruppert S, Donahue CJ, Moore A, Ashkenazi A (1996) Induction of apoptosis by Apo-2 ligand, a new member of the tumor necrosis factor cytokine family. J Biol Chem 271: 12687–12690
205. Pizzuti A, A.L. E (1996) Human homologue sequences to the Drosophila dishevelled segment-polarity gene are deleted in the DiGeorge syndrome. Am J Hum Genet 58: 722–729
206. Pulkki KJ (1997) Cytokines and cardiomyocyte death. Ann Med 29: 339–343
207. Raff M (1998) Cell suicide for beginners. Nature 396: 119–122
208. Raff MC (1992) Social controls on cell survival and cell death. Nature 356: 397–400
209. Rajah R, Valentinis B, Cohen P (1997) Insulin-like growth factor- binding protein-3 induces apoptosis and mediates the effects of transforming growth factor-β1 on programmed cell death through a p53- and IGF-independent mechanism. J Biol Chem 272: 12181–12188
210. Rajaram S, Baylink DJ, Mohan S (1997) Insulin-like growth factor-binding proteins in serum and other biological fluids: regulation and functions. Endocrine Rev 18: 801–831
211. Rankin AJ, V. SF (1990) The inotropic effect of atrial natriuretic factor in the anesthetized rabbit. Pflügers Arch 417: 353–359
212. Rao L, White E (1997) Bcl-2 and the ICE family of apoptotic regulators: making a connection. Curr Opin Genet Dev 7: 52–58
213. Rattner A, Hsieh JC, Smallwood PM, Gilbert DJ, Copeland NG, Jenkins NA, Nathans J (1997) A family of secreted proteins contains homology to the cysteine-rich ligand-binding domain of frizzled receptors. Proc Natl Acad Sci 94: 2859–2863
214. Ray CA, Black RA, Kronheim SR, Greenstreet TA, Sleath PR, Salvesen GS, Pickup DJ (1992) Viral inhibitors of inflammation: cowpox virus encodes an inhibitor of the interleukin-1β converting enzyme. Cell 69: 597–604
215. Rechler MM (1997) Editorial: Growth inhibition by insulin-like growth factor (IGF) binding protein-3 – Whats IGF got to do with it? Endocrinology 138: 2645–2647
216. Reed JC (1997) Double identity for proteins of the Bcl-2 family. Nature 387: 773–776
217. Reiss K, Cheng W, Ferber A, Kajstura J, Li P, Li B, Olivetti G, Homcy CJ, Baserga R, Anversa P (1996) Overexpression of insulin-like growth factor-1 in the heart is coupled with myocyte proliferation in transgenic mice. Proc Natl Acad Sci 93: 8630–8635

218. Reiss K, Kajstura J, Zhang X, Li P, Szoke E, Olivetti G, Anversa P (1994) Acute myocardial infarction leads to upregulation of the IGF-1 autocrine system, DNA replication, and nuclear mitotic division in the remaining viable cardiac myocytes. Experimental Cell Research 213: 463–472

219. Reiss K, Meggs LG, Li P, Olivetti G, Caspasso JM, Anversa P (1994) Upregulation of IGF_1, IGF_1-receptor, and late growth related genes in ventricular myocytes acutely after infarction in rats. J Cell Physiol 158: 160–168

220. Revilla Y, Cebrian A, Baixeras E, Martinez C, Vinuela E, Salas ML (1997) Inhibition of apoptosis by the African swine fever virus Bcl-2 homologue: role of the BH1 domain. Virology 228: 400–404

221. Richter C (1995) Oxidative damage to mitochondrial DNA and its relationship to ageing. Int J Biochem Cell Biol 27: 647–653

222. Robledo O, Chevalier S, Froger J, Barthelaix-Pouplard A, Pennica D, Gascan H (1997) Regulation of interleukin 6 expression by cardiotrophin 1. Cytokine 9: 666–671

223. Robledo O, Fourcin M, Chevalier S, Guillet C, Auguste P, Pouplard-Barthelaix A, Pennica D, Gascan H (1997) Signaling of the cardiotrophin-1 receptor: evidence for a third receptor component. J Biol Chem 272: 4855–4863

224. Roy N et al. (1995) The gene for neuronal apoptosis inhibitory protein is partially deleted in individuals with spinal muscular atrophy. Cell 80: 167–178

225. Roy N, Deveraux QL, Takahashi R, Salvesen GS, Reed JC (1997) The c-IAP-1 and c-IAP-2 proteins are direct inhibitors of specific caspases. Embo J 16: 6914–6925

226. Rubinfeld B, Albert I, Porfiri E, Munemitsu S, Polakis P-R (1997) Loss of β-catenin regulation by the APC tumor suppressor protein correlates with loss of structure due to common somatic mutations of the gene. Cancer Res 57: 4624–4630

227. Russell-Jones DL, Leach RM, Wak JPT, Thomas CK (1993) Insulin-like growth factor-I gene expression is increased in the right ventricular hypertrophy induced by chronic hypoxia in the rat. J Mol Endocrinol 10: 99–102

228. Sadoshima J, Izumo S (1993) Molecular characterization of angiotensin II-induced hypertrophy of cardiac myocytes and hyperplasia of cardiac fibroblasts: a critical role of the AT1 receptor subtype. Circ Res 73: 413–423

229. Sadoshima J, Izumo S (1993) Signal transduction pathways of angiotensin II induced c-fos gene expression in cardiac myocytes in vitro: roles of phospholipid-derived second messengers. Circ Res 73: 424–438

230. Sadoshima J, Izumo S (1997) The cellular and molecular response of cardiac myocytes to mechanical stress. Ann Rev Physiol 59: 551–571

231. Sadoshima J, Xu Y, Slayter HS, Izumo S (1993) Autocrine release of angiotensin II mediates stretch-induced hypertrophy of cardiac myocytes in vitro. Cell 75: 977–984

232. Sakahira H, Enari M, Nagata S (1998) Cleavage of CAD inhibitor in CAD activation and DNA degradation during apoptosis. Nature 391: 96–99

233. Santos AC, Uyemura SA, Santos NAG, Mingatto FE, Curti C (1997) Hg(II)-induced renal cytotoxicity: in vitro and in vivo implications for the bioenergetic and oxidative status of mitochondria. Mol Cell Biochem 177: 53–59

234. Saraste A, Pulkki K, Kallajoki M, Henriksen K, Parvinen M, Voipio-Pulkki LM (1997) Apoptosis in human acute myocardial infarction. Circulation 95: 320–323

235. Satoh T, Enokido Y, Aoshima H, Uchiyama Y, Hatanaka H (1997) Changes in mitochondrial membrane potential during oxidative stress-induced apoptosis in PC12 cells. J Neurosci Res 50: 413–420

236. Schneider P, Bodmer JL, Thome M, Hofmann K, Holler N, Tschopp J (1997) Characterization of two receptors for TRAIL. FEBS Lett 416: 329–334

237. Schoenbeck U, Herzberg M, Petersen A, Wohlenberg C, Gerdes J, Flad HD, Loppnow H (1997) Human vascular smooth muscle cells express interleukin-1β-converting enzyme (ICE), but inhibit processing of the interleukin-1β precursor by ICE. J Exp Med 185: 1287–1294

238. Schulze-Osthoff K, Ferrari D, Los M, Wesselborg S, Peter ME (1998) Apoptosis signaling by death receptors. Eur J Biochem 254: 439–459

239. Schumacher R, Soos MA, Schlessinger J, Brandenburg D, Siddle K, Ullrich A (1993) Signaling-competent receptor chimeras allow mapping of major insulin binding domain determinants. J Biol Chem 268: 1087–1094

240. Schumann H, Morawietz H, Hakim K, Zerkowski HR, Eschenhagen T, Holtz J, Darmer D (1997) Alternative splicing of the primary Fas transcript generating soluble Fas antagonists is suppressed in the failing human ventricular myocardium. Biochem Biophys Res Comm 239: 794–798

241. Scorrano L, Petronilli V, Bernardi P (1997) On the voltage dependence of the mitochondrial permeability transition pore: a critical appraisal. J Biol Chem 272: 12295–12299

242. Screaton GR, Monkolsapaya J, Xu XN, Cowper AE, McMichael AJ, Bell JL (1997) TRICK2, a new alternatively spliced receptor that transduces the cytotoxic signal from TRAIL. Curr Biol 7: 693–696

243. Screaton GR, Xu XN, Olsen AL, Cowper AE, Tan R, McMichael AJ, Bell JI (1997) LARD: a new lymphoid-specific death domain containing receptor regulated by alternative pre-mRNA splicing. Proc Natl Acad Sci 94: 4615–4619
244. Shadel GS, Clayton DA (1997) Mitochondrial DNA maintenance in vertebrates. Ann Rev Biochem 66: 409–435
245. Sheng Z, Knowlton K, Chen J, Hoshijima M, Brown JH, Chien KR (1997) Cardiotrophin 1 (CT-1) inhibition of cardiac myocyte apoptosis via a mitogen-activated protein kinase-dependent pathway: divergence from downstream CT-1 signals for myocardial cell hypertrophy. J Biol Chem 272: 5783–5791
246. Sheng Z, Pennica D, Wood WI, Chien KR (1996) Cardiotropin-1 displays early expression in the murine heart tube and promotes cardiac myocyte survival. Development 122: 419–428
247. Sheridan JP, Marsters SA, Pitti RM, Gurney A, Skubatch M, Baldwin D, Ramakrishnan L, Gray CL, Baker K, Wood WI, Goddard AD, Godowski P, Ashkenazi A (1997) Control of TRAIL-induced apoptosis by a family of signaling and decoy receptors. Science 277: 818–821
248. Shier P, Watt VM (1989) Primary structure of a putative receptor for a ligand of the insulin family. J Biol Chem 264: 14605–14608
249. Shigenaga MK, Hagen TM, Ames BN (1994) Oxidative damage and mitochondrial decay in aging. Proc Natl Acad Sci 91: 10771–10778
250. Shirozu M, Tashiro K, Nakamura T, Lopez ND, Nazarea M, Hamada T, Sato T, Nakano T, Honjo T (1996) Characterization of novel secreted and membrane proteins isolated by the signal sequence trap method. Genomics 37: 273–280
251. Shizukuda Y, Buttrick PB, Geenen DL, Borczuk AC, Kitsis RN, Sonnenblick EH (1998) β-Adrenergic stimulation causes cardiocyte apoptosis: influence of tachycardia and hypertrophy. Am J Physiol 275: H961–H968
252. Skulachev PV (1998) Uncoupling. New approaches to an old problem of bioenergetics. Biochim Biophys Acta 1363
253. Steare SE, Yellon DM (1995) The potential for endogenous myocardial antioxidants to protect the myocardium against ischaemia-reperfusion injury: refreshing the parts exogenous antioxidants cannot reach? J Mol Cell Cardiol 27: 65–74
254. Steemans M, Goossens V, Van de Craen M, Van Heereweghe F, Vancompernolle K, De Vos K, Vandenabeele P, Groten J (1998) A caspase-activated factor (CAF) induces mitochondrial membrane depolarization and cytochrome c release by a nonproteolytic mechanism. J Exp Med 188: 2193–2198
255. Stephanou A, Brar B, Heads R, Knight RD, Marber MS, Pennica D, Latchman DS (1998) Cardiotrophin-1 induces heat shock protein accumulation in cultured cardiac cells and protects them from stressful stimuli. J Mol Cell Cardiol 30: 849–855
256. Susin SA, Zamzami N, Castedo M, Hirsch T, Marchetti P, Macho A, Daugas E, Geuskens M, Kroemer G (1996) Bcl-2 inhibits the mitochondrial release of an apoptogenic protease. J Exp Med 184: 1331–1341
257. Svrzic D, Schubert D (1990) Insulin-like growth factor 1 supports embryonic nerve cell survival. Biochem Biophys Res Comm 172: 54–60
258. Tajima M, Bartunek J, Weinberg EO, Ito N, Lorell BH (1998) Atrial natriuretic peptide has different effects on contractility and intracellular pH in normal and hypertrophied myocytes from pressure-overloaded hearts. Circulation 98: 2760–2764
259. Takahashi T, Honda H, Hirai H, Tsujimoto Y (1997) Overexpressed Bcl-x$_L$ prevents bacterial superantigen-induced apoptosis of thymocytes in vitro. Cell Death Diff 4: 159–165
260. Takahashi T, Taniguchi T, Takahashi A, Oda A, Kawasaki S, Domoto K, Ishikawa Y, Yokoyama M (1998) Activation of Akt/protein kinase B following stimulation with angiotensin II in vascular smooth muscle cells (abstr). Circulation 98 (suppl-I): I-462
261. Takemoto M, Egashira K, Tomita H, Usui M, Okamoto H, Kitabatake A, Shimokawa H, Sueishi K, Takeshita A (1997) Chronic angiotensin-converting enzyme inhibition and angiotensin II type 1 receptor blockade: effects on cardiovascular remodeling in rats induced by the long-term blockade of nitric oxide synthesis. Hypertension 30: 1621–1627
262. Takemoto M, Egashira K, Usui M, Numaguchi K, Tomita H, Tsutsui H, Shimokawa H, Sueishi K, Takeshita A (1997) Important role of tissue angiotensin-converting enzyme activity in the pathogenesis of coronary vascular and myocardial structural changes induced by long-term blockade of nitric oxide synthesis in rats. J Clin Invest 99: 278–287
263. Tanaka M, Kovalenko SA, Gong JS, Borgeld HJ, Katsumata K, M. H, Yoneda M, Ozawa T (1996) Accumulation of deletions and point mutations in mitochondrial genome in degenerative diseases. Ann N Y Acad Sci 786: 102–111
264. Tartaglia LA, Ayres TM, Wong GHW, Goeddel DV (1993) A novel domain within the 55 kd TNF receptor signals cell death. Cell 74: 845–853
265. Teiger E, Dam TV, Richard L, Wisnewsky C, Tea BS, Gaboury L, Tremblay J, Schwartz K, Hamet P (1996) Apoptosis in pressure overload-induced heart hypertrophy in the rat. J Clin Invest 97: 2891–897
266. Testi R (1996) Sphingomyelin breakdown and cell fate. Trends Biochem Sci 21: 468–471

267. Thatte U, Dahanukar S (1997) Apoptosis: clinical relevance and pharmacological manipulation. Drugs 54: 511–532
268. Thome M, Schneider P, Hofmann K, Fickenscher H, Meinl E, Neipel F, Mattmann C, Burns K, Bodmer JL, Schroeter M, Scaffidi C, Krammer PH, Peter ME, Tschopp J (1997) Viral FLICE-inhibitory proteins (FLIPs) prevent apoptosis induced by death receptors. Nature 386: 517–521
269. Thornberry NA, Lazebnik Y (1998) Caspases: enemies within. Science 281: 1313–1316
270. Thornberry NA, Rano TA, Peterson EP, Rasper DM, Timkey T, Garcia-Calvo M, Houtzager VM, Nordstrom PA, Roy S, Vaillancourt JP, Chapman KT, Nicholson DW (1997) A combinatorial approach defines specificities of members of the caspase family and granezyme B: functional relationships established for key mediators of apoptosis. J Biol Chem 272: 17907–17911
271. Tomlinson A, Strapps W, Heemskerk J (1997) Linking Frizzled and Wnt signaling in Drosophila development. Development Suppl 124: 4515–4521
272. Turrens JF (1997) Superoxide production by the mitochondrial respiratory chain. Biosci Reports 17: 3–8
273. Uren AG, Vaux DL (1997) Viral inhibitors of apoptosis. Vitam Horm 53: 175–193
274. Van den Eijnde SM, Luijsterburg AJM, Boshart L, De Zeeuw CI, van Dierendonck JH, Reutelingsperger CPM, Vermeij-Keers C (1997) In situ detection of apoptosis during embryogenesis with annexin V: from whole mount to ultrastructure. Cytometry 29: 313–320
275. Van Engeland M, Nieland LJW, Ramaekers FCS, Schutte B, Reutelingsperger CPM (1998) Annexin V-affinity assay: a review on an apoptosis detection system based on phosphatidylserine exposure. Cytometry 31: 1–9
276. Vanags DM, Porn-Ares MI, Coppola S, Burgess DH, Orrenius S (1996) Protease involvement in fodrin cleavage and phosphatidylserine exposure in apoptosis. J Biol Chem 271: 31075–31085
277. Vercesi AE, Kowaltowski AJ, Grijalba MT, Meinicke AR, Castilho RF (1997) The role of reactive oxygen species in mitochondrial permeability transition. Biosci Reports 17: 43–52
278. Vinson CR, Conover S, Adler PN (1989) A Drosophila tissue polarity locus encodes a protein containing seven potential transmembrane domains. Nature 338: 263–264
279. Wahlander H, Isgaard J, Jennische E, Friberg P (1992) Left ventricular insulin-like growth factor I increases in early renal hypertension. Hypertension 19: 25–32
280. Wallace DC (1992) Diseases of the mitochondrial DNA. Ann Rev Biochem 61: 1175–1212
281. Wallace DC (1992) Mitochondrial genetics: a paradigm for aging and degenerative disease. Science 256: 628–632
282. Wang G-H, Bertin J, Wang Y, Martin DA, Wang J, Tomaselli KJ, Armstrong RC, Cohen JI (1997) Bovine herpesvirus 4 BORFE2 protein inhibits Fas and Tumor Necrosis Factor Receptor 1-induced apoptosis and contains death effector domains shared with other gamma-2 herpesviruses. J Virol 71: 8928–8932
283. Wang L, Ma W, Markovich R, Wang PH (1997) Insulin-like growth factor I inhibits activation of apopain/CPP32 pathway and induction of apoptosis in cardiomyocytes (abstr). Circulation 96: I-553
284. Wang S, Krinks M, Lin K, Luyten FP, Moos M (1997) Frzb, a secreted protein expressed in the Spemann organizer, binds and inhibits Wnt-8. Cell 88: 757–766
285. Wang S, Souza RF, Kong D, Yin J, Smolinski KN, Zou TT, Frank T, Young J, Flanders KC, Sugimura H, Abraham JM, Meltzer SJ (1997) Deficient transforming growth factor-beta1 activation and excessive insulin-like growth factor II (IGFII) expression in IGFII receptor-mutant tumors. Cancer Res 57: 2543–2546
286. Wang Y, Macke JP, Abella BS, Andreasson K, Worley P, Gilbert DJ, Copeland NG, Jenkins N, Nathans J (1996) A large family of putative transmembrane receptors homologous to the Drosophila tissue polarity gene frizzled. J Biol Chem 271: 4468–4476
287. White E (1996) Life, death, and the pursuit of apoptosis. Genes Dev 10: 1–15
288. Wickman A, Isgaard J, Adams MA, Friberg P (1997) Inhibition of nitric oxide in rats. Regulation of cardiovascular structure and expression of insulin-like growth factor I and its receptor messenger RNA. J Hypertens 15: 751–759
289. Wollert KC, Taga T, Saito M, Narazaki M, Kishimoto T, Glembotski CC, Vernallis AB, Heath JK, Pennica D, Wood WI, Chien KR (1996) Cardiotrophin-1 activates a distinct form of cardiac muscle cell hypertrophy: assembly of sarcomeric units in series via gp130/leukemia inhibitory factor receptor-dependent pathways. J Biol Chem 271: 9535–9545
290. Wong LL, Adler PN (1993) Tissue polarity genes of Drosophila regulate the subcellular location of prehair initiation in pupal wing cells. J Cell Biol 123: 209–221
291. Wu CF, Bishopric NH, Pratt RE (1997) Atrial natriuretic peptide induces apoptosis in neonatal rat cardiac myocytes. J Biol Chem 272: 14860–14866
292. Yagi T, Hatefi Y (1984) Thiols in oxidative phosphorylation: inhibition and energy-potentiated uncoupling by monothiol and dithiol modifiers. Biochemistry 23: 2449–2455
293. Yagi T, Hatefi Y (1987) Thiols in oxydative phosphorylation: thiols in the FO of ATPsynthase essential for ATPase activity. Arch Biochem Biophys 254: 102–109

294. Yang-Snyder J, Miller JR, Brown JD, Lai CJ, Moon RT (1996) A frizzled homolog functions in a vertebrate WNT signaling pathway. Curr Biol 6: 1302–1306

295. Yoshida K, Taga T, Saito M, Suematsu S, Kumanogoh A, Tanaka T, Fujiwara H, Hirata M, Yamagami T, Nakahata T, Hirabayashi T, Yoneda Y, Tanaka K, Wang WZ, Mori C, Shiota K, Yoshida N, Kishimoto T (1996) Targeted disruption of gp130, a common signal transducer for the interleukin 6 family of cytokines, leads to myocardial and hematological disorders. Proc Natl Acad Sci 93: 407–411

296. Yost C, Torres M, Miller JR, Huang E, Kimelman D, Moon RT (1996) The axis-inducing activity, stability, and subcellular distribution of β-catenin is regulated in Xenopus embryos by glycogen synthase kinase 3. Genes Dev 10: 1443–1454

297. Zamzami N, Marchetti P, Castedo M, Hirsch T, Susin SA, Masse B, Kroemer G (1996) Inhibitors of permeability transition interfere with the disruption of the mitochondrial transmembrane potential during apoptosis. FEBS Lett 384: 53–57

298. Zamzami N, Susin SA, Marchetti P, Hirsch T, I G-M, Castedo M, Kroemer G (1996) Mitochondrial control of nuclear apoptosis. J Exp Med 183: 1533–1544

299. Zhang X, Dostal DE, Reiss K, Cheng W, Kajstura J, Li O, Huang H, Sonnenblick EH, Meggs LG, Baker KM, Anversa P (1995) Identification and activation of autocrine renin-angiotensin system in adult ventricular myocytes. Am J Physiol 269: H1791–H1802

300. Zoratti M, Szabo I (1995) The mitochondrial permeability transition. Biochim Biophys Acta 1241: 139–176

301. Zou H, Henzel WJ, Liu X, Lutschg A, Wang X (1997) Apaf-1, a human protein homologous to c. elegans CED-4, participates in cytochrome c-dependent activation of caspase-3. Cell 90: 405–413

302. Zumkeller W, Schwab M (1999) Insulin-like growth factor system in neuroblastoma tumorigenesis and apoptosis: potential diagnostic and therapeutic perspectives. Horm Metab Res 31: 138–141

Author's address:
Dedicated to Prof. Dr. H. J. Just on the occasion of his 65th birthday
Institut für Pathophysiologie
Medizinische Fakultät
Martin-Luther-Universität Halle-Wittenberg
Magdeburger-Str. 18
06097 Halle/Saale
E-mail: juergen.holtz@medizin.uni-halle.de

Analysis of inherited causes of hypertrophic cardiomyopathy as part of clinical practice

H.-P. Vosberg[1], J. Moolman[2], C. Döhlemann[3], P. McKeown[4], S. Reith[5]

[1] Max-Planck-Institut für physiologische und klinische Forschung, Abt. Experimentelle Kardiologie, 61231 Bad Nauheim, Germany
[2] University of Stellenbosch, Division of Medical Physiology, Tygerberg 7505, RSA
[3] Universitäts-Kinderklinik LMU München, 80337 München, Germany
[4] Regional Medical Cardiology Centre, Royal Victoria Hospital, Belfast BT12 6BA, UK
[5] Medizinische Klinik I der Rheinisch-Westfälischen Technischen Hochschule, Abteilung Kardiologie, Aachen, Germany

Abstract

One of the major goals in human molecular genetics is the identification of mutations causing heritable disease. Genetic data do not only improve theoretical knowledge of pathogenic causes and mechanisms, but they also penetrate into clinical practice, first, by introducing new diagnostic tools and, second, by gradually setting up improved standards of prognosis, counseling and ultimately therapy. A case in question in cardiology is hypertrophic cardiomyopathy (HCM), a dominant disease of the cardiac sarcomere traced to mutations in seven different heart muscle genes. Current goals in research on HCM are – at least in part – targetted at determining the extent of causes and to collect data regarding clinical phenotypes (expressivity) as a function of specific mutations. Here we report about the genetic and clinical analysis of three cases of HCM caused by inherited or de novo mutations in two of the seven known HCM-related genes.

One of the most important results of recent developments in genetics and in particular in molecular human genetics was the identification of mutations responsible for numerous inherited diseases. Among them were the widely known Duchenne muscular dystrophy, cystic fibrosis or Huntington's disease, but many other disorders summarily classified as Mendelian (or single gene) diseases have also been successfully analyzed, including several cardiac disorders.

A corollary of growing knowledge about causes of disease is a shift in the role of medical genetics. In the past, this discipline was essentially theoretical and descriptive, mainly providing post festum conclusions. Now it is rapidly becoming part of clinical practice by introducing new diagnostic concepts and by contributing to an improved understanding of pathogenic mechanisms.

Genetic analysis in the area of primary heart diseases has recently been focused predominantly on two different categories, cardiomyopathies and diseases associated with arrhythmia, particularly torsade de pointes, traced to dysfunctional ion channels (long QT syndromes). The term "cardiomyopathy" collectively refers to a number of disorders which affect morphology and function of the myocard. Causes and clinical manifestations vary between different groups of cardiomyopathies. The following discussion will be restricted to hypertrophic cardiomyopathies (HCM).

Regarding DNA analysis, the genetic laboratory can offer diagnostic support as to assessment of causes in cases of doubt, for instance in sporadic patients with no family history, or in early preclinical stages in members of families known to transmit inherited conditions. It can further be expected that the systematic evaluation of increasing amounts of genetic data obtained through "genetic field work" from many patients and many families will afford improved risk stratification, which in turn may lead to efficient preventive measures or even new therapies. To summarize the attitude of many scientists and clinicians, one may anticipate that DNA analysis will become sort of a "gold standard" in clinical medicine aimed at more accurate diagnosis and improved management.

HCM is a primary disorder of the myocardium. It was observed long ago that it is usually associated with an asymmetrical increase in myocardial muscle mass, most frequently in the interventricular septum (9). Typical manifestations are altered cardiac contraction and relaxation, and arrhythmic disorders associated with chest pain, dyspnoe, and syncopes (5). Previously HCM was characterized as a disease of young adults with a concomitant high tendency of risk carriers to become sick. It is now realized that symptoms may develop at any age, however, rarely in children. Patients may be asymptomatic for most of their lifes (7, 8). The considerable phenotypic variability implies that a familial disposition is not always recognized.

Progression is usually slow. The most dreadful complication is that of sudden cardiac death, in most instances as a consequence of ventricular fibrillation. The annual mortality rate among carriers is about 1 % (8). Occasionally sudden death may be the only manifestation of the disease in the absence of symptoms otherwise characteristic for HCM. The prevalence in the general population has recently been calculated to be in the range of 1 in 500 (4). If this estimate is correct, HCM would belong to the frequent inherited diseases in man.

The dominant transmission of HCM has been known long since. The molecular causes known today indicate a considerable degree of heterogeneity. More than hundred mutations in seven genes have been reported. All of these genes code for proteins functioning in cardiac sarcomeres. Thus, the primary dysfunction in HCM impairs cardiac contraction. The mutated proteins are β-myosin heavy chain (on chromosome 14), cardiac troponin T and I (chromosome 1 and 19, resp.), α-tropomyosin (chromosome 15), the essential and regulatory myosin light chains (chromosome 3 and 12, resp.), and myosin binding protein-C (chromosome 11). The single most frequently mutated gene is the β-myosin heavy chain gene expressed in the muscle of the ventricles and also in slow skeletal muscle. Up to 30 % or more of all cases of HCM with known mutations can be traced to this gene (for further details see 10).

These results have led to an increasing demand for genetic diagnosis by cardiologists or by human geneticists who are consulted by members of HCM families. One may expect that it is easy – at least in principle, technical difficulties notwithstanding – to apply DNA analysis as the presumed "gold standard". In fact it is easy in some cases, but not in others. In a candidate gene test run with 31 index cases, we were able to identify mutations presumed to be related to HCM in 9 of them (11).

Here we wish to discuss that the identification of a mutation is not only a technical problem (techniques are not considered here), but it may also require reasoning about clinical and pathogenic relevance of the finding. A mutation may by itself explain the disorder, but it may also be unrelated to the disease, or it may be part of a complex set of unknown factors responsible for the pathologic process.

Table 1. Phenotype relations of HCM mutations in three study families.

Family	Gene affected	Transmission	Type of mutation	Position in mRNA	Phenotype
SM	β-MHC[1]	(co-dominant)[3]	missense	codon 349	non-related to disease
	β-MHC[1]	de novo	missense	codon 719	severe disease
WF	β-MHC[1]	dominant	missense	codon 1205	mild disease, incomplete penetrance
EA	MyBP-C[2]	dominant	insertion of one G	codon 791	mild disease, late onset, incomplete penetrance

[1] β-myosin heavy chain; [2] myosin binding protein-C; [3] co-dominant indicates a neutral mutation which is expressed without changing the phenotype

Genetic analysis seems justified if a patient suffers from sporadic HCM with no family history known (a frequent case), or if he or she is member of a family with an identified risk of disease (less frequent). The clinical diagnosis based on conventional major and minor criteria (6) should ideally be known, but often it is only suspected and comes with a notice to the genetic lab, asking for confirmation of the diagnosis (according to our experience a common request).

The goal of the genetic analysis is the determination of a cause. If a mutation has been identified, the question arises whether it is sufficient to explain the cause. The conclusion of sufficiency is straightforward if the diagnosis has clearly been confirmed on clinical grounds and if the mutation has been described before as a disease factor, preferably in large families. A number of mutations responsible for HCM have been detected repeatedly in the genes coding for β-myosin heavy chain (missense mutations in position 403, 606, 719, and others), troponin T (missense mutation in position 92, mutations in this gene have in general a high tendency to cause a severe form of HCM), and myosin binding protein-C (e.g., the G insertion demonstrated below, or other mutations which disrupt the translational reading frame).

If the clinical diagnosis is only suspected but not confirmed in an unequivocal manner (the disease may be mild), the chances are high that no mutation will be detected. If one finds a genetic change in one of the HCM genes, one will immediately resort to the known list of mutations. What if the mutation is not part of that list?

A consequence of the extensive heterogeneity of HCM-related mutations is the frequent discovery of new mutations not reported before. (Findings of this kind will be obtained more often once rapid and affordable screening methods will become available.) In these cases conclusions may be difficult. They bear on the presumed disease relation of a single gene mutation (the truly Mendelian case), or alternatively on the possibility that causes are complex and a given mutation is only one of several factors (strictly speaking a non-Mendelian case).

We wish to present a summary of three studies, done on request by cardiologists, in the course of which mutations in established HCM-genes were identified. In all three cases we had reasons to assume, or we could even show, that conclusions derived from DNA analyses require second thoughts. The three study cases are listed in Table 1.

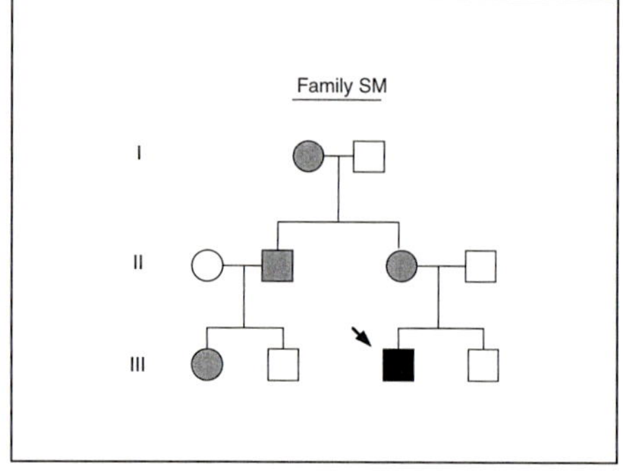

Fig. 1. Family SM. Squares and circles indicate males and females, resp. Only one member, a boy of 6 1/2 years, was affected by HCM (arrow). Four other members (shaded) were carriers of a β-myosin heavy chain missense mutation (in codon 349) unrelated to disease. The patient had two mutations, one in codon 349 and a de novo mutation in codon 719.

The main subject of the first study (family SM) was a sporadic patient. The pedigree is depicted in Fig. 1. A child (arrow) suffered cardiac arrest at the age of 6 1/2 years. He could be resuscitated because an ambulance with an emergency doctor was incidentally nearby. No symptoms had been previously reported. And no one in the family was known to be carrier of a cardiac risk. To be sure in this case, we even confirmed paternity. Screening of the β-myosin heavy chain gene led to the discovery of two missense mutations in this gene, one in codon 349 (Met-Thr) and one in position 719 (Arg-Trp). The first mutation (349) has not previously been seen; the second one (719) had been described several times. Albeit information about clinical phenotypes were incomplete in the published cases, one could safely conclude from the literature that this mutation causes, as a rule, a severe form of HCM.

Analysis of family SM showed co-dominant transmission of the 349 mutation through the maternal grandmother. Careful investigation predominantly based on echocardiography of four carriers who only had this mutation (but not the 719 change of the proband) failed to produce evidence of a disease disposition in any of them. We, therefore, concluded that the 349 mutation was a rare genetic variant unrelated to disease. The second mutation (719) was interpreted as a new mutation (de novo) which presumably occured in a single parental germ cell. Since the affected boy was a carrier of both mutations, we were interested to know whether the new mutation and the variant were located in cis (both mutations on one allele) or in trans (both mutations on either allele). By cloning and sequencing we found that the distribution was in trans (3). Thus, the boy had no intact β-myosin heavy chains. This finding was taken by us to hypothesize that the 349 mutation is per se silent (no phenotype). However, in a complex genotype with a clearly disease-related mutation in the opposite allele, such a silent mutation may contribute to the phenotype at least to a degree by possibly aggravating the clinical condition. We note that the manifestation in the case of this boy was particularly severe.

We cannot prove that our assumption is correct. But from this study we can safely conclude that de novo mutations occur (thus, it is worthwhile to search for mutations in sporadic cases) and that not all mutations which may be found (here: 349) are explanatory.

The second study (family WF) indicated a different type of genetic complexity. The pedigree is shown in Fig. 2. Only two, possibly three adult members of this family were clearly symptomatic (II-1, II-3, II-9), and cardiac hypertrophy was demonstrated by echocardiography in only two of them (II-1, II-2). Only one case (II-2) was severe. This patient had undergone surgery (myectomy) because of leftventricular outflow obstruction and had later a defibrillator implanted because of episodes of nonsustained ventricular tachycardia.

A molecular analysis of the β-myosin heavy chain gene as a candidate led to the identification of a mutation in an unusual position of the protein (codon 1205): an amino acid

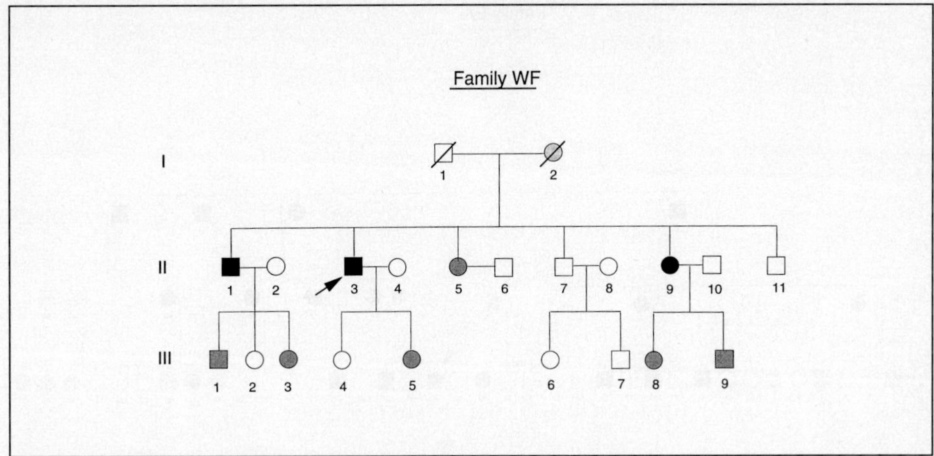

Fig. 2. Family WF. Symbols as in Fig. 1. Slashes indicate deceased family members. The index patient (58 y) is marked by the arrow. He was the only severely affected patient. Two other members had mild (II-1) or borderline (II-9) symptoms of HCM. Of nine living carriers of the mutation, six (shaded) were asymptomatic.

exchange (Glu-Lys) was found in the "hinge" of the filamentous rod of β-myosin. No mutations have ever been reported in the rod before, except for some in the direct vicinity of the globular head. The hinge is located in a clear distance to the head domain of myosin. By investigating the entire family, we found nine carriers of the mutation, all first or second degree relatives. This mutation was not detected in the general population (200 individuals were studied), it is therefore unlikely that it is a neutral genetic polymorphism. The biochemistry of the exchange (a negatively charged glutamic acid was replaced by a positively charged lysine) was highly nonconservative in a region of the molecule otherwise strictly preserved in the evolution of myosins. Thus, this change seemed to have a certain a priori probability of being significant for the phenotype. Since the structure of the filamentous rod of myosins is still not fully understood, the consequences of this type of change in electrochemical charge are open to discussion.

Considering these results we cannot draw a strong conclusion about the phenotype relation of this mutation despite the biochemical evidence of a significant change. One interpretation would regard this nonconservative exchange as causing a mild form of HCM, with late onset, moderate courses, and incomplete penetrance (penetrance = propensity of the mutation to produce an identifiable phenotype). Alternatively, it cannot be excluded that this mutation is a neutral genetic variant, and the real mutation (possibly restricted to those who clearly have symptoms) has not become known yet. Thirdly, both explanations could be right. The few patients in this family may have a composite phenotype with more than one deficiency (not necessarily in contractility genes), and those, who are virtually free of symptoms, may only have the Glu-Lys exchange in position 1205. This exchange would then be qualified as relatively harmless. The case is open to further investigation.

The third study (family EA) was focused on a different mutation in another HCM gene coding for the myosin binding protein-C gene (MyBP-C). The pedigree is shown in Fig. 3. The function of this protein is not completely understood. It may be involved in the structural organization of thick filaments of the sarcomeres. It is also possible that it contributes to the control of myosin activities by β-adrenergic agonists (for further references see 7).

Family EA was large. Altogether 49 members were available for study. Since 10 symptomatic patients were readily identified, the path to the gene was through analyzing link-

Family EA

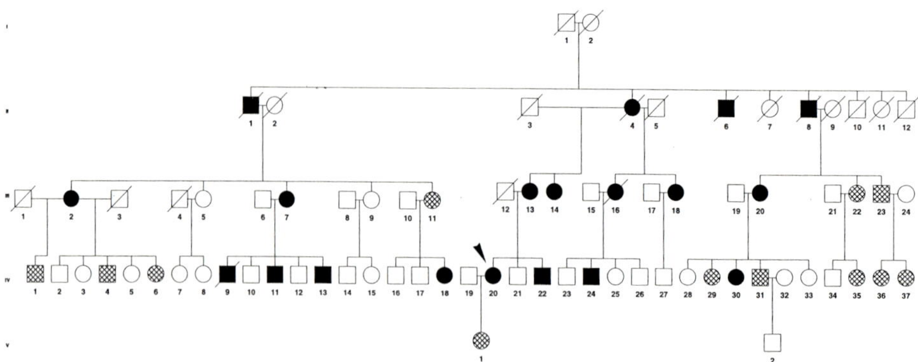

Fig. 3. Family EA. Symbols as in Fig. 2. The index patient is marked by the arrow. Black symbols indicate symptomatic or borderline patients, or deceased family members with documented cardiac disease. Cross-hatching denotes asymptomatic carriers of the mutation in the MyBP-C gene.

age of polymorphic markers and the disease. The gene was mapped to chromosome 11 where the MyBP-C gene had been localized before (1, 12). By screening this gene as a likely candidate using blood and myocardial tissue, a mutation was found in exon 24. The change consisted of an insertion of a single base (G) following codon 791 of the gene. This insertion generated a new splice donor site within exon 24 which caused the formation of an incomplete mRNA. This altered message was actually identified – as predicted – in cardiac tissue of one of the patients (myectomy material was used). Details of this analysis will be published (Moolman et al. manuscript in preparation).

The major point of this investigation was that – similar to the results of the two preceding studies – the number of gene carriers by far exceeded the number of patients. Of 49 individuals tested, 27 had the mutation. Only 10 of them were clearly symptomatic. Five members were listed as "borderline cases". They had minor signs compatible with the diagnosis of a HCM in a very early, almost preclinical stage. Twelve members were completely asymptomatic. Thus, the disease in this family is on the average mild (however, two cases of premature sudden cardiac death were also reported). Age of onset showed a large spread between 19 years (a borderline case) and 68 years. Our analysis is in good agreement with data of others suggesting that mutations in this gene cause mild disease with highly variable age of onset. With this conclusion the case could be regarded as solved.

However, by careful inspection of clinical data in relation to pedigree positions it was noticed that the mild character was not evenly shared by the different branches of this 5 generation pedigree. The gene carriers in one branch were more often symptomatic than carriers in other branches (see Fig. 3: progeny of family member II-4; this proband was herself a patient). We cannot exclude that this skewed distribution of expressivities of the disease is fortuitous. But it may also indicate that the patients in one branch are carriers of an unidentified genetic condition, similar to what we have discussed in family WF (see above). No data exist as yet which could support this notion, but respective genetic investigations will be initiated.

Summary

The techniques for analysing HCM candidate genes are available; however, they are slow, expensive, and still too labor intensive. Automated analysis will eventually take over (most notably DNA chip technologies of different kinds). Today most laboratories involved in molecular studies of HCM causes operate selectively by restricting the number of genes tested and by using indirect screening methods rather than sequencing entire genes (but this may change). Despite these obstacles, mutations are detected in both, patients of families and sporadic cases at a reasonable rate. Here we have discussed the point that mutations are not always easily interpreted in terms of their relation to HCM. Genetic changes may be neutral and of no selective value, or they may cause disease only in connection with other – aquired or inherited – factors. The clearcut Mendelian mutation which acts by itself does exist, but in considering the suggested high prevalence of HCM (1 in 500), this seemingly single gene disorder may in the majority of cases rather be a multifactorial phenomenon.

References

1. Bonne G, Carrier L, Bercovici J, Cruaud C, Richard P, Hainque B, Gautel M, Labeit S, James M, Beckman J, Weissenbach J, Vosberg HP, Fiszman M, Komajda M, Schwartz K (1995) Cardiac myosin binding protein-C gene splice acceptor site mutation is associated with familial hypertrophic cardiomyopathy. Nature Genet 11: 438–440
2. Carrier L, Bonne G, Bährend E, Yu B, Richard P, Niel F, Hainque B, Cruaud C, Gary F, Labeit S, Bouhour JB, Dibourg O, Desnos M, Hagege A, Trent RJ, Komajda M, Fiszman M, Schwartz K (1997) Organization and sequence of human cardiac myosin binding protein C gene (MYBPC3) and identification of mutations predicted to produce truncated proteins in familial hypertrophic cardiomyopathy. Circ Res 80: 427–434
3. Jeschke B, Uhl K, Weist B, Schröder D, Meitinger T, Döhlemann C, Vosberg HP (1998) A high risk phenotype of hypertrophic cardiomyopathy associated with a compound genotype of two mutated β-myosin heavy chain genes. Hum Genet 102: 299–304
4. Maron BJ, Gardin JM, Flack JM, Gidding SS, Kurosaki TT, Bild ED (1995) Prevalence of hypertrophic cardiomyopathy in a general population of young adults. Echocardiographic analysis of 4,111 subjects in the CARDIA study. Circulation 92: 785–789
5. Maron BJ, Bonow RO, Cannon III RO, Leon MB, Epstein SE (1987) Hypertrophic cardiomyopathy. Interrelations of clinical manifestation, pathophysiology, and therapy. N Engl J Med 316: 780–789, 844–852
6. McKenna WJ, Spirito P, Desnos M, Dubourg O, Komajda M (1997) Experience from clinical genetics in hypertrophic cardiomyopathy: Proposal for new diagnostic criteria in adult members of affected families. Heart 77: 130–132
7. Niimura H, Bachinski LL, Sangwatanaroj S, Watkins H, Chudley AE, McKenna WJ, Kristinnson A, Roberts R, Sole M, Maron BJ, Seidman JG, Seidman CE (1998) Mutations in the gene for cardiac myosin binding protein C and late-onset familial hypertrophic cardiomyopathy. N Engl J Med 338: 1248–1257
8. Spirito P, Seidman CE, McKenna WJ, Maron BJ (1997) The management of hypertrophic cardiomyopathy. N Engl J Med 336: 775–785
9. Teare D (1958) Asymmetrical hypertrophy of the heart in young adults. Br Heart J 20: 1–8
10. Vosberg HP, Haberbosch W (1998) Kardiomyopathien – genetische Ursachen und Pathogenese. In: Ganten D, Ruckpaul K (eds) Handbuch der Molekularen Medizin, Band 3 Herz-Kreislauferkrankungen. Springer Verlag, Berlin Heidelberg, pp 61–110
11. Vosberg HP, Weist B, Uhl K, Schulz O, Trojani A, Schlepper M, McKeown P (1998) Molecular diagnosis of causes of dominantly inherited hypertrophic cardiomyopathy. In: Schmacher G, Sauer U (eds) Herzfehler und Genetik/Genetics of cardiopathies. Wissenschaftliche Verlagsgesellschaft Stuttgart, (in press)
12. Watkins H, Conner D, Thierfelder L, Jarcho JA, MacRae C, McKenna WJ, Maron BJ, Seidman JG, Seidman CE (1995) Mutations in the cardiac myosin binding protein-C gene on chromosome 11 cause familial hypertrophic cardiomyopathy. Nature Genet 11: 434–437

Author's address:
H.-P. Vosberg
Benekestraße 2
61231 Bad Nauheim, Germany

Molecular genetics of arrhythmogenic right ventricular cardiomyopathy

A. Rampazzo[1], A. Nava[2], M. Miorin[1], N. Tiso[1], G. Thiene[3], G. A. Danieli[1]

[1] Department of Biology, [2] Department of Cardiology and [3] Department of Pathology, University of Padova, Italy

Abstract

Arrhythmogenic right ventricular cardiomyopathy/dyspalsia (ARVD), a familial cardio-myopathy, is characterized by fibro-fatty replacement of the right ventricular myocardium. Clinical manifestations include structural and functional abnormalities of the right ventricle and arrhythmias.

It is inherited as an autosomal dominant trait. Four loci have been mapped so far: ARVD1 on chromosome 14q24.3, ARVD2 on chromosome 1q42-q43, ARVD3 on chromosome 14q12-q22, and ARVD4 on chromosome 2q32.1-q32.3. A rare form with an autosomal recessive mode of inheritance, associated with diffuse nonepidermolytic palmoplantar keratoderma and wooly hair (Naxos disease) was mapped to chromosome 17q21.

Although no gene has yet been identified, the identification of ARVD loci and the availability of several DNA polymorphic markers in their close proximity, open the way to the pre-symptomatic detection of ARVD carriers by DNA analysis.

Arrhythmogenic right ventricular cardiomyopathy/dysplasia is an important cause of sudden death in young adults (11). This heart muscle disease is characterized by myocardial distrophy, mostly of the right ventricle, with massive fibro-fatty infiltration accounting for ventricular electrical instability at risk of severe arrhythmias and even cardiac arrest.

The typical clinical presentation of the disease is ventricular tachycardia, often on exercise, and left bundle branch block pattern (4). Ventricular tachycardia are thought to be due to re-entry between the abnormal and normal areas of the right ventricle. A recent multi-centered study revealed that ARVD is a progressive heart muscle disease with different clinico-pathological patterns: a) "silent" cardiomyopathic abnormalities localized to the right ventricle in asymptomatic victims of sudden death; b) "overt" disease characterized by segmental or global right ventricular structural changes, often associated with only histological evidence of left ventricular involvement and underlying symptomatic ventricular arrhythmias; c) "end-stage" biventricular cardiomyopathy mimicking dilated cardiomyopathy, which leads to progressive heart failure and may require heart transplantation (2).

The prevalence rate of ARVD, estimated in a population sample of about 800,000 subjects on the Venetian mainland, was higher than 6/10,000 inhabitants. A recent study, aiming at identifying cardiac cause of death in otherwise negative medico-legal autopsies, revealed that in 1,000 adults under 65 years of age, who suffered a sudden death, 50 (5 %) were affected with ARVD, although they had no previous cardiac symptoms (3).

ARVD is in general inherited as an autosomal dominant trait with incomplete penetrance (5). A rare form with an autosomal recessive mode of inheritance, associated with diffuse nonepidermolytic palmoplantar keratoderma and woolly hair was reported on Naxos island (Greece) (6).

In recent years, the availability of polymorphic DNA markers mapped along every human chromosome made the identification of disease loci relatively simple. In principle, the linkage study detects a conserved haplotype (i.e., a series of alleles at different loci in a given chromosomal region) transmitted associated with the disease from generation to generation. The different alleles of polymorphic markers are due to variation in the number of internal repeats, and they are identified by polyacrilamide gel electrophoresis.

At the beginning of our genetic study it was unclear whether or not ARVD was a genetically heterogeneous disease. Therefore, we decided to focus our study on a very large Italian family showing recurrence of ARVD in four different branches. Eighty-two subjects were clinically evaluated and 19 were found to be affected; juvenile sudden death has occurred in three cases. The clinical findings were typical of ARVD; the clinical aspect was polymorphous: severe, moderate and mild manifestations were reported. After having screened different markers on chromosomes 1, 2, 6, 12, and 17, we obtained positive lod scores with markers of chromosome 14, thus, providing statistically significant evidence of linkage with the region 14q23–q24 and demonstrating that ARVD was indeed a genetic disease (7).

Three other families available for the genetic study at that time, analyzed with markers linked to ARVD1 locus failed to show linkage. Therefore, genetic heterogeneity of ARVD was assumed.

In one three generation family with 23 subjects (11 of which were affected), where ARVD was peculiarly characterized by effort-induced polymorphic tachycardias, significantly positive lod scores (above 4 at $\Theta=0$) were obtained for the region 1q42–q43 (where ACTN2 was mapped). In particular, significantly high lod scores were obtained for a polymorphism within one intron of the gene ACTN2 and for three additional flanking markers. These findings provided evidence for the existence of a second ARVD locus (ARVD2, MIM 600996), mapped to 1q42–q43 (8).

An independent study, performed on three small families in a different Italian laboratory, provided a cumulative lod score of 3.26 for the marker D14S252, located in the region 14q12–q22, suggesting the existence of a third ARVD locus. Mistakenly this locus, mapped on 14q12–q22, was named by the authors ARVD2 instead of ARVD3 (10).

Evidence in favor of a fourth ARVD locus (ARVD4) was obtained in 1997 in our laboratory. In a North American three generation family, the haplotype defined by seven polymorphic DNA markers of the chromosome 2 long arm (2q32.1–q32.3) was found to be invariably transmitted associated with the disease. The linkage was confirmed in two additional unrelated families (cumulative lod score 3.46 at $\Theta=0$) (9). In these three families, the clinical features of ARVD are typical of the disease, however, the left ventricle always appears partially affected, thus, supporting the hypothesis that a different gene is involved.

Up to now, we have analyzed 19 families with the sets of markers associated with the different ARVD loci. Linkage with a specific locus was proved in 11 families. In particular, in 5 families the disease resulted associated with markers of the ARVD1 locus, in 4 with ARVD4, and in 2 with markers of ARVD2 locus. In no one there was evidence of association with the ARVD3 locus.

The genetic heterogeneity of the disease correlates with the clinical heterogeneity. In the five families in which the disease was linked to ARVD1 locus, the clinical findings are typical of arrhythmogenic right ventricular cardiomyopathy and the clinical aspect is polymorphous: severe, moderate, and mild manifestations are reported. In the two families linked to ARVD2 locus, all the affected subjects exhibit effort polymorphous ventricular arrhythmias. In the four families linked to ARVD4 locus, the affected subjects are characterized by an early localized involvement of the left ventricle.

Other families with recurrent ARVD did not show linkage with any of the markers associated to ARVD1, ARVD2, ARVD3, and ARVD4. Therefore the existence of at least another ARVD gene, independently involved in the genetic determination of the disease should be postulated.

Very recently, the gene involved in the Naxos disease was mapped to chromosome 17q21 by a British group (1). Therefore, to date five ARVD loci have been identified.

Both the identification of ARVD loci and the availability of several DNA polymorphic markers in their close proximity, open the way to pre-symptomatic detection of ARVD carriers ARVD by DNA analysis. This opportunity will greatly facilitate early prophylaxis of life-threatening complications in the at risk subjects in the affected families. However, the real focus of the problem in molecular genetics of ARVD is the identification and cloning of the involved genes.

In the last two years we focused our attention on the ARVD1 locus. We constructed a YAC contig of the chromosome 14q23–q24, and on it we established the relative position of the known markers, since the fine map of the region was not fully established. The YAC contig spans an interval 3 Mb long. Clones were assembled by STS content by using 16 polymorphic DNA markers whose map position was re-established. Linkage analysis performed on three independent Italian families succeeded in refining the localization of the ARVD1 gene by detecting recombinants with flanking markers. In one of these families, an affected subject showed recombinations between the ARVD1 locus and markers of the candidate region. These recombinations confine the position of the ARVD1 locus to the region defined by the markers D14S254-D14S42-D14S279, in the region 14q24.3. These three markers are included in a YAC 450 Kb long. This YAC does not include any of the known genes of the region; α-actinin1 gene was mapped outside the critical region, thus, excluding its involvement in the genetic determination of the disease.

A search in the databases succeeded in detecting 28 ESTs (Expressed Sequence Tags) mapping in the region 14q24.3. Twenty-four of them corresponded to still uncharacterized genes. Three YACs of the critical region were tested for amplification with specific primers of such ESTs. The results showed that 4 ESTs map within the critical region and could be considered candidate genes for the ARVD1 locus. The expression of the genes corresponding to the four ESTs detected in the critical region will be tested in the cardiac tissue and the corresponding cDNA will be screened for mutations in an ARVD1 patient.

A similar approach is presently in progress in our lab for the locus ARVD2. We already constructed the YAC contig, reduced the critical interval to 1.5 Mb, and are mapping the potentially interesting ESTs in this interval.

In the present phase of the study the systematic collection of clinical information and of DNA specimens in ARVD families is still of paramount importance, both for identifying new ARVD loci and refining the genetic localization of known loci. Moreover, the collection of a large number of ARVD families and their genetic characterization would allow the establishment of relative frequency of each ARVD type and the prevalence in the population. It is important to stress the great importance of linkage studies in ARVD families; for the first time a reliable tool is available for the predictive DNA testing, which discloses the perspective of an early treatment of the affected subjects, even before the manifestation of the clinical symptoms.

References

1. Coonar AS, Protonotarios N, Tsatsopoulou A, Needham EWA, Houlston RS, Cliff S, Otter MI, Murday VA, Mattu RK, McKenna WJ (1988) Gene for arrhythmogenic right ventricular cardiomyopathy with diffuse nonepidermolytic palmoplantar keratoderma and woolly hair (Naxos disease) maps to 17q21. Circulation 97: 2049–2058

2. Corrado D, Basso C, Thiene G, McKenna WJ, Davies MJ, Fontaliran F, Nava A, Silvestri F, Blomstrom-Lundqvist C, Wlodarska E, Fontaine, Camerini F (1997) Spectrum of clinicopathologic manifestations of arrhythmogenic right ventricular cardiomyopathy/dysplasia: a multicenter study. J Am Coll Cardiol 6: 1512–152.

3. Loire R, Tabib A (1996) Unexpected sudden cardiac death. An evaluation of 1,000 autopsies. Arch Mal Coeur Vaiss 89: 13–18

4. McKenna WJ, Thiene G, Nava A, Blomstrom-Lundqvist C, Fontaine G, Camerini F (1994) Criteria for the diagnosis of arrhythmogenic right ventricular cardiomyoapthy (dysplasia). Brit Heart J 71: 215–218

5. Nava A, Thiene G, Canciani B, Scognamiglio R, Daliento L, Buja G, Martini B, Stritoni P, Fasoli G (1988) Familial occurrence of right ventricular dysplasia. A study involving nine families. J Am Coll Cardiol 12: 1222–1228

6. Protonotarios NI, Tsatsopoulou AA (1997) The Naxos disease. In: Nava A, Rossi L, Thiene G (eds) Arrhythmogenic Right Ventricular Cardiomyopathy/Dysplasia. Elsevier, pp 454–462

7. Rampazzo A, Nava A, Danieli GA, Buja GF, Daliento L, Fasoli G, Scognamiglio R, Corrado D, Thiene G (1994) The gene for arrhythmogenic right ventricular cardiomyopathy maps to chromosome 14q23–q24. Human Molecular Genetics 3: 959–962

8. Rampazzo A, Nava A, Erne P, Eberhard M, Vian E, Slomp P, Tiso N, Thiene G, Danieli GA (1995) A new locus for arrhythmogenic right ventricular cardiomyoapthy (ARVD2) maps to chromosome 1q42–q43. Human Molecular Genetics 4: 2151–215

9. Rampazzo A, Nava A, Miorin M, Fonderico P, Pope B, Tiso N, Livolsi B, Zimbello R, Thiene G, Danieli GA (1997) ARVD4, a new locus for arrhythmogenic right ventricular cardiomyopathy maps to chromosome 2 long arm. Genomics 45: 259–263

10. Severini GM, Krajinov M, Pinamonti B, Sinagra G, Fioretti P, Brunazzi MC, Falaschi, Camerini F, Giacca M, Mestroni L (1996) A new locus for arrhythmogenic right ventricular dysplasia on the long arm of chromosome 14. Genomics 31: 193–200

11. Thiene G, Nava A, Corrado D, Rossi L, Pennelli L (1988) Right ventricular cardiomyopathy and sudden death in young people. N Engl J Med 318:129–133

Autor's address:
Dr. A. Rampazzo
Department of Biology
University of Padova
Via G. Colombo 3
I-35131 Padova, Italy

Cardiomyopathy: Genetics in muscular dystrophies

C. Rocco[1], S. Miocic[2], L. Mestroni[3]

[1]Department of Cardiology, Ospedale Maggiore, Trieste, Italy; [2]International Center for Genetic Engineering and Biotechnology, Trieste; [3]Division of Cardiology, University of Colorado Health Science Center, Denver, CO, USA

Abstract

Dilated cardiomyopathy (DC) presents high mortality and morbidity and is a leading indication to heart transplantation; among etiopathological hypotheses the existence of genetic defects has recently become consistent. However, genetic studies are complicated by the genetic heterogeneity of the disease. A skeletal muscle involvement (by definition subclinical) was present in 18 % of our cases belonging to families with X-linked DC (XLDC) or autosomal dominant inheritance (MDDC). Different mutations/deletions of the gene codifying for dystrophin, a protein that plays a critical role in membrane stability, force transduction, and organizing membrane specialization, have been identified in XLDC. The absence of clinical signs of skeletal muscle involvement in patients with XLDC could be explained by the compensatory production of the brain and Purkinje isoforms in the muscles, which assures a lower but still sufficient expression of dystrophin and a clinically normal phenotype. In the MDDC form, no disease gene has been identified so far, however, genes codifying for cytoskeletal proteins, such as the components of the DAG complex, appear to be excellent candidates. This hypothesis is supported by the recent findings of involvement of these genes in muscular dystrophies associated with cardiomyopathy as well as in DC in animal models and humans. In conclusion, DC is frequently inherited and heterogeneous. Among the different subgroups of patients with FDC, skeletal muscle involvement can be present even if subclinical and, therefore, should always be carefully investigated.

Dilated cardiomyopathy (DC) presents high mortality and morbidity and is a leading indication to heart transplantation. By definition, the disease, characterized by dilatation and impaired contractility, is of unknown origin, and, in recent decades, a large series of studies has been performed to identify its etiopathological mechanisms. Among the hypothesized factors, the existence of genetic defects leading to DC has recently become consistent, based on the demonstration of familial cases. In the past, retrospective studies reported a frequency of familiarity of only 2 % (6), but in more recent prospective surveys based on systematic family screening, the frequency of familiarity raised to at least 30 % (2, 3, 7).

Genetic studies are complicated by the genetic heterogeneity of familial dilated cardiomyopathy (FDC), meaning that different genes can cause similar phenotypes. In our family population of 39 kindreds with FDC, six different types of FDC have been be identified, based on different pattern of transmission, clinical features, and, when available,

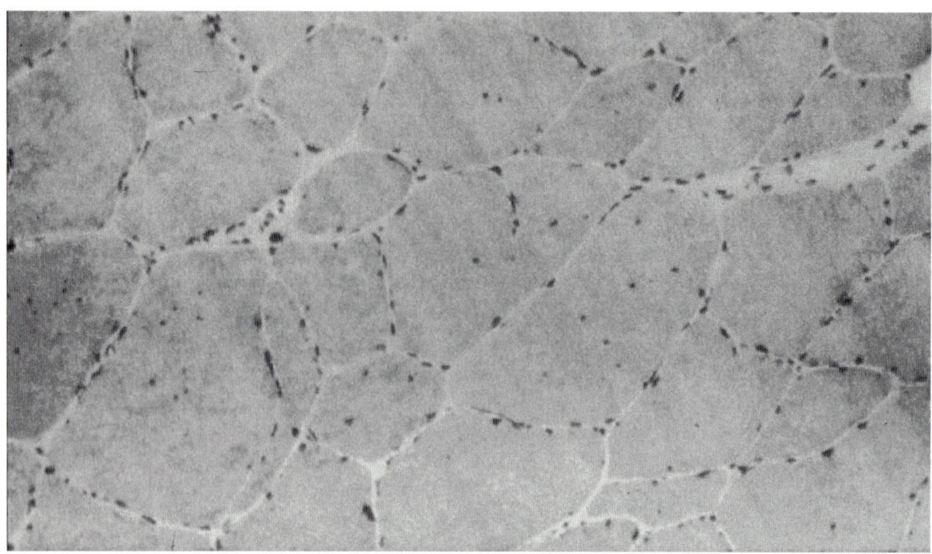

Fig. 1. Skeletal muscle biopsy of a patient with MDDC. Non-specific myopathic changes: variability in fiber size due to the presence of atrophic (< 20 um) and hypertrophic fibers (> 90 um), fiber splitting, and increase in internal nuclei.

molecular genetic data. Among them, FDC with skeletal muscle involvement (by definition subclinical) was present in 18 % of cases, belonging to families with X-linked DC (XLDC) or autosomal dominant inheritance (MDDC) (13).

Absence of male-to-male transmission, early onset, and rapid progression in males and late development and slow evolution in female carriers characterize XLDC. The skeletal muscle involvement is usually suggested by a slight and inconstant increase of serum CK, while no clinical evidence of myopathy can generally be demonstrated.

The disease gene responsible of this form of FDC has been identified in the dystrophin gene. Dystrophin is a huge cytoskeletal protein that resides in the inner part of the sarcolemma and is associated with a large transmembrane glycoprotein complex (the DAG complex) which binds elements of extracellular matrix. Thus, it plays a critical role in membrane stability, force transduction, and organizing membrane specializations. Molecular genetic studies, performed by different groups, have recently demonstrated that mutations (8, 12), deletions (9, 14), and rearrangements of the gene codifying for dystrophin are responsible for DC. Our group, in particular, identified a point mutation in the region of the first muscle exon-first intron junction of the dystrophin gene, which leads to the absence of dystrophin transcripts in the cardiac muscle. Conversely, in the skeletal muscles of these patients, a compensatory production of the brain and Purkinje isoforms assures a lower but still sufficient expression of dystrophin and a clinically normal phenotype (8).

In another family with X-linked transmission of DC, a deletion involving the 48–49 exons was identified by multiplex PCR. This mutation was previously reported in Becker's muscle dystrophy patients with severe cardiomyopathy. These data suggest a critical role of the 5' end and the exon 48 regions of the dystrophin gene in the myocardial function (9).

A clinically similar form of FDC identified in our family population is characterized by autosomal dominant inheritance and, like XLDC, subclinical muscular involvement

(Fig. 1) (5). No disease gene has been identified so far for this subgroup of patients; however, genes codifying for cytoskeletal proteins, such as the components of the DAG complex, appear to be excellent candidates. This hypothesis is supported by the recent findings of involvement of these genes in muscular dystrophies associated with cardiomyopathy as well as in DC in animal models and humans (1, 4, 10). In particular, a missense mutation of the cardiac actin gene has very recently been demonstrated to cosegregate with DC in two families (11).

In conclusion, DC is frequently inherited and heterogeneous. Among the different subgroups of patients with FDC, skeletal muscle involvement can be present even if subclinical and, therefore, should always be carefully investigated. The dystrophin gene is the first gene identified in association with DC, but other cytoskeletal proteins appear to be involved in the pathogenesis of the disease.

It can be expected that, by understanding the genetic mechanisms underlying DC, molecular genetics will allow us in the future to reach an early diagnosis, to define the correlation within the clinical features and outcome, and to identify new therapeutic targets and gene therapies for the disease.

References

1. Fadic R, Sunada Y, Waclawik AJ, Buck S, Lewandoski PJ, Campbell KP, Lotz BP (1996) Brief report: deficiency of a dystrophin-associated glycoprotein (adhalin) in a patient with muscular dystrophy and cardiomyopathy. N Engl J Med 334: 362–366
2. Gregori D, Rocco C, Di Lenarda A, Sinagra G, Miocic S, Camerini F, Mestroni L (1996) Estimating the frequency of familial dilated cardiomyopathy and the risk of misclassification errors. Circulation 94: 1–270
3. Keeling PJ, Gang G, Smith G, Seo H, Bent SE, Murday V, Caforio ALP, McKenna WJ (1995) Familial dilated cardiomyopathy in the United Kingdom. Br Heart J 73: 417–421
4. Maeda M, Holder E, Lowes B, Bies RD (1997) Dilated cardiomyopathy associated with deficiency of the cytoskeletal protein metavinculin. Circulation 95: 17–20
5. Mestroni LMF, Milasin J, Di Lenarda A, Sinagra G Rocco C, Vatta M, Matulic M, Falaschi A, Camerini F, Giacca M (1996) Familial dilated cardiomyopathy with subclinical skeletal involvement. Circulation 94: I-271
6. Michels VV, Driscoll DJ, Miller FA (1985) Familial aggregation of idiopathic dilated cardiomypathy. Am J Cardiol 55: 1232–1233
7. Michels VV, Moll PP, Miller FA, Tajik AJ, Chu JS, Driscoll DJ, Burnett JC, Rodeheffer RJ, Chesebro JH, Tazelaar H (1992) The frequency of familial dilated cardiomyopathy in a series of patients with idiopathic dilated cardiomyopathy. N Engl J Med 326: 77–82
8. Milasin J, Muntoni F, Severini GM, Bartoloni L, Vatta M, Krajinovic M, Mateddu A, Angelini C, Camerini F, Falaschi A, Mestroni L, Giacca M (1996) A point mutation in the 5' splice site of the dystrophin gene first intron responsible for X-linked dilated cardiomyopathy. Hum Mol Genet 5: 73–79
9. Muntoni F, Cau M, Ganau A, Congiu R, Arvedi G, Mateddu A, Morrosu MG, Cianchetti C, Realdi G, Cao A, Melis MA (1993) Deletion of the dystrophin muscle-promoter region associated with X-linked dilated cardiomyopathy. N Engl J Med 329: 921–925
10. Nigro V, Okasaki Y, Belsito A, Piluso G, Matsuda Y, Politano L, Nigro G, Ventura C, Abbondanza C, Molinari AM, Acampora DMM, Hayashizaki Y, Puca GA (1997) Identification of the syrian Hamster cardiomyopathy gene. Hum Mol Genet 6: 601–607
11. Olson TM, Michels VV, Thibodeau SN, Tai Y, Keating MT (1998) Actin mutation in dilated cardiomyopathy, a heritable form of heart failure. Science 280: 750–752
12. Ortiz-Lopez R, Li H, Su J, Goytia V, Towbin JA (1997) Evidence for a dystrophin missense mutation as a cause of X-linked dilated cardiomyopathy (XLCM). Circulation 95: 2434–2440
13. Rocco C, Gregori D, Miocic S, Di Lenarda A, Sinagra G, Caforio AL, Vatta M, Matulic M, Zerial T, Giacca M, Mestroni L (1997) New insight into the gentic of dilated cardiomyopathy. Circulation 96 (8): I-696

14. Yoshida K, Ikeda SI, Nakamura A, Kagoshima M, Takeda S, Shoji S, Yanagisawa N (1993) Molecular analysis of the Duchenne muscular dystrophy gene in patients with Becker muscular dystrophy presenting with dilated cardiomyopathy. Muscle & Nerve 16: 1161–1166

Author's adress:
Chiara Rocco, MD
Area di Emerggenza
Ospedale Civile di Tolmezzo
via Morgagni
I-33028 Tolmezzo, Italy
or
Department of Cardiology
Ospedale Maggiore
p.zza Ospedale 1
I-34100 Trieste, Italy
e-mail: chiara.rocco@iol.it

Molecular impact of ion channel mutations for the pathogenesis of long-QT (LQT) syndromes

E. Schulze-Bahr[1,2], H. Wedekind[1,2], W. Haverkamp[1], M. Borggrefe[1,2], G. Breithardt[1,2], H. Funke[3]

[1] Department of Cardiology and Angiology, Hospital of the University of Münster, Münster, Germany
[2] Section Molecular Cardiology, Institute for Arteriosclerosis Research at the University of Münster, Münster, Germany
[3] Section Molecular Genetics, Institute for Arteriosclerosis Research at the University of Münster, Münster, Germany

Abstract

Molecular genetics of inherited cardiac arrhythmias had a late onset compared to the advances of genetics achieved in other inherited cardiac disorders. This was related to the high mortality and early disease onset of these arrhythmias resulting in mostly small nucleus families. Thus, traditional linkage studies that are based on the genetic information obtained from large multi-generation families were made more difficult.

In 1991, the first chromosomal locus for congenital long-QT (LQT) syndrome was identified by linkage analysis on chromosome 11p15.5 (LQT1). Meanwhile, the disease-causing gene at the LQT1 locus, a gene encoding a K+ channel subunit of the IKs channel, and three other major genes, all encoding cardiac ion channel components, were identified. Taken together, LQT syndrome turned out to be a heterogeneous channelopathy. Moreover, the power of linkage studies to reveal the genetic causes of the LQT syndrome were also important to identify unknown, but fundamental channel components that contribute to the ion currents tuning the ventricular repolarization. In vitro expression of the altered ion channel genes demonstrated in each case that the altered ion channel function produces prolongation of the action potential and the propensity to ventricular arrhythmias. Since these ion channels are pharmacological targets of many antiarrhythmic (and other) drugs, individual and potentially deleterious drug responses may be related to genetic variation in ion channel genes. In acquired LQT a genetic basis has also been recently proposed in part, since single mutations in LQT genes have been specifically found (see Table 2).

The discovery of ion channel defects in the LQT syndrome represents the major achievement in the understanding and implies potential therapeutic management. The knowledge of the genomic structure of the LQT genes now offers the possibility to detect the underlying genetic defect in appoximately 80 % of all patients. With this specific information, containing the type of ion channel (Na+ versus K+ channel) and electrophysiological alteration by the mutation (loss-of-function versus change-of-function mutation), gene-directed, elec-

With technical assistance of E. Morhofer and T. Wißling. Supported by DFG (Schu 1082/2-1) and IMF (Sc 1-1-II/97-15) and the Alfried-Krupp-Stiftung, Essen, and the European Union (BIOMED 2 programme; BMT 4-CT96-0028)

tive drug therapies have been initiated in genotyped LQT patients. Based on preliminary data that were supported by in-vitro models of LQT syndromes, this approach may be useful in re-compensating the phenotype in some LQT patients.

Mutation detection is a new diagnostic tool which may become more important in patients with a normal QTc or just a borderline prolongation of the QTc interval at presentation. These patients represent approximately 30–40 % of all familial cases. Moreover, LQT3 syndrome and idiopathic ventricular fibrillation are allelic disorders and genetically overlap. In both, mutations in the LQT3 gene SCN5A encoding Na+ channel subunit for I_{Na} have been reported. Thus, the clinical nosology of inherited arrhythmias may be reconsidered after elucidation of the underlying molecular bases.

Meanwhile, genotype-phenotype correlations in large families are on the way to evaluate intergene, interfamilial, and intrafamilial differences in the clinical phenotype reflecting gene specific, gene-site specific, and individual consequences of a given mutation. The LQT syndrome is phenotypically heterogeneous due to the reduced penetrance and variable expressivity associated with a LQT mutation.

The current data on molecular genetics and genotype-phenotype correlations and the implications for diagnosis and treatment are discussed.

Introduction

More than 300,000 people in the United States die suddenly each year. Ventricular arrhythmias are responsible for most of these deaths, since cardiac arrhythmias account for more

Table 1. Conditions associated with a prolongation of the heart rate-corrected QT (QTc) interval in the surface ECG. According to (20, 21) and (1)

Clinical forms of long-QT syndromes		
Inherited	Romano-Ward syndrome	Autosomal dominant, normal hearing
	Jervell and Lange-Nielsen syndrome	Autosomal recessive, mute-deafness
	LQT + syndactyly	Autosomal dominant
	Sporadic	Non-familial
Acquired	Antiarrhythmics	Class IA and III drugs
	Antidepressants	Tricyclics
	Antidiabetics	Glibenclamide
	Antifungals	Itraconazole, Ketaconazole
	Antihistaminics	Astemizole, Terfenadine
	Antimicrobials	Erythromycin, Trimethoprim, Chloroquine, Halofantrine
	Electrolyte disturbances	Depletion of K+, Mg++
	Neuroleptics	Phenothiazines
	Other conditions	Sick-sinus syndrome, AV block, severe bradycardia hyperparathyroidism, hypothyroidism, pheochromocytoma, anorexia, starvation, liquid protein diet cerebrovascular accident, encephalitis, subarachnoidal hemorrhage
	Prokinetics	Cisapride

than 10 % of all natural deaths. The congenital long-QT (LQT) syndrome is characterized by a marked prolonged repolarization in surface ECG, recurrent syncopes and sudden death resulting from ventricular arrhythmias, especially of the torsades-de-pointe-type (20, 49). The incidence of the congenital LQT syndrome has been estimated as 1:10,000 to 1:15,000 of live births (71). The two inherited forms of the LQT syndrome are autosomal recessive in the Jervell and Lange-Nielsen (JLN) syndrome (23), in which the QTc prolongation is co-inherited with sensoneurinal deafness or deaf-mutism, and, more frequently, autosomal dominant in the Romano-Ward (RWS) syndrome. Once considered a rare entity, genetic analyses facilitate recognition of congenital LQT syndromes with increasing frequency. Additionally, families have been described in which both syndromes occurred together (31, 40, 59).

The numerous causes of QTc prolongation in the surface ECG are listed in Table 1. Besides familial (inherited) forms of the LQT syndrome, the incidence of acquired LQT syndrome and torsade-de-pointe tachyarrhythmias is higher, since many exogenous factors may cause QTc prolongation by exerting their deleterious effects on the same ion channels that were altered in congenital LQT syndrome (Fig. 1). Most notable, quinidine causes QTc prolongation in 1.8 – 8.8 % of cases (21, 38). Acquired LQT syndrome may still be an important side effect when antiarrhythmics of the class IA or class III, frequently prescribed antimicrobials or neuroleptics are used. The prolongation of action potential and repolarization changes in surface ECG caused by specific drug actions may be phenotypically indistinguishable from inherited forms of QTc prolongation. Although a history of familial LQT syndrome and the patient's ECG without exposure to the specific drug are useful in differentiating between these two forms of LQT syndromes, a genetic ion channel variant may still predispose to deleterious drug response in acquired LQT syndrome (14, 43, 46). We recently found in 23 % of patients with acquired LQT syndrome mutations by screening the complete coding sequence of the LQT genes. Taken together, acquired LQT syndrome is in part a pharmacogenetic disease that is characterized by the drug's enhancement of a subclinical, inherited ion channel defect (46).

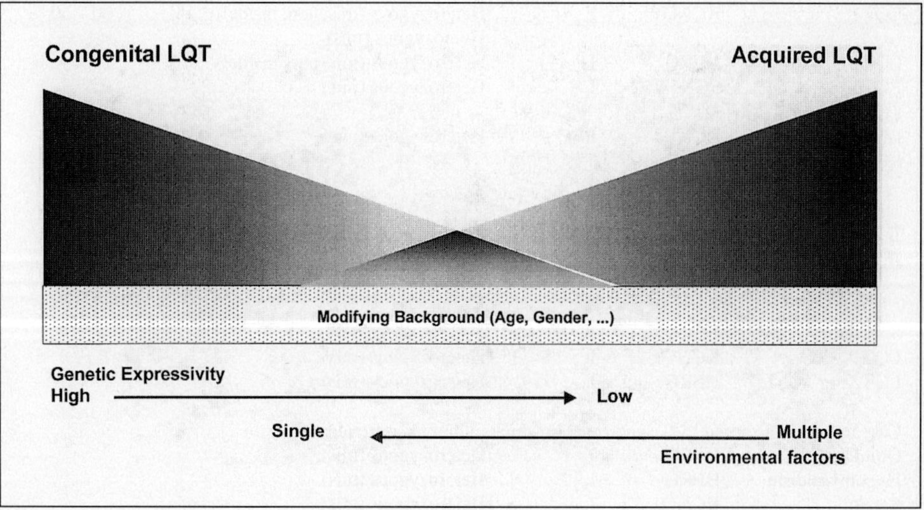

Fig. 1. Genetic and environmental factors causing QTc prolongation – clinical overlap between inherited and acquired LQT syndromes.

Molecular genetics of the LQT syndromes

In 1991, the first landmark article reported tight genetic linkage of the Romano-Ward syndrome to chromosome 11p15.5 in an exceptionally large Utah pedigree (26, 27). Within this candidate region, several genes including the Harvey ras1 (HRAS1) gene, could be excluded (12, 19, 47, 50) and the disease causing gene at the LQT1 locus, therefore, remained unknown for the next five years. Meanwhile, genetic heterogeneity has been demonstrated by linkage analyses in other LQT families and new loci have been identified on chromosomes 7q35-q36 (LQT2), 3p24-p27 (LQT3), and 4q25-q27 (LQT4) (9, 45) (see Table 2).

With the localization of the human *eag*-related gene (HERG) at the LQT2 locus (63, 64), this K+ channel gene became an interesting candidate for LQT2, since expression in the human heart was demonstrated. Importantly, Sanguinetti and co-workers showed that the HERG encoded polypeptide strongly resembles the properties of the rapidly-activating component of delayed rectifier (I_{Kr}) channel in the human heart (41, 43, 57, 58). Moreover, blockade of the IKr channel during phase 3 of the cardiac action potential is one of the important mechanisms of action of class III antiarrhythmics and other drugs (28, 29, 63) associated with acquired LQT syndrome suggesting a functional link between both forms of the LQT syndrome (43). Subsequently, in nine families with linkage to the LQT2 locus,

Table 2. Mutated genes and types of mutations found in the different forms of long-QT syndrome

Genetic forms of long-QT syndromes				
Nomenclature	Gene	Current	Type of mutation	Distribution of mutations
Romano-Ward syndrome				
LQT1	KCNQ1	I_{Ks}	Heterozygous (mis, non, ins/del)	30 – 50 %
			Homozygous (mis)	< 1 %
LQT2	HERG	I_{Kr}	Heterozygous (mis, non, ins/del)	20 – 40 %
LQT3	SCN5A	I_{Na}	Heterozygous (mis)	< 5 %
LQT4	?!			< 1 %
LQT5	KCNE1	I_{Ks}	Heterozygous (mis)	< 3 %
LQTx	?!			?!
Jervell and Lange-Nielsen syndrome				
JLN1	KCNQ1	I_{Ks}	Homozygous (mis, non, ins/del)	80 %
JLN2	KCNE1	I_{Ks}	Compound heterozygote (mis), Homozygous (mis)	20 %
Sporadic LQT syndrome				
LQT1	KCNQ1	I_{Ks}	Heterozygous (mis)	?
LQT2	HERG	I_{Kr}	Heterozygous (mis)	?
Case reports in acquired LQT syndrome, in which mutations were identified				
Quinidine	HERG	I_{Kr}	Heterozygous (mis)	
Hypothyroidism	HERG	I_{Kr}	Heterozygous (mis)	
Sotalol	KCNQ1	I_{Kr}	Heterozygous (mis)	
Halofantrine	KCNQ1	I_{Ks}	Heterozygous (mis)	

mis = missense mutation; non = nonsense mutation; ins/del = insertion or deletion

mutations in HERG were clearly associated with the LQT2 syndrome (10, 47, 50). Also, sporadic cases of LQT syndromes, in which the patient's parents are healthy, have been shown to result from newly occurring (de-novo) mutations in HERG (10) and support the causative role of HERG in the LQT2 syndrome. Mutations in HERG reduce the I_{Kr} current and, thus, prolong the action potential duration and ventricular repolarization. Based on our data from the LQTS Database Münster, approximately 30 – 40 % of all patients belong to the LQT2 subgroup.

At the LQT3 locus on chromosome 3p21-p24, the β-subunit of the cardiac Na+ channel has been localized by in-situ hybridization. Wang and co-workers found in three families with LQT3 syndrome mutations in SCN5A that were localized in functionally important domains of channel inactivation or voltage sensing (71, 72). Different from the LQT1, LQT2, and LQT5 types in which a reduction of repolarization currents resume the action potential prolongation, LQT3 syndrome later turned out to be related to a delayed activation or incomplete inactivation of the Na+ channel that acts through initial, rapid depolarization phase of action potential (phase 0) (5, 70). Mutations in SCN5A at least represent rare forms of the congenital LQT syndrome.

The LQT1 gene remained concealed until 1996. Using positional cloning techniques, Wang and co-workers analyzed three other ion channel genes in the candidate gene region before mutations in the gene KCNQ1 (formerly KVLQT1) were identified (70). Recently, the full-length clone of KCNQ1 containing 129 additional (for a total of 676) amino acids was published (74). Furthermore, a truncated isoform (so-called isoform 2) exits that is co-localized in cardiac tissue and exhibits a dominant negative effect on isoform 1 when co-expressed in cos-7 cells (13, 24). At present, the I_{Ks} channel is composed by three different proteins in a specific ratio, expressed KCNQ1 isoform 1 and 2, and minK (13). A given mutation in the KCNQ1 gene will have different effects depending on its exonic position in the gene (e.g., an exon 1B-mutation will only occur in its specific isoform 2, whereas an exon 4-mutation will alter both, isoform 1 and 2). The probably different functional effects by a mutation within the isoform interplay and the specific expression pattern of isoforms may explain in part the widespread phenotypic variation found in LQT1 patients.

From linkage data of other collaborating groups (18, 69, 70) as well as from our own data, 30 – 50 % of all LQT mutations are expected in the KCNQ1 gene. The KCNQ1 gene product is most likely a pore-forming α-subunit that interacts together with the β-subunit minK (minimal potassium channel) to form the slowly-activating component of the delayed rectifier (I_{Ks}) channel (4, 7, 13, 39, 42). The loss of channel function decreases the I_{Ks} current, resulting in prolongation of the action potential duration and delayed repolarization.

Very recently, the phenotypic and genetic heterogeneity of the LQT syndrome became more complex by a candidate gene approach in families without linkage to LQT1-4 locus. Mutations in the KCNE1 gene that encodes minK have been shown to reduce the I_{Ks} current and therefore cause autosomal dominant LQT5 (60). Because this gene is also expressed in the cochlea and labyrinth of the inner ear and because null mutant (–/–) mice for minK have collapsed labyrinths, similar to those found in JLN syndrome autopsies (cited from 16), KCNE1 appeared to be a good candidate gene for autosomal recessive Jervell and Lange-Nielsen (JLN) syndrome. Recently, we and others identified KCNE1 mutations in JLN families after linkage to the LQT1-4 loci was excluded (15, 48, 51, 65). Parents of patients with the JLN2 syndrome have normal hearing and mostly normal surface ECG; affected individuals are expected to have two mutant alleles. Such patients (with two mutant alleles) have a more adverse course and a higher rate of sudden cardiac death.

The physiological co-operation of the KCNE1 gene (minK) and the KCNQ1 gene products in the formation of the I_{Ks} channel, also suggested a possible role of the KCNQ1

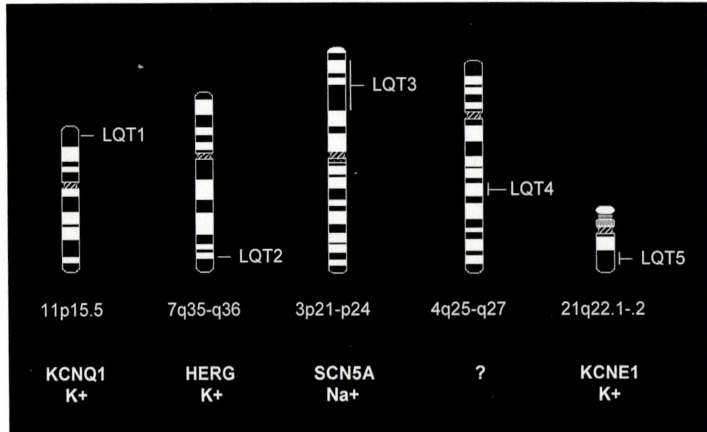

Fig. 2. Chromosomal assignment of the five known LQT loci after linkage analysis. At the LQT4 locus, the causative gene is still unknown. Another unidentified LQT locus (LQT6) exists by linkage exclusion of the LQT1–LQT5 loci.

gene in the non-LQT5-linked JLN syndrome (62; Fig. 2). Independently, two groups demonstrated linkage of the disease locus to the LQT1 locus and, subsequently, detected mutations in this gene (34, 59). Again, parents and relatives of JLN1 patients, who were (obligate) heterozygotes (with a single mutant allele), were clinically unaffected.

In families with congenital LQT syndrome, a variable clinical expressivity of the disease can be observed and may even include patients without prolongation of the QTc interval (66). Data obtained from an analysis of 199 LQT1 family members suggested a QTc cut-off value of $440ms^{1/2}$ could lead to a misclassification of 11 % of family members. No affected gene carriers had a QTc of $410ms^{1/2}$ or less and no normal male person had a QTc of $470ms^{1/2}$ or more (females: $480ms^{1/2}$ or more) (66).

In addition, single LQT families have been reported in which the typical pattern of inheritance (dominant, in Romano-Ward syndrome; recessive, in JLN syndrome) has been interfered by variable gene expressivity. In 1972, Mathews and co-workers already reported a LQT family with an autosomal dominant co-inheritance of QTc prolongation and deafness ("autosomal dominant JLN syndrome") (31). Very recently, Priori and co-workers reported a LQT1 patient with a homozygous KCNQ1 mutation, but without inner ear deafness (36). These rare observations may raise again the question of disease nosology, e.g., whether Romano-Ward syndrome has to be classified according to the initial ("historic") description of symptoms (QTc prolongation, but lack of inner ear deafness) or according to its mode of genetic transmission (autosomal dominant, i.e., single mutant allele; autosomal recessive, i.e., two mutant alleles, as in the JLN syndrome). In the latter case, the family reported by Mathews and co-workers would have been classified as Romano-Ward syndrome, because of the missing inner ear deafness of their patients.

Genotype-phenotype correlation in LQT syndromes

After disease gene identification and establishment of the genomic structures of the LQT genes, systematic mutation screening has now started to identify mutations in large LQT families and to correlate the genetic, gene-specific finding with the clinical features of the affected family members. The identification of the mutations is made more difficult, since genetic heterogeneity exists. A complete gene analysis is recommended because each nucleotide position may harbor the genetic alteration, and by the fact that this analysis implies more than 24,000 base pairs per patient. The use of single-strand conformation polymorphisms (SSCP) techniques, therefore, accelerates analysis speed, but has a lower sensitivity and specificity in mutation detection compared with sequencing techniques. Here, a mutation within a PCR-amplified gene fragment can be recognized on the basis of an altered migration pattern during electrophoresis. An example is shown in Fig. 3.

An early report by Moss and co-workers suggested a gene-specific phenotype in the repolarization pattern of the surface ECG (32); these data were limited in the number of families per gene locus as well as in the number of investigated mutations per gene (e.g., in SCN5A one mutation). In contrast, other reports on genotyped families propose that these phenotypic findings are likely to be private rather than gene-specific characteristics in a given family (11, 45). Recent data of mutant LQT channels which were expressed in vitro demonstrated different mechanisms of mutation actions on wildtype channel and resulted at least in a broad phenotypic spectrum of current reduction and different current characteristics (41, 53, 73).

Besides specific ECG phenotypes in LQT families, LQT3 patients have a differential response in Na+ channel blockade compared to LQT2 patients, who have a defective K+ channel (35). Moreover, LQT3 patients shortened their QTc intervals more than other LQT

Fig. 3. Fluorescent curves obtained after gel electrophoresis of fluorescent-labeled and PCR-amplified exon 8 of HERG (LQT2 gene). Compared with the wildtype DNA fragments, a mobility shift (i.e., a different peak characteristic in the curve) is caused by a mutation, as seen in codon 611 (Thy611End, middle panel) and in codon 613 (Thr613Met, lower panel).

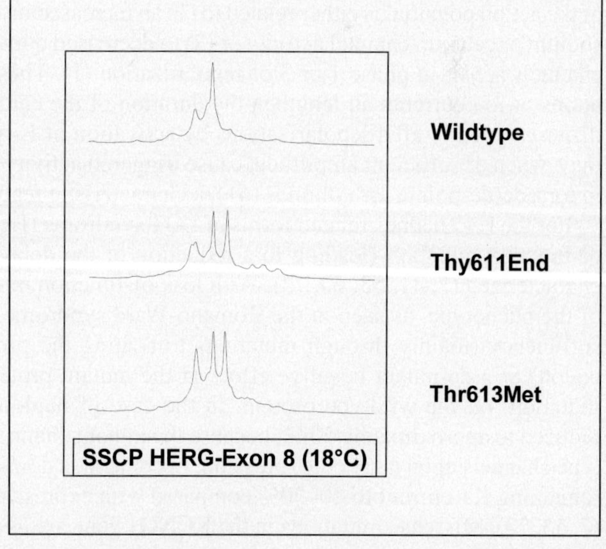

patients with an increase in heart beat; cardiac events occurred more at rest or sleep in LQT3 patients. Taken together, LQT3 patients may have a different physiological behavior based on the defective (Na+) ion channel when compared with defective K+ channel. This may result, in the future, in gene-directed pharmacological therapies (35, 55, 56).

The localization of a specific mutation within a LQT gene has different phenotypic effects that seem to be related to the functional importance of the mutated domain (e.g., the transmembraneous and the pore domains are major functional domains) (14). Truncating mutations may here be an exception, since they may result in a retention of heteromeric channel complexes in the endoplasmatic reticulum independent to their position of truncation (17). Donger and co-workers found a significant difference in QTc prolongation, frequency, and severity of clinical symptoms when misense mutations of the transmembraneous channel domains were compared with a C-terminal missense mutations in codon 555 (14).

The presence of one or two mutant alleles has a gene-dosage effect on the value of the QTc interval as has been demonstrated in JLN syndrome families. Carriers of two mutant alleles had a more pronounced QTc prolongation in JLN1 (33, 34, 59, 65) and in JLN2 (15, 48, 51, 65). This relationship to QTc prolongation was independent whether the patient was homozygous for a truncation or a missense mutation.

In-vitro phenotypes of LQT syndromes

The knowledge of the genes causing for the LQT syndromes leads to a broader understanding of the generation of the cardiac action potential, since the encoded ion channel components are the fundamental class of proteins for generating and tuning the electrical signals during each heart beat through the cell membranes. Moreover, each molecular defect in the LQT syndrome opens the possibility for topological structure-function relationships.

The finding that the LQT syndrome resembles a heterogeneous class of channelopathies supports the "intracellular hypothesis of LQT syndrome" (37, 61), in which a prolongation of the action potential is either related to (1) an increased inward current through maintained sodium or calcium channel activity or (2) to decreased outward currents through potassium channels active in phase 1 or 3 of repolarization (1). These genetically determined alterations of ion currents all lengthen the duration of the cardiac action potential which predisposes to early afterdepolarizations by activation of L-type Ca++ channels (22). These may, when of sufficient amplitude, cause triggered activity that is the initiating mechanism in torsade-de-pointe arrhythmias (61), a characteristic feature of the LQT syndrome.

For the K+ channel-related forms of LQT syndrome (LQT1, –2, and –5), so-called loss-of-function mutation (leading to a reduction of the delayed-rectifier current) have been characterized (7, 41, 53, 60, 73). With loss-of-function mutations, a dominant inheritance of the phenotype, as seen in the Romano-Ward syndrome, may be explained by haploinsufficiency (mainly through mutations truncating the protein by introduction of a stop codon) or a dominant negative effect of the mutant protein (mainly through a missense mutation) on the wildtype protein. In the case of haploinsufficiency, the K+ current is reduced to approximately 50 %, because the mutant channels do not interact with the wildtype channels upon a 1:1 co-expression. In contrast, a dominant negative effect reduces the remaining K+ current to 20–30% compared with expression of the wildtype channel only (7, 53, 73). Missense mutations in the KCNQ1 gene are associated with various degrees of

I_{Ks} reduction when co-expressed with the wildtype protein; this may be related to the broad phenotypic spectrum seen in LQT1 patients (7, 14). Not every missense mutation still exhibits a severe dominant negative effect and dramatically reduces the K+ current; the LQT1 mutation Arg555Cys has been found to form homomeric functional channels (which most of all mutations do not) and probably represents an electrophysiologically "mild" mutation (7) that was, additionally, associated with a low clinical expressivity (14).

Expression of JLN1 mutations exhibit no dominant effects by reducing the wildtype current only to approximately 50 % (7, 73) and, most likely, result from haploinsufficiency. This is compatible with the recessive mode of genetic transmission in the JLN syndrome, in which a single mutant allele (as obligate for JLN patients) is not sufficient enough for high disease expressivity, but two mutant alleles (as obligate for JLN patients) causes severe and early disease onset.

Like in the KCNQ1 gene, mutations in HERG decrease either the density of expressed K+ channel current (dominant negative effect) or the prevention of assembly of a functional channel protein (haploinsufficiency) (41, 56). Most of the by in-vitro expression characterized missense mutations did not form functional channels in homomeric state, but suppressed wildtype HERG function, indicating that mutant and wildtype subunits form heteromeres which are functional in part by reducing the wildtype current density to 20 – 30 % (41).

In contrast to the LQT1, –2, and –5 forms, mutations in the Na+ channel SCN5A (LQT3) primarily lead to a gain-of-function with altered ion channel properties (3, 5, 16, 29, 30, 67, 70). In 1995, Bennett and co-workers first characterized mutant SCN5A channels responsible for the rapid upstroke current I_{Na} of the phase 0; three different mutations located in a domain for channel inactivation or voltage sensing were studied by heterologous expression. Expression of one mutation, ΔKPQ, resulted in a tiny, but sustained inward Na+ current during membrane depolarization by dispersed re-openings and long-standing bursts of channel activity. Therefore, the balance in maintaining homeostasis between inward and outward currents through channel inactivation was disturbed and, subsequently, prolonged the action potential in LQT3 patients (5). Still other mechanisms may underlie the pathophysiology of the LQT3 syndrome (16). Recently, Makita and co-workers characterized a missense mutation (R1623Q) in SCN5A that had normal inactivation properties, but substantially differed by a delayed channel activation as determined by prolonged open times with bursting behavior (30). An and co-workers recently suggested that spatial changes in the interplay of α- and β-subunits also may influence channel inactivation. A novel missense mutation (D1790G) had no significant effect on the biophysical properties of monomeric SCN5A channels, but heteromeric channels composed of these two subunits showed a shift in steady-state inactivation without the detection of a sustained inward current, as found in other LQT3 mutant channels (3).

Pharmacological targeting in LQT syndromes, "re-compensation" of the phenotypes

Attempts in targeting the LQT phenotypes to "re-compensate" its pathophysiological properties in-vitro were performed by several groups after the genetic information was obtained, classifying LQT syndrome as a disorder of defective ion channels. These preliminary, encouraging results have been transmitted in part into in-vivo trials. The expression data from in vitro analyses of mutant LQT channels at least demonstrated that the molecular mechanisms even within a single LQT gene clearly vary because of different, underlying mutations and, consequently, may require specified medical approaches. LQT1 patients with a dominant negative effect caused by the mutation may benefit from K+ channel openers, whereas LQT1 patients with a haploinsufficient effect due to the mutation may not. In the future, a clear electrophysiological characterization of a found mutation is essential before starting gene-directed therapies and before therapeutical rationales are given.

In LQT3 mutant channels, application of mexiletine has been efficiently shown to suppress selectively the mutant phenotype by inhibition of late-openings (68). The drug's affinity to mutant channels in the inactivated state was similar to wildtype channels. Recently, Priori and co-workers were able to show a significant reduction of QTc prolongation in LQT3 patients carrying mutant Na+ channels (35) that were known to be influenced by mexiletine in vitro (68). Also lidocaine in vitro showed comparable effects as mexiletine (2).

Patients with LQT2 may be particularly susceptible to adrenergic-triggered events, hypokalemia, respond poorly to cardiac pacing and may benefit from β-blocker therapy (52). The unique feature of the I_{Kr} channel, to increase paradoxically the outward current by increasing extracellular K+, was used to attempt to improve the channel dysfunction in LQT2 patients; a 24 % reduction in the QTc was observed by elevating serum K+ and, T-wave dysmorphologies resolved (8). Potassium channel openers (e.g., pinacidil, nicorandil) that have been previously shown in animal models to suppress delayed repolarization and early afterdepolarizations (6) may be therapeutical options for LQT1, LQT2 and LQT5 patients. A case report of a 17-year-old boy with LQT syndrome refractory to β-blocker therapy demonstrated the beneficial effect of therapy with nicorandil (44); long-term treatment markedly reduced early afterdepolarizations from 17 % to 4 %, normalized the patient's ECG, and abolished recurrent syncopes. Shimizu and co-workers recently reported shortening of the QTc interval, decreased dispersion of $MAPD_{90\%}$ and abolishing of early afterdepolarizations in LQT1 patients, and gave first evidence for a putative therapeutical role of potassium channel openers in patients with this genotype (55).

These exciting, gene-directed therapeutical approaches await further confirmation and detailed, prospective investigations; they strongly suggest a new management of genotyped LQT patients.

Future Directions

LQT syndrome has reached the era of molecular genetics. This disorder is through its heterogeneity meanwhile more complex than previously thought; analysis of DNA is a new diagnostic tool that may be helpful in recognition of patients with a low or borderline clinical expressivity. Acquired LQT syndrome, in which a part of the population is at risk towards an excessive drug response seems to have in part a genetic predisposition and, therefore, is a novel pharmacogenetic disease. It is very likely that other gene defects and/or modifying factors that control expression and translation of these genes will be involved in the pathogenesis of LQT syndromes, since the phenotypic variability even in a single family may be high. The combination of established techniques in molecular genetics and in electrophysiology turned to be out a powerful tool to provide insights into the mechanistic factors in the LQT syndrome and into the basis in the generation of the action potential. With this exciting and still growing information, the therapeutical management of patients will hopefully be improved.

References

1. Ackerman MJ (1998) The long QT syndrome: Ion channel diseases of the heart. Mayo Clin Proc 73: 250–269
2. An RH, Bangalore R, Rosero SZ, Kass RS (1996) Lidocaine block of LQT-3 mutant human Na+ channels. Circ Res 79: 103–108
3. An RH, Wang XL, Kerem B, Benhorin J, Medina A, Goldmit M, Kass RS (1998) Novel LQT-3 mutation affects Na+ channel activity through interactions between alpha- and beta1-subunits. Circ Res 83: 141–146
4. Barhanin J, Lesage F, Guillemare E, Fink M, Lazdunski M, Romey G (1996) K(V)LQT1 and lsK (minK) proteins associate to form the I(Ks) cardiac potassium current. Nature 384: 78–80
5. Bennett PB, Yazawa K, Makita N, George ALJ (1995) Molecular mechanism for an inherited cardiac arrhythmia. Nature 376: 683–685
6. Carlsson L, Abrahamsson C, Drews L, Duker G (1992) Antiarrhythmic effects of potassium channel openers in rhythm abnormalities related to delayed repolarization. Circulation 85: 1491–1500
7. Chouabe C, Neyroud N, Guicheney P, Lazdunski M, Romey G, Barhanin J (1997) Properties of KvLQT1 K+ channel mutations in Romano-Ward and Jervell and Lange-Nielsen inherited cardiac arrhythmias. EMBO J 16: 5472–5479
8. Compton SJ, Lux RL, Ramsey MR, Strelich KR, Sanguinetti MC, Green LS, Keating MT, Mason JW (1996) Genetically defined therapy of inherited long-QT syndrome. Correction of abnormal repolarization by potassium. Circulation 94: 1018–1022
9. Curran M, Atkinson D, Timothy K, Vincent GM, Moss AJ, Leppert M, Keating M (1993) Locus heterogeneity of autosomal dominant long QT syndrome. J Clin Invest 92: 799–803
10. Curran ME, Splawski I, Timothy KW, Vincent GM, Green ED, Keating MT (1995) A molecular basis for cardiac arrhythmia: HERG mutations cause long QT syndrome. Cell 80: 795–803
11. Dausse E, Berthet M, Denjoy I, Andre-Fouet X, Cruaud C, Bennaceur M, Faure S, Coumel P, Schwartz K, Guicheney P (1996) A mutation in HERG associated with notched T waves in long QT syndrome. J Mol Cell Cardiol 28: 1609–1615
12. Dausse E, Denjoy I, Kahlem P, Bennaceur M , Faure S, Weissenbach J, Coumel P, Schwartz K, Guicheney P (1995) Readjusting the localization of long QT syndrome gene on chromosome 11p15. C R Acad Sci III 318: 879–885
13. Demolombe S, Baro I, Pereon Y, Bliek J, Mohammad-Panah R, Pollard H, Morid S, Mannens M, Wilde A, Barhanin J, Charpentier F, Escande D (1998) A dominant negative isoform of the long QT syndrome 1 gene product. J Biol Chem 273: 6837–6843
14. Donger C, Denjoy I, Berthet M, Neyroud N, Cruaud C, Bennaceur M, Chivoret G, Schwartz K, Coumel P, Guicheney P (1997) KVLQT1 C-terminal missense mutation causes a forme fruste long-QT syndrome. Circulation 96: 2778–2781
15. Duggal P, Vesely MR, Wattanasirichaigoon D, Villafane J, Kaushik V, Beggs AH (1998) Mutation of the gene for IsK associated with both Jervell and Lange-Nielsen and Romano-Ward forms of Long-QT syndrome. Circulation 97: 142–146
16. Dumaine R, Wang Q, Keating MT, Hartmann HA, Schwartz PJ, Brown AM, Kirsch GE (1996) Multiple mechanisms of Na+ channel-linked long-QT syndrome. Circ Res 78: 916–924
17. Folco E, Mathur R, Mori Y, Buckett P, Koren G (1997) A cellular model for long QT syndrome. Trapping of heteromultimeric complexes consisting of truncated Kv1.1 potassium channel polypeptides and native Kv1.4 and Kv1.5 channels in the endoplasmic reticulum. J Biol Chem 272: 26505–26510
18. Guicheney P (1998) Personal communication
19. Guicheney P, Denjoy I, Kahlem P, Dausse E , Roy N, Komajda M, Schwartz K, Coumel P (1994) Families with long qt syndrome linked to chromosome 11-phenotypic heterogeneity. J General Physiol 104: A11–A11
20. Haverkamp W, Schulze-Bahr E, Hördt M, Wedekind H, Borggrefe M, Assmann G, Funke H, Breithardt G (1997) QT-Syndrome – Aspekte zur Pathogenese, Molekulargenetik, Diagnose und Therapie. Deut Ärztebl: 667–672
21. Haverkamp W, Shenasa M, Borggrefe M, Breithardt G (1995) Torsade de pointes. From cell to bedside. Cardiac Electrophysiology. Philadelphia, WB Saunders, pp 885–899
22. January CT, Riddle JM (1989) Early afterdepolarizations: Mechanism of induction and block. A role for L-type Ca2+ current. Circ Res 64: 977–990

23. Jervell A, Thingstad R, Endsjo TO (1966) The surdo-cardiac syndrome: Three new cases of congenital deafness with syncopal attacks and Q-T prolongation in the electrocardiogram. Am Heart J 72: 582–593

24. Jiang M, Tseng-Crank J, Tseng GN (1997) Suppression of slow delayed rectifier current by a truncated isoform of KvLQT1 cloned from normal human heart. J Biol Chem 272: 24109–24112

25. Kambouris NG, Nuss HB, Johns DC, Tomaselli GF, Marban E, Balser JR (1998) Phenotypic characterization of a novel long-QT syndrome mutation (R1623Q) in the cardiac sodium channel. Circulation 97: 640–644

26. Keating M, Atkinson D, Dunn C, Timothy K, Vincent GM, Leppert M (1991) Linkage of a cardiac arrhythmia, the long QT syndrome, and the Harvey ras-1 gene. Science 252: 704–706

27. Keating M, Dunn C, Atkinson D, Timothy K, Vincent GM, Leppert M (1991) Consistent linkage of the long-QT syndrome to the Harvey ras-1 locus on chromosome 11. Am J Hum Genet 49: 1335–1339

28. Kiehn J, Lacerda AE, Wible B, Brown AM (1996) Molecular physiology and pharmacology of HERG. Single-channel currents and block by dofetilide. Circulation 94: 2572–2579

29. Kiehn J, Wible B, Ficker E, Taglialatela M, Brown AM (1995) Cloned human inward rectifier K+ channel as a target for class III methanesulfonanilides. Circ Res 77: 1151-1155

30. Makita N, Shirai N, Nagashima M, Matsuoka R, Yamada Y, Tohse N, Kitabatake A (1998) A de novo missense mutation of human cardiac Na+ channel exhibiting novel molecular mechanisms of long QT syndrome. FEBS Lett 423: 5–9

31. Mathews ECJ, Blount AW, Blount AW Jr, Townsend JI (1972) Q-T prolongation and ventricular arrhythmias, with and without deafness, in the same family. Am J Cardiol 29: 702–711

32. Moss AJ, Zareba W, Benhorin J, Locati EH, Hall WJ, Robinson JL, Schwartz PJ, Towbin JA, Vincent GM, Lehmann MH (1995) ECG T-wave patterns in genetically distinct forms of the hereditary long QT syndrome. Circulation 92: 2929–2934

33. Neyroud N, Denjoy I, Donger C, Gary F, Villain E, Leenhardt A, Benali K, Schwartz K, Coumel P, Guicheney P (1998) Heterozygous mutation in the pore of potassium channel gene KvLQT1 causes an apparently normal phenotype in long QT syndrome. Eur J Hum Genet 6: 129–133

34. Neyroud N, Tesson F, Denjoy I, Leibovici M, Donger C, Barhanin J, Faure S, Gary F, Coumel P, Petit C, Schwartz K, Guicheney P (1997) A novel mutation in the potassium channel gene KVLQT1 causes the Jervell and Lange-Nielsen cardioauditory syndrome. Nat Genet 15: 186–189

35. Priori SG, Napolitano C, Cantu F, Brown AM, Schwartz PJ (1996) Differential response to Na+ channel blockade, beta-adrenergic stimulation, and rapid pacing in a cellular model mimicking the SCN5A and HERG defects present in the long-QT syndrome. Circ Res 78 : 1009–1015

36. Priori SG, Schwartz PJ, Napolitano C, Bianchi L, Dennis A, De FM, Brown AM, Casari G (1998) A recessive variant of the Romano-Ward long-QT syndrome? Circulation 97: 2420–2425

37. Roden DM, Lazzara R, Rosen M, Schwartz PJ, Towbin J, Vincent GM (1996) Multiple mechanisms in the long-QT syndrome. Current knowledge, gaps, and future directions. The SADS Foundation Task Force on LQTS. Circulation 94: 1996–2012

38. Roden DM, Woosley RL, Primm RK (1986) Incidence and clinical features of the quinidine-associated long QT syndrome: implications for patient care. Am Heart J 111: 1088–1093

39. Romey G, Attali B, Chouabe C, Abitbol I, Guillemare E, Barhanin J, Lazdunski M (1997) Molecular mechanism and functional significance of the MinK control of the KvLQT1 channel activity. J Biol Chem 272: 16713–16716

40. Sanchez Cascos A, Sanchez Pernaute R, Cifuentes S (1990) A child affected by the Romano-Ward syndrome born of a mother with the Jervell and Lange-Nielsen syndrome. Rev Esp Cardiol 43: 406–407

41. Sanguinetti MC, Curran ME, Spector PS, Keating MT (1996) Spectrum of HERG K+-channel dysfunction in an inherited cardiac arrhythmia. Proc Natl Acad Sci USA 93: 2208–2212

42. Sanguinetti MC, Curran ME, Zou A, Shen J, Spector PS, Atkinson DL, Keating MT (1996b) Coassembly of K(V)LQT1 and minK (IsK) proteins to form cardiac I(Ks) potassium channel. Nature 384: 80–83

43. Sanguinetti MC, Jiang C, Curran ME, Keating MT (1995) A mechanistic link between an inherited and an acquired cardiac arrhythmia: HERG encodes the IKr potassium channel. Cell 81: 299–307

44. Sato T, Hata Y, Yamamoto M, Morita H, Mizuo K, Yamanari H, Saito D, Ohe T (1995) Early afterdepolarization abolished by potassium channel opener in a patient with idiopathic long QT syndrome. J Cardiovasc Electrophysiol 6: 279–282

45. Schott JJ, Charpentier F, Peltier S, Foley P, Drouin E, Bouhour JB, Donnelly P, Vergnaud G, Bachner L, Moisan JP (1995) Mapping of a gene for long QT syndrome to chromosome 4q25-27. Am J Hum Genet 57: 1114–1122

46. Schulze-Bahr E et al. (1998) Submitted for publication

47. Schulze-Bahr E, Haverkamp W, Funke H (1995) The long-QT syndrome. N Engl J Med 333: 1783–1784

48. Schulze-Bahr E, Haverkamp W, Wedekind H, Rubie C, Hordt M, Borggrefe M, Assmann G, Breithardt G, Funke H (1997) Autosomal recessive long-QT syndrome (Jervell Lange-Nielsen syndrome) is genetically heterogeneous. Hum Genet 100: 573–576

49. Schulze-Bahr E, Haverkamp W, Wiebusch H, Schulte H, Hördt M, Borggrefe M, Breithardt G, Assmann G, Funke H (1996) Molekulare Differenzierung des Romano-Ward-Syndroms. Herzschrittmacherther Elektrophys 7 (1): 21–26

50. Schulze-Bahr E, Haverkamp W, Wiebusch H, Schulte H, Hördt M, Borggrefe M, Breithardt G, Assmann G, Funke H (1995) Molecular analysis at the Harvey-Ras 1 gene in patients with long-QT syndrome. J Mol Med 73: 565–569

51. Schulze-Bahr E, Wang Q, Wedekind H, Haverkamp W, Chen Q, Sun Y, Rubie C, Hördt M, Towbin JA, Borggrefe M, Assmann G, Qu X, Somberg JC, Breithardt G, Oberti C, Funke H (1997) KCNE1 mutations cause Jervell and Lange-Nielsen syndrome. Nat Genet 17: 267–268

52. Schwartz PJ, Priori SG, Locati EH, Napolitano C, Cantu F, Towbin JA, Keating MT, Hammoude H, Brown AM, Chen LS (1995) Long QT syndrome patients with mutations of the SCN5A and HERG genes have differential responses to Na+ channel blockade and to increases in heart rate. Implications for gene-specific therapy. Circulation 92: 3381–3386

53. Shalaby FY, Levesque PC, Yang WP, Little WA, Conder ML, Jenkins-West T, Blanar MA (1997) Dominant-negative KvLQT1 mutations underlie the LQT1 form of long QT syndrome. Circulation 96: 1733–1736

54. Shimizu W, Antzelevitch C (1997) Sodium channel block with mexiletine is effective in reducing dispersion of repolarization and preventing torsade de pointes in LQT2 and LQT3 models of the long-QT syndrome. Circulation 96: 2038–2047

55. Shimizu W, Kurita T, Matsuo K, Suyama K, Aihara N, Kamakura S, Towbin JA, Shimomura K (1998) Improvement of repolarization abnormalities by a K+ channel opener in the LQT1 form of congenital long-QT syndrome. Circulation 97: 1581–1588

56. Smith P.L, Baukrowitz T, Yellen G (1996) The inward rectification mechanism of the HERG cardiac potassium channel. Nature 379: 833–836

57. Spector PS, Curran ME, Keating MT, Sanguinetti MC (1996) Class III antiarrhythmic drugs block HERG, a human cardiac delayed rectifier K+ channel. Open-channel block by methanesulfonanilides. Circ Res 78: 499–503

58. Spector PS, Curran ME, Zou AR, Sanguinetti MC (1996) Fast inactivation causes rectification of the IKr channel. J Gen Physiol 107: 611–619

59. Splawski I, Timothy KW, Vincent GM, Atkinson DL, Keating MT (1997) Molecular basis of the long-QT syndrome associated with deafness. N Engl J Med 336: 1562–1567

60. Splawski I, Tristani-Firouzi M, Lehmann MH, Sanguinetti MC, Keating MT (1997) Mutations in the hminK gene cause long QT syndrome and suppress IKs function. Nat Genet 17: 338–340

61. Tan HL, Hou CJ, Lauer MR, Sung RJ (1995) Electrophysiologic mechanisms of the long QT interval syndromes and torsade de pointes. Ann Intern Med 122: 701–714

62. Tesson F, Donger C, Denjoy I, Berthet M, Bennaceur M, Petit C, Coumel P, Schwartz K, Guicheney P (1996) Exclusion of KCNE1 (IsK) as a candidate gene for Jervell and Lange- Nielsen syndrome. J Mol Cell Cardiol 28: 2051–2055

63. Trudeau MC, Warmke JW, Ganetzky B, Robertson GA (1995) HERG, a human inward rectifier in the voltage-gated potassium channel family. Science 269: 92–95

64. Trudeau MC, Warmke JW, Ganetzky B, Robertson GA (1996) HERG sequence correction. Science 272: 1087–1087

65. Tyson J, Tranebjaerg L, Bellman S, Wren C, Taylor JF, Bathen J, Aslaksen B, Sorland SJ, Lund O, Malcolm S, Pembrey M, Bhattacharya S, Bitner-Glindzicz M (1997) IsK and KvLQT1: Mutation in either of the two subunits of the slow component of the delayed rectifier potassium channel can cause Jervell and Lange-Nielsen syndrome. Hum Mol Genet 6: 2179–2185

66. Vincent GM, Timothy KW, Leppert M, Keating M (1992) The spectrum of symptoms and QT intervals in carriers of the gene for the long-QT syndrome. N Engl J Med 327: 846–852

67. Wang DW, Yazawa K, George ALJ, Bennett PB (1996) Characterization of human cardiac Na+ channel mutations in the congenital long QT syndrome. Proc Natl Acad Sci USA 93: 13200–13205

68. Wang DW, Yazawa K, Makita N, George ALJ, Bennett PB (1997) Pharmacological targeting of long QT mutant sodium channels. J Clin Invest 99: 1714–1720

69. Wang Q (1997) Personal communication

70. Wang Q, Curran ME, Splawski I, Burn TC, Millholland JM, Van Raay TJ, Shen J, Timothy KW, Vincent GM, De JT, Schwartz PJ, Toubin JA, Moss AJ, Atkinson DL, Landes GM, Connors TD, Keating MT (1996) Positional cloning of a novel potassium channel gene: KVLQT1 mutations cause cardiac arrhythmias. Nat Genet 12: 17–23

71. Wang Q, Shen J, Li Z, Timothy K, Vincent GM, Priori SG, Schwartz PJ, Keating MT (1995a) Cardiac sodium channel mutations in patients with long QT syndrome, an inherited cardiac arrhythmia. Hum Mol Genet. 4: 1603–1607

72. Wang Q, Shen J, Splawski I, Atkinson D, Li Z, Robinson JL, Moss AJ, Towbin JA, Keating MT (1995b) SCN5A mutations associated with an inherited cardiac arrhythmia, long QT syndrome. Cell 80: 805–811

73. Wollnik B, Schroeder BC, Kubisch C, Esperer HD, Wieacker P, Jentsch TJ (1997) Pathophysiological mechanisms of dominant and recessive KVLQT1 K+ channel mutations found in inherited cardiac arrhythmias. Hum Mol Genet. 6: 1943–1949
74. Yang WP, Levesque PC, Little WA, Conder ML, Shalaby FY, Blanar MA (1997) KvLQT1, a voltage-gated potassium channel responsible for human cardiac arrhythmias. Proc Natl Acad Sci USA 94: 4017–4021

Author's address:
Eric Schulze-Bahr, M.D.
Department of Cardiology and Angiology
Hospital of the University of Münster
D-48129 Münster, Germany
E-mail heart@uni-muenster.de

Acquired abnormal QT prolongation and torsade de pointes – clinical significance of genetic information from congenital long QT syndrome

W. Haverkamp[1,2], G. Mönnig[1,2], L. Eckhardt[1], P. Kirchhof[1], H. Wedekind[1,2], E. Schulze-Bahr[1,2], H. Funke[2], M. Borggrefe[1,2], G. Breithardt[1,2]

[1]Hospital of the Westfälische Wilhelms-University, Department of Cardiology and Angiology, and [2]Institut for Arteriosclerosis Research, Münster, Germany

Abstract

The long QT syndrome (LQTS) is an either inherited or acquired disorder, characterized primarily by prolongation of the QT interval, by recurrent syncope, and sudden cardiac death. The congenital variant which has recently been identified as a genetic channelopathy typically becomes clinically manifest in childhood or early adulthood. The frequencies of syncope and sudden death vary from family to family. The so-called acquired form of the syndrome is largely an iatrogenic disease, most cases being related to the administration of drugs that prolong the QT interval often in combination with other environmental factors like hypokalemia. This includes not only antiarrhythmic drugs but also several other non-cardiac drugs generally not thought to have significant electrophysiologic effects. Only in response to these triggers does the QT interval become abnormally prolonged and do ventricular tachyarrhythmias of the torsade de pointes type occur. Evidence that the majority of patients with acquired abnormal QT prolongation has mutations in the genes causing congenital LQTS is so far lacking. Recent studies suggest that acquired LQTS is a multifactorial disorder. Genetic factors, an increased sensitivity to specific triggers, and environmental factors seem to play a role.

Introduction

The congenital long QT syndrome (LQTS) is an inherited disorder, characterized primarily by prolongation of the QT interval, by recurrent syncope, and sudden cardiac death, particularly in association with emotional or physical stress (33, 37, 42). The syndrome which has recently been identified as a genetic channelopathy (Table 1) usually becomes clinically manifest during childhood or early adulthood and shows a clear female preponderance. The frequencies of syncope and sudden death vary from family to family. However, among untreated symptomatic patients, mortality is high, with 20 % in the first year after an initial

Table 1. Genetic characterization of congenital long QT syndrome

LQT locus	Location	Gene	Gene product
LQT1	11p15.5	KCNQ1	α-subunit of potassium channel (I_{Ks})
LQT2	7q35–36	HERG	α-subunit of potassium channel (I_{Kr})
LQT3	3p21–24	SCN5A	α-subunit of sodium channel (I_{Na})
LQT4	4q25–27	Unknown	Unknown
LQT5	21q22.1–22	KCNE1	β-subunit of potassium channel (I_{Ks})
LQT6	Unknown	Unknown	Unknown
JNL1	11p15.5	KCNQ1	α-subunit of potassium channel (I_{Ks})
JNL2	21q22.1–22	KCNE1	β-subunit of potassium channel (I_{Ks})

LQT: long QT syndrome; JNL: Jervell-and-Lange-Nielsen syndrome; I_{Kr}: rapidly activating component of the delayed rectifier potassium current I_K; I_{Ks}: slowly activating component of the delayed rectifier potassium current I_K; I_{Na}: rapid sodium inward current

syncope and approximately 50 % within 10 years. Prognosis can be substantially improved by the use of β-blocking agents which reduce long-term mortality to less than 5 % (33). However, compared to healthy individuals, mortality remains elevated.

The cause of syncope in patients with LQTS is polymorphic ventricular tachycardia of the torsade de pointes type (Fig. 1). The term "torsade de pointes" (TDP) was coined in the 1960s by the French cardiologist Dessertenne in order to individualize this particular form of tachyarrhythmia which is characterized by QRS complexes of progressively changing amplitude and contour that seem to revolve around the isoelectric line (8). TDP is commonly non-sustained but sometimes may also degenerate into ventricular fibrillation.

The congenital form of LQTS is not the only disorder associated with the occurrence of TDP. The arrhythmia is also typical for the so-called acquired variant of LQTS which mimics several aspects of the congenital form (19, 36). However, in contrast to the latter, patients with acquired LQTS and their family members (!) usually have a normal QT interval. Only in response to specific triggers does it become abnormally prolonged. In parallel, the propensity to develop TDP markedly increases. Triggers which may result in abnormal QT prolongation and recurrent TDP are either drugs that prolong the QT interval (Table 2)

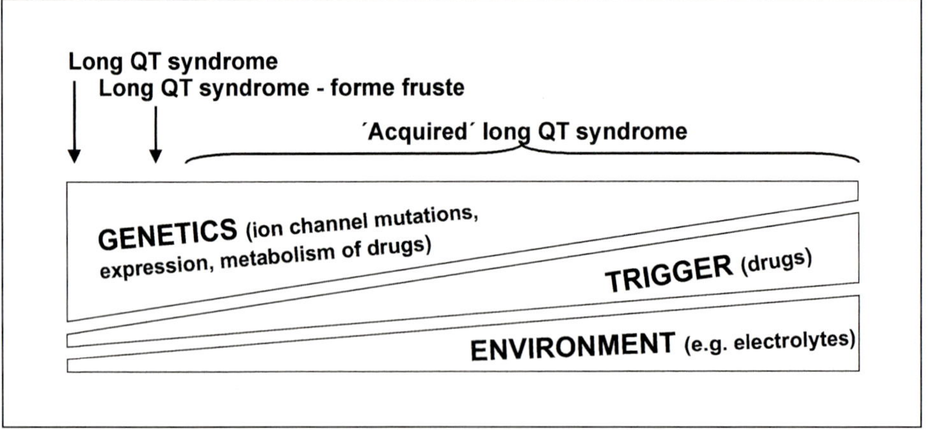

Fig. 1. The concept of multifactorial origin of acquired abnormal QT prolongation and TDP. See text for discussion.

Table 2. Drugs associated torsade de pointes

	Estimated incidence of TDP
Antiarrhythmic drugs	
– Quinidine	2–8.8 %
– Disopyramide	2–3 %
– Procainamide	2–3 %
– Ajmaline	*
– Propafenone	*
– d,l-sotalol	1.8–4.8 %
– Amiodarone (rare)	0.5–1 %
– Dofetilide	1.5–4 %
– Semantalide	*
– Almokalant	≥ 8 %
– Ibutilide	6 %
Calcium-channel blockers	
– Bepridil	*
– Lidoflazine	*
Tri- and tetracyclic antidepressants	
– Amitryptiline	*
– Imipramine	*
– Doxepin	*
– Maprotiline	*
Phenothiazines	*
– Thioridazine	*
– Chlorpromazine	*
Butyrophenone antipsychotics	
– Droperidol	*
– Haloperidol	*
Other psychotropic drugs	
– Cloral hydrate	*
Antihistaminics	
– Astemizole	*
– Terfenadine	*
Antibiotics	
– Erythromycin	*
– Clarithromycin	*
– Spiramycin	*
– Trimethoprim-sulfamethoxazole	*
– Pentamidine	*
– Halofantrine	*
– Quinine	*
Promotility agents	
– Cisapride	*
Serotonin antagonists	
– Ketanserin	*
– Zimeldine	*
Ionic contrast media	
– Ketanserin	*
Miscellaneous	
– Terodiline	*
– Probucol	*
– Arsenic poisoning, poisoning with organo-phosphorus insecticides	*
* only case reports available	

Table 3. Risk factors for drug-induced torsade de pointes

- Prolonged baseline QT
- Abnormally prolonged QT interval during drug
- T wave lability
- T wave morphology changes during drug
- Recent cardioversion from atrial fibrillation
- Hypokalemia, hypomagnesemia
- Diuretic use
- Bradycardia
- High drug doses or concentrations
- Use of drugs interfering with the metabolism of drugs known to cause torsade de pointes
  (e.g., inhibitors of cytochrome P450 enzymes like erythromycin, ketoconazole, and grapefruit juice)
- Rapid intravenous infusion
- Female gender
- Cardiac hypertrophy
- Altered nutritional states (anorexia nervosa, diets, starvation)
- Cerebrovascular diseases (e.g., intracranial hemorrhage)

and/or other factors and circumstances which delay repolarization (e.g., hypokalemia, severe bradycardia) (Table 3). The QT interval remains prolonged as long as the drug and/or other causative factors are active. After withdrawal of the QT-prolonging drug and correction of other causative factors, the QT interval normalizes and the propensity to the development of TDP disappears. In contrast to the congenital form, arrhythmias occurring in the acquired form are not precipitated by heightened sympathetic tone.

The purpose of the present article is to summarize the many causes and circumstances which may result in acquired abnormal QT prolongation and TDP, to discuss the potential electrophysiologic mechanisms underlying this particular form of drug-induced tachyarrhythmia, to discuss the relevance of so-called risk factors for its occurrence, and, last but not least, to answer the question whether recent progress made toward our understanding of the molecular mechanisms underlying the congenital LQTS may help to understand why TDP occurs in patients with acquired abnormal QT prolongation, i.e., individuals with otherwise normal myocardial repolarization.

Causes and incidence of acquired abnormal QT prolongation and torsade de pointes

TDP secondary to acquired abnormal QT prolongation has been described under a variety of circumstances (Table 1) (17, 19, 35). The most common cause of the arrhythmia seems to be the administration of antiarrhythmic drugs that prolong the action potential, i.e., class IA and class III agents. The incidence of TDP in patients treated with quinidine has been estimated to range between 2.0 and 8.8 % (26, 39). Although TDP preferentially occurs shortly after initiation of therapy, it may also develop during long-term treatment. The late occurrence of TDP has been linked to changes in dose, reinitiation of the drug after short discontinuation, and transient electrolyte disorders like hypokalemia and/or hypomagnesemia. TDP has also been described to occur during therapy with disopyramide and procainamide which both have effects on repolarization similar to quinidine (26, 46).

The incidence of torsade de pointes associated with sotalol which, besides its class III activity, possesses significant beta-blocking activity has been estimated to range between 1.8 % and 4.8 % (18, 21). In a series of 396 patients who underwent serial drug testing because of either sustained ventricular tachyarrhythmias or aborted sudden death at our institution, the incidence of TDP was 1.8 % (7 patients) (18). Although several cases with TDP due to treatment with amiodarone have been published, an analysis by Hohnloser and coworkers suggest that, despite QT interval prolongation, the development of TDP seems to be relatively rare (incidence < 1 %) (20, 21). The complex electrophysiological profile of the drug which, besides its action potential prolonging effect, exhibits noncompetitive beta-sympatholytic, calcium antagonistic, and lidocaine-like local anesthetic effects seems to be responsible for this phenomenon.

TDP secondary to exposure to newer so-called "pure" class III agents (e.g., dofetilide, sematalide, d-sotalol, almokalant, ibutilide) and treatment with N-acetyl-procainamide, the major metabolite of procainamide, has been well documented (11, 21, 25, 43). As with other drugs known to prolong myocardial repolarization, the incidence of TDP is dose-dependent, i.e., it increases with higher dosages/drug concentrations (see section Risk factors). Patients who initially developed TDP during therapy with a class IA antiarrhythmic agent and then developed the arrhythmia again on a second or third class IA agents ("cross-reactivity") have been reported (3, 26, 45). Individual cases of cross-reactivity have also been reported for class IA drugs and amiodarone, for a class IA agent and lidoflazine, and for sotalol and amiodarone (7, 27).

As already pointed out, TDP have not only been reported to occur secondary to treatment with cardiac or antiarrhythmic drugs, but also during treatment with several other drugs not generally thought to have significant effects on myocardial repolarization. Non-cardiovascular drugs which have been shown to be potentially associated with abnormal QT prolongation and TDP include, e.g., phenothiazines, antidepressants, other psychotropic drugs, antihistamines of the H1 blocking type, the promotility agent cisapride, and some antibiotics, most notably erythromycin (19). It is noteworthy that these apparently harmless drugs can create life-threatening ventricular arrhythmias and that physicians can unwittingly expose their patients to risk. Estimation of the incidence of TDP during treatment with non-cardiovascular drugs is difficult. A large number of reported case reports and individual small series suggest that the occurrence of this particular form of drug-related proarrhythmia is not a trivial problem. One factor which renders estimation of the true incidence of TDP difficult is that making the diagnosis of TDP is far from being easy. This seems to be particularly true for the non-cardiologist. A proper diagnosis largely depends on a proper electrocardiographic documentation. This includes the simultaneous recording of several electrocardiographic leads which is essential to recognize the twisting action of the QRS complexes, which may not be recognized in all leads. Furthermore, much misunderstanding has been created by including any polymorphic form of ventricular tachycardia under the term "torsade de pointes". Taking these considerations into account, it is easily conceivable that a large number of misdiagnosed, drug-induced cases exist which have never been reported.

Several cases with acquired abnormal QT prolongation and TDP in the absence of action potential prolonging drugs have been reported. In these cases, the occurrence of TDP has been attributed to the presence of severe hypokalemia, hypomagnesemia and/or bradycardia resulting from heart block. These factors (particularly hypokalemia and bradycardia) also very often accompany drug-induced TDP (19, 26). Other rare causes of acquired LQTS include ionic contrast media (14), some poisons (30), and even a Chinese herbal remedy (4). The development of TDP in patients with altered nutritional states, e.g., anorexia nervosa or during treatment with "liquid protein" diets and other fat weight-reducing diets has been reported (23, 44). However, QT prolongation and eventually TDP secondary to these conditions have been attributed to marked metabolic disturbances (e.g., hypokalemia).

Mechanisms of torsade de pointes in acquired abnormal QT prolongation

Recently, in vitro and in vivo experimental studies have suggested that early afterdepolarizations (EADs) and triggered activity may play an important role in the genesis of ventricular tachyarrhythmias of the TDP type. EADs are cellular depolarizations occurring either during phase 2 and 3 of the transmembrane potential before repolarization is completed (12). These depolarizations may give rise to a premature action potential or a train of action potentials when the threshold for activation is reached. The resulting depolarization has been referred to as "triggered activity" since it is caused by a second nondriven upstroke induced by an afterdepolarization. The induction of EADs in in vitro preparations has been demonstrated for almost all drugs listed in Table 2 (12). Most of them exert their QT prolonging effect which can be considered as a prerequisite for the development of EADs, by blocking the rapidly activating component of the delayed rectifier potassium current I_{Kr}. Some of the drugs also block other potassium channels (e.g., quinidine also blocks I_{Ks}, I_{to}, I_{K1} (48). However, usually the concentration necessary are at least an order of magnitude higher than those required to block I_{Kr}. Only a few drugs mainly inhibit the slowly activation component of the current (I_{Ks}) (e.g., azimilide). It has been suggested that the incidence of TDP is lower with the latter drugs; however, the development of TDP has been described (15) and prospective data comparing the incidence with blockers of I_{Kr} and I_{Ks} are not available.

Some investigators have suggested that TDP may be initiated and also maintained by triggered activity simultaneous originating at several independent competing foci. However, others have suggested that TDP may be initiated by triggered activity but maintained by a circus movement reentry mechanism. El-Sherif and coworkers (13) recently developed a canine in vivo model of LQTS using anthopleurin-A, an agent that prolongs action potential duration by slowing inactivation of the sodium current. Using high resolution three dimensional isochronal maps of activation and repolarization patterns, they showed that the initial beat of all episodes of polymorphic ventricular tachycardia consistently arose as a subendocardial focal activity, whereas subsequent beats were due to successive reentrant excitation in the form of rotating scrolls. Increased transmural electrical heterogeneity resulting from spatial differences in action potential duration and morphology has been suggested as the substrate underlying reentrant activation.

Risk factors for the occurrence of acquired abnormal QT prolongation and torsade de pointes

Several risk factors for the development of drugs-related TDP have been proposed (Table 3). Most of them have been derived from case reports or databases accumulating patients who developed TDP associated with particular drugs. Only recently systematic attempts to identify risk factors for TDP in larger cohorts of patients have been made.

In most series, patients developing drug-related TDP were found to have a borderline or prolonged (>0.44 ms$^{1/2}$) rate-corrected QT interval at baseline (before drug administration). An increased dispersion of QT intervals compared to individuals who never experienced the arrhythmia has been documented. The fact that the QT interval is usually longer in women compared to man has been suggested to, at least in part, account for the higher prevalence of abnormal QT prolongation and TDP in females. In almost all series of patients with drug-induced TDP, a 2–3 fold higher incidence of the arrhythmia in women has been demonstrated (29, 32). New T wave morphologic changes, particularly biphasic T waves, developing independently of pre-existing disturbances of repolarization during therapy with class III agents also seem to represent risk factors for the occurrence of TDP. This has recently been demonstrated by Houltz et al. (22) in a study where almokalant was administered intravenously in 100 patients with atrial fibrillation. In this study, six patients (6 %) developed TDP. Even in the absence of a congenital LQTS, these findings suggest an increased lability of repolarization in patients with acquired LQTS.

Instability of repolarization may also result from interventions affecting cardiac memory. We recently reported on a patient who developed QT prolongation and new changes in T wave morphology after catheter ablation of AV-reentrant tachycardia (16). As described by others, these repolarization abnormalities persisted and were suggested to represent 'cardiac memory'. Two days after ablation, sotalol therapy was started because of paroxysms of atrial fibrillation. After the second sotalol dose, recurrent episodes of TDP developed. Serum potassium concentration was normal. The drug had led to a substantial further prolongation of the QT interval. Most interestingly, before ablation the patient had tolerated oral sotalol for many years.

As discussed above, bradycardia (e.g., sinus bradycardia, high degree AV block) and/or low potassium serum concentrations are common among patients who develop drug-induced TDP. There is a bulk of evidence demonstrating that action potential prolongation and the appearance of EADs in in vitro preparations is favored by bradycardia and hypokalemia. Many reports demonstrating that these factors alone are capable of inducing TDP exist. More importantly, it has been demonstrated that the I_{Kr} blocking properties of quinidine and dofitilide are strikingly dependent on extracellular potassium concentration (48). An marked increase in drug block of I_{Kr} is observed when potassium is lowered. A marked decrease in drug concentrations necessary to produce blockade of 50 % of the resulting current (IC_{50}) results. On the other hand, channel block resulting from dofitilide decreased when potassium is elevated.

Although drug-induced TDP may occur at subtherapeutic dosages and concentrations (preferentially in combination with low potassium, see above), high drug dosages and concentrations constitute an important risk factor for TDP. This is best exemplified by the available experience with most of the non-cardiovascular drugs listed in Table 2. In most of the cases of TDP secondary to drugs like cisapride or terfenadine (47), factors that had led to substantial accumulation of the drug were present. In some patients, concomitant hepatic and/or renal disease resulting in elevated plasma levels due to increases in the elimination half-life of the drug has been found. However, an even more important factor which may lead to excessive increases in plasma concentration is the coadministration of drugs that inhibit the biotransformation of the TDP-causing agent to noncardioactive metabolites. With regard to this problem, inhibition of the cytochrome P450 enzyme system seems to be particularly important (2). Many of the drugs listed in Table 2 are metabolized by specific hepatic cytochrome P450 enzymes (especially the CYP2D6 and CYP3A/4 isoenzymes) in the gut and liver. The interference of drugs with the P450 enzyme system is to some extent complex. As an example, quinidine is both an inhibitor and a substrate for the system: it is a potent inhibitor of the CYP2D6 isoenzyme, but it is metabolized by CYP3A4. The coadministration of substrates and inhibitors of this enzyme or even the daily intake of grapefruit juice (the exact chemical responsible for enzyme inhibition within grapefruit juice is not entirely clear) may lead to up to 5- to 20-fold increases in the plasma concentration of the parent compound. In addition, recent studies show that, presumably due to genetic polymorphism, individually different levels of activity of certain P450 enzymes exist. So-called poor metabolizers with absent or substantially diminished enzyme activity may also show drug accumulation (2).

High plasma concentrations of a drug may also result from rapid intravenous application (5). The development of TDP after rapid intravenous infusion of class III agents has been reported. However, as already pointed out, high drug concentrations are not an absolute preerequisite for TDP since its occurrence at low plasma quinidine and sotalol concentrations has been reported (1, 39).

The importance of underlying structural heart as a potential risk factor for TDP is not clear. Acquired abnormal QT prolongation associated with TDP has been observed in patients with various types of heart diseases as well as in patients without detectable heart disease. Thus, it seems that structural myocardial changes are at least not a prerequisite for this particular form of proarrhythmia. However, in larger series arterial hypertension was present in a significant proportion of patients (19, 39). In several studies, it was the most represented type of cardiovascular disease. Experimental studies have demonstrated that myocardial hypertrophy results in action potential prolongation (34). In isolated myocytes from cats with right ventricular hypertrophy due to pulmonary banding, the delayed rectifier potassium current (I_K) was found to be reduced in hypertrophied cells (28). Similar findings have been obtained in felines with left ventricular hypertrophy due to abdominal aortic obstruction (15). No study discriminating the two components of the delayed rectifier, I_{Kr} and I_{Ks}, are available. Thus, it seems conceivable that hypertrophy resulting from arterial hypertension increases the propensity to the development of TDP. It has also been suggested that the presents of heart failure represents a risk factor for TDP. As in cardiac hypertrophy, action potential prolongation has been demonstrated experimentally. However, not the delayed rectifier potassium current I_K but the transient outward current I_{to} seems to be predominantly affected. To date, the role of I_{to} in the pathogenesis of TDP is not clear.

A rather special clinical situation where the propensity to the development of TDP can be considered to be increased is immediately following cardioversion from atrial fibrillation. Several reports on the development of TDP after cardioversion exist (6, 19). In almost all cases, patients were treated with either class IA or class III agents and in most cases additional hypokalemia was present. In this particular situation, bradycardia which is a common finding after cardioversion can be suggested to further contribute to the lability of repolarization present in this particular situation.

Molecular biology of the congenital LQTS: implications for acquired LQTS

More than 30 years after its first detailed description, the congenital LQTS has now become the focus of considerable scientific attention. This is primarily due to the recent discovery that the disorder is a genetic channelopathy (38, 41). Mutations causing the disease have been identified in four genes (LQT1, LQT2, LQT3, and LQT5), each encoding a cardiac ion channel protein (Table 1). The SCN5A mutations (LQT3) result in defective sodium channel inactivation, whereas KNCQ1 (LQT1), KCNE1 (LQT5), and HERG mutations (LQT2) result in decreased outward potassium current. Either mutation decreases net outward current during repolarization and, thereby, accounts for abnormally prolonged QT intervals on the surface electrocardiogram. So far, the mutant gene for LQT4, which has been mapped to chromosome 4 (4q25–27), has not yet been discovered.

The fact that the rapidly activating potassium current I_{Kr} is involved in both the pathogenesis of the congenital as well as the acquired form of LQTS has led to the suggestion that there may be a genetic predisposition for acquired LQTS. Mutations in HERG have been found to account for approximately 20 % of all cases of congenital LQTS. However, recent studies in patients with drug-induced QT prolongation and TDP have yield only a small number of individual cases in whom the clinical setting had suggested an acquired form of the syndrome and genetic analysis revealed a familial form. In our own series of 17 patients with drug-induced LQTS who underwent SSCP analysis and direct sequencing of the 4 genes known to cause congenital LQTS, a mutation was found in only 4 patients (23 %) (40). Although these findings do not exclude that other channels are involved, they favor a multifactorial origin of acquired LQTS. It is conceivable that modifier genes that influence the pattern and clinical manifestation of the disease and other factors that control the expression and translation of genes may play a role. This has also been suggested to account for two major clinical aspects of congenital LQTS, namely the female preponderance (which can be found in both the congenital and the acquired form of the disease) and the marked heterogeneity of the clinical manifestation (phenotypic heterogeneity) of the disorder (31, 33).

Although only a small segment of the population seems to be at risk for acquired abnormal QT prolongation and TDP, experimental data suggest that, the adequate circumstances and the presence of triggers provided, the ability to develop TDP is an intrinsic property of almost any heart (9). We have recently studied the ability of clofilium, d,l-sotalol and erythromycin to produce TDP in the isolated rabbit heart (10, 24). Animals of both sex were studied. The experimental model was designed to reproduce conditions that are clinically known to be associated with an increased propensity to the development of TDP: the drugs were infused in the presence of either normal (5.88 mM) or low (1.5 mM) potassium concentration in sinus-driven or atrioventricular (AV)-blocked hearts. None of the drugs alone did produce TDP. However, episodes of TDP established in almost all hearts when AV-block and potassium was lowered and sufficiently high drug concentrations were present. A rather high incidence of experimentally-induced TDP-like arrhythmias in otherwise normal animals has been reported by several other groups.

The concept of multifactorial origin of acquired abnormal QT prolongation and TDP is further illustrated in Fig. 2. In patients with the congenital form of the syndrome, ion channel mutations form the major substrate for abnormal QT prolongation and the development of TDP. Activation of the adrenergic system is the prominent trigger for arrhythmias in most patients. Presumably due to the presence of modifier genes, the frequency of syncope, i.e., arrhythmia, varies from patients to patients. Many patients have a lot of events because the substrate dominates. However, some patients have ion channel mutations which, under normal conditions, do not significantly affect channel function and, thus, do not result in QT prolongation. In these patients who can be suggested to have a form 'fruste' of the congenital long QT syndrome, abnormal QT prolongation only becomes manifest in the presence of active triggers. The majority of individuals (with 'acquired' QT syndrome) does not have mutations in genes encoding ion channels involved in the repolarization process. However, for example, female gender and other genetic factors may increase their propensity to the development of TDP to a level higher than that of the majority of the population. The adequate triggers (e.g., treatment with erythromycin) and environmental factors (administration of an inhibitor of the cytochrome P450 system and bradycardia) provided, TDP may develop. Since these patients form a spectrum with varying degree of propensity to TDP, it takes very little in some of them to develop TDP while others need high drug concentration, bradycardia, and hypokalemia. However, the situation in which the arrhythmia become manifest is usually very unique and in most patients it occurs only once during a life-time. If this hypothesis would be true, genetic screening of the genes known to be causative for a congenital QT syndrome would be able to identify a subgroup of patients with an increased propensity to TDP (i.e., those patients with a 'forme fruste' of the congenital long QT syndrome) but it would not allow to identify all patients at risk for acquired TDP, and, more importantly, it would not allow to exclude an increased propensity to develop this particular form of proarrhythmia prior to drug exposure.

Implications for future drug development

The often complex and multifactorial origin of acquired abnormal QT prolongation and TDP has important implications for future drug development. The experience made with the available QT prolonging drugs (particularly those made with the 'non-cardiac' drugs) has alerted the authorities and has led to the suggestion of several new guidelines that might be applied to future development of other drugs. It has been suggested that every new drug should be screened for effects on potassium channels and/or for in vitro and in vivo effects on the QT interval. If a drugs prolongs repolarization comprehensive dose-response studies should be performed. It has also been suggested that metabolic evaluations should be conducted in order to identify the types of patients likely to have increased drug levels resulting from either decreased clearance or decreased metabolism. More extensive drug interaction screening has been requested, particularly for agents that are metabolized by one of the P450 enzymes. It seems conceivable that for the identification of slow metabolizers who have an inherited decreased level of activity of certain P450 enzymes, genetic screening may be helpful.

Conclusions and future directions

Despite the improvement in our understanding which the recent identification of the genes causing congenital LQTS has made, many aspects of the mechanisms underlying abnormal QT prolongation and TDP are not yet elucidated. The initial hope that most cases of acquired LQTS, like individuals with the congenital variant of the syndrome, have mutations of ion channel genes, has not come true. Currently, there is no evidence to suggest that the majority of patients with acquired LQTS suffer from a subclinical variant (from fruste) of the congenital form of the syndrome, although this may be the case in individual patients.

However, this does not exclude that acquired LQTS has a genetic background. Current evidence suggests that the disease has a multifactorial origin with environmental factors significantly modulating the genetic basis. A better understanding of the mechanisms underlying acquired LQT will require integration of molecular genetic data with cellular electrophysiological information that can relate the phenomenon of drug-induced abnormal QT prolongation and TDP to changes in presumably both environmental and genetically determined ion channel structure, expression, and/or regulation.

From the clinical point of view, the major problem continues to be the identification of the patients at increased risk of acquired abnormal QT prolongation development of TDP. As long as effective screening for an increased propensity to acquired abnormal QT prolongation is not possible, the physician prescribing drugs which may result in QT prolongation must be aware of the problem of acquired TDP and must try to control all the risk factors from which we know that they may increase the propensity to TDP. This is strongly recommended not only during iniation of therapy but also during long-term treatment.

Acknowledgment   This work was supported in part by the Franz-Loogen-Stiftung, Düsseldorf, Germany, by research grants from the Center of Innovative Medical Research (IMF) of the Westfälische Wilhelms University of Münster, by the Deutsche Forschungsgemeinschaft (Schu 1082/2–1), and by the BIOMED2 program (ERB BMH4-CT96–0028) of the European Union.

References

1. Bauman JL, Bauernfeind RA, Hoff JV, Strasberg B, Swiryn S, Rosen KM (1984) Torsade de pointes due to quinidine: Observations in 31 patients. Am Heart J 107: 425–430
2. Baumann JL, Sanoski CA, Lingtak-Neander C (1997) Pharmacokinetic and pharmacodynamic drug interactions with antiarrhythmic agents. Cardiol Rev 5: 292–304
3. Breithardt G, Seipel L, Haerten K (1980) Paradoxic response to disopyramide and quinidine. Z Kardiol 69: 556–561
4. Bryer-Ash M, Zehnder J, Angelchik P, Maisel A (1987) Torsade de pointes precipitated by a chinese herbal remedy. Am J Cardiol 60: 1186–1187
5. Carlsson L, Abrahamsson C, Andersson B, Duker G, Schiller LG (1993) Proarrhythmic effects of the class III agent almokalant: Importance of infusion rate, QT dispersion, and early afterdepolarisations. Cardiovasc Res 27: 2186–2193
6. Choy AMJ, Darbar D, Dell'Orto S, Roden DM (1996) Increased sensitivity to QT prolonging drug therapy immediately after cardioversion to sinus rhythm. Circulation 94: I-202
7. Clark M, Friday K, Anderson J et al. (1985) Drug induced torsades de pointes: High concordance rate among type IA antiarrhythmic drugs and amiodarone. J Am Coll Cardiol 5: I-450
8. Dessertenne F, Fabiato A, Coumel P (1966) Un chapitre nouveau délectrocardiographie: les variations progressive de lamplitude de lélectrocardiogramme. Actual Cardiol Angeiol Int 15: 241–258
9. Eckardt L, Haverkamp W, Borggrefe M, Breithardt G (1998) Experimental models of torsade de pointes. Cardiovasc Res 39: 178–183
10. Eckardt L, Haverkamp W, Mertens H, Johna R, Clague JR, Borggrefe M, Breithardt G (1998) Drug-related torsades de pointes in the isolated rabbit heart: comparison of clofilium, d,l-sotalol, and erythromycin. J Cardiovasc Pharm 32: 425–434
11. Ellenbogen KA, Stambler BS, Wood MA, Sager PT, Wesley-RC J, Meissner MC, Zoble RG, Wakefield LK, Perry KT, Vander-Lugt JT (1996) Efficacy of intravenous ibutilide for rapid termination of atrial fibrillation and atrial flutter: A dose-response study. J Am Coll Cardiol 28: 130–136
12. El-Sherif N (1991) Early afterdepolarizations and arrhythmogenesis. Experimental and clinical aspects. Arch Mal Coeur Vaiss 84: 227–234
13. El-Sherif N, Chinushi M, Caref EB, Restivo M (1997) Electrophysiological mechanism of the characteristic electrocardiographic morphology of torsade de pointes tachyarrhythmias in the long-QT syndrome: Detailed analysis of ventricular tridimensional activation patterns. Circulation 96: 4392–4399
14. Emori T, Fujieda H, Ohe T (1996) Polymorphic ventricular tachycardia induced by intracoronary injection of ioxaglate in a patient with borderline QT prolongation. J Cardiovasc Electrophysiol 7: 962–966
15. Furukawa T, Myerburg R, Furukawa N, Kimura S, Bassett AL (1994) Metabolic inhibition if ICa,L and IK differs in feline left ventricular hypertrophy. Am J Physiol 266: H1121–H1131

16. Haverkamp W, Hördt M, Breithardt G, Borggrefe M (1998) Torsade de pointes secondary to d,l-sotalol after catheter ablation of incessant atrioventricular reentrant tachycardia-evidence for a significant contribution of the "cardiac memory". Clin Cardiol 21: 55–58

17. Haverkamp W, Hördt M, Chen X, Hindricks G, Willems S, Kottkamp H, Rotman B, Brunn J, Borggrefe M, Breithardt G (1993) Torsade de pointes. Z Kardiol 82: 763–774

18. Haverkamp W, Martinez RA, Hief C, Lammers A, Mühlenkamp S, Wichter T, Breithardt G, Borggrefe M (1997) Efficacy and safety of d,l-sotalol in patients with ventricular tachycardia and in survivors of cardiac arrest. J Am Coll Cardiol 30: 487–495

19. Haverkamp W, Shenasa M, Borggrefe M, Breithardt G (1995) Torsade de pointes. In: Zipes DP, Jalife J (eds) Cardiac Electrophysiology. From Cell to Bedside. WB Saunders Company, Philadelphia, pp 885–899

20. Hohnloser SH, Klingenheben T, Singh BN (1994) Amiodarone-associated proarrhythmic effects. A review with special reference to torsade de pointes tachycardia. Ann Intern Med 121: 529–535

21. Hohnloser SH, Singh BN (1995) Proarrhythmia with class III antiarrhythmic drugs: Definition, electrophysiologic mechanisms, incidence, predisposing factors, and clinical implications. J Cardiovasc Electrophysiol 6: 920–936

22. Houltz B, Darpo B, Edvardsson N (1998) Electrocardiographic and clinical predictors of torsades de pointes induced by almokalant infusion in patients with chronic atrial fibrillation or flutter. PACE 21: 967–969

23. Isner JM, Roberts WC, Heymsfield SB et al. (1985) Anorexia nervosa and sudden death. Ann Intern Med 102: 49–52

24. Johna R, Mertens H, Haverkamp W, Eckardt L, Niederbröcker T, Borggrefe M, Breithardt G (1998) Clofilium in the isolated perfused rabbit heart: A new model to study proarrhythmia induced by class III antiarrhythmic agents. Bas Res Cardiol 93: 127–135

25. Karam R, Marcello S, Brooks RR, Corey AE, Moore A (1998) Azimilide dihydrochloride, a novel antiarrhythmic agent. Am J Cardiol 81: 40D–46D

26. Kay GN, Plumb VJ, Arciniegas JG, Henthorn RW, Waldo AL (1983) Torsade de pointes: The long-short initiating sequence and other clinical features: observations in 32 patients. J Am Coll Cardiol 2: 806–817

27. Kennelly BM (1977) Comparison of lidoflazine and quinidine in prophylactic treatment of arrhythmias. Br Heart J 39: 540–545

28. Kleiman RB, Houser SR (1989) Outward currents in normal and hypertrophied feline ventricular myocytes. Am J Physiol 256: H1540–H1561

29. Lehmann MH, Hardy S, Archibald D, Quart B, MacNeil DJ (1996) Sex difference in risk of torsade de pointes with d,l-sotalol. Circulation 94: 2535–2541

30. Little RE, Kay GN, Cavender JB, Epstein AE, Plumb VJ (1990) Torsade de pointes and T-U wave alternans associated with arsenic poisoning. Pacing Clin Electrophysiol 13: 164–170

31. Locati EH, Zareba W, Moss AJ, Schwartz PJ, Vincent GM, Lehmann MH, Towbin JA, Priori SG, Napolitano C, Robinson JL, Andrews M, Timothy K, Hall WJ (1998) Age- and sex-related differences in clinical manifestations in patients with congenital long-QT syndrome: Findings from the International LQTS Registry. Circulation 97: 2237–2244

32. Makkar RR, Fromm BS, Steinman RT, Meissner MD, Lehmann MH (1993) Female gender as a risk factor for torsades de pointes associated with cardiovascular drugs. JAMA 270: 2590–2597

33. Moss AJ, Schwartz PJ, Crampton RS, Tzivoni D, Locati EH, MacCluer J, Hall WJ (1991) The long QT syndrome. Prospective longitudinal study of 328 families. Circulation 84: 1136–1144

34. Nähbauer M, Kääb S (1998) Potassium channel down-regulation in heart failure. Cardiovasc Res 37: 324–334

35. Roden DM (1997) A practical approach to torsade de pointes. Clin Cardiol 20: 285–290

36. Roden DM (1998) Taking the "idio" out of "idiosyncratic": Predicting torsades de pointes. Pacing Clin Electrophysiol 21: 1029–1034

37. Roden DM, George ALJ, Bennett PB (1995) Recent advances in understanding the molecular mechanisms of the long QT syndrome. J Cardiovasc Electrophysiol 1023–1031

38. Roden DM, Lazzara R, Rosen M, Schwartz PJ, Towbin J, Vincent GM (1996) Multiple mechanisms in the long-QT syndrome. Current knowledge, gaps, and future directions. The SADS Foundation Task Force on LQTS. Circulation 94: 1996–2012

39. Roden DM, Woosley RL, Primm RK (1986) Incidence and clinical features of the quinidine-associated long QT syndrome: Implications for patient care. Am Heart J 111: 1088–1093

40. Schulze-Bahr E, Guicheney P, Szafranski P, Richard P, Haverkamp W, Chen Q, Wedekind H, Assmann G, Borggrefe M, Breithardt G, Coumel P, Hördt M, Mergenthaler J, Mönnig G, Neyround N, Rubie C, Towbin J, Zhang D, Denjoy I, Wang Q, Funke H (1998) Mutations in cardiac ion channel genes associated with acquired long-QT-syndrome, submitted.

41. Schulze-Bahr E, Haverkamp W, Funke H (1995) The long-QT syndrome. N Engl J Med 333: 1783–1784

42. Schwartz PJ, Moss AJ, Vincent GMCRS (1993) Diagnostic criteria for the long QT syndrome. An update. Circulation 88: 782–784

43. Sedgwick ML, Lip G, Rae AP, Cobbe SM (1995) Chemical cardioversion of atrial fibrillation with intravenous dofetilide. Int J Cardiol 49: 159–166

44. Siegel RJ, Cabeen WR, Roberts WC (1981) Prolonged QT interval-ventricular tachycardia syndrome from massive rapid weight loss utilizing the liquid-protein-modified-fast diet: sudden death with sinus node ganglionitis and neuritis. Am Heart J 102: 121–123
45. Soffer J, Dreifus LS, Michelson EL (1982) Polymorphous ventricular tachycardia with normal and long Q-T intervals. Am J Cardiol 49: 2021–2029
46. Tzivoni D, Keren A, Stern S, Gottlieb S (1981) Disopyramide-induced torsade de pointes. Arch Intern Med 141: 946–947
47. Woosley RL (1996) Cardiac actions of antihistamines. Annu Rev Pharmacol Toxicol 36: 342–346
48. Yang T, Roden DM (1996) Extracellular potassium modulation of drug block of IKr. Implications for torsade de pointes and reverse use-dependence. Circulation 93: 407–411

Author's address:
Wilhelm Haverkamp, MD
Medizinische Klinik und Poliklinik,
Innere Medizin C (Kardiologie, Angiologie)
Westfälische Wilhelms-Universität Münster
48129 Münster
Germany
Email: haverkw@uni-muenster.de

Molecular genetic approaches to human hypertension

F. C. Luft

Franz Volhard Clinic and Max Delbrück Center for Molecular Medicine, Medizinische-Fakultät der Charite, Campus-Buch, Humboldt University of Berlin, Germany

Abstract

For the past decade, hypertension research has shifted strongly in the direction of molecular genetics. The success stories are the monogenic hypertensive syndromes. Classic linkage analyses have located the responsible genes and three the genes for glucocorticoid-remediable aldosteronism, Liddle syndrome, and apparent mineralocorticoid excess have been cloned and their functions elucidated. Other monogenic syndromes are currently being intensively studied However, in the area of primary hypertension, the successes have relied on the candidate gene approach. Allelic variants in the genes for angiotensinogen, α-adducin, β-2 adrenergic receptor, the G-protein beta3 subunit, and the T594M mutation in the β subunit of the epithelial sodium channel have been identified; however, the importance of these allelic variants to primary hypertension as a whole is not yet clear. A variant in the angiotensin converting enzyme gene could initially not be convincingly associated with hypertension, but more recent analyses suggest an influence of the deleted allele on blood pressure in men, but apparently not in women. In all likelihood we are dealing with many genes with small effects. Affected sibling pair linkage analyses will probably not be successful in identifying the loci of these genes. To find new genes, novel approaches will be necessary, including searching for quantitative trait loci linked to blood pressure in normotensive persons, haplotype sharing methodology in trios and family units, the use of better study designs, and the investigation of isolated populations.

Introduction

Over a decade ago, with the introduction of restriction fragment-length polymorphism technology as a relatively routine laboratory procedure, the National Heart Lung and Blood Institute of the National Institutes of Health, USA decided to place major emphasis on molecular genetics in terms of supporting research grant applications (24). Similar emphasis was placed on this area of research in France, Great Britain, and elsewhere. Nongeneticists (such as yours truly) shifted their research emphasis to the new area in a process termed "retooling". As has the field of molecular genetics in general, the molecular genetics of hypertension has rapidly expanded if not exploded. It is hard to pick up an issue of any hypertension-related journal without encountering reports on this or that polymorphism, the confirmation of this association study, or the refutation of that association study. Nevertheless, the results of this heady area of research are a little more sobering. Exactly how many genes have been found that are important to primary hypertension? How have these findings facilitated diagnosis? More importantly, what new therapeutic insights have been developed from these findings? Funding for this area of research has been generous to the detriment of other investigative areas. Sooner or later, we shall be called to account for where all the money went. Perhaps, we should start thinking of the answers, if for no other reason than to formulate better questions. After all, we do not want molecular genetics to be regarded as "the god that failed".

Monogenic hypertension

Monogenic hypertension is the bright spot in the area of molecular genetics of human hypertension. The attitude here is that by elucidating rare monogenic diseases, we shall come to understand mechanisms of disease applicable to primary hypertension (25). This promise has been kept largely through the efforts and successes of Lifton and colleagues. Glucocorticoid-remediable aldosteronism (GRA) is a good example.

Glucocorticoid-remediable aldosteronism

Patients with GRA have an autosomal dominant monogenic hypertension and are usually suspected of having primary aldosteronism. They have a volume expansion, salt-sensitive, form of hypertension, tend toward metabolic alkalosis with hypokalemia (not invariably), and respond to both thiazide diuretics and spironolactone. The latter fact is a clinical clue that mineralocorticoid products may be involved. Their renin values are low while the aldosterone values are both elevated. The patients also have 18-hydroxy and 18-oxocortisol, steroids not normally found in appreciable amounts, in their urine. Recognizing these abnormal products (an intermediate phenotype) led to solving the mystery. Replacement amounts of prednisone ameliorate the hypertension, cause the abnormal steroids to disappear, and give the syndrome its name. The abnormal cortisol derivatives and the favorable effects of glucocorticoid treatment suggested that inner cortical zones, which express the gene for 17 α-hydroxylase (CYP17) and are ACTH-responsive, were the source of the excess mineralocorticoids. Two distinct gene products (11 β-hydroxylase and aldosterone synthase) perform the terminal steps in glucocorticoid and mineralocorticoid biosynthesis, respectively. A linkage analysis in a large pedigree localized the responsible gene to chromosome 8, exactly at the site where the genes for 11 β-hydroxylase and aldosterone synthase also reside (23). This fact suggested that a chimeric gene might be responsible, which indeed proved to be the case. Aldosterone synthase (CYP11B2) and 11 β-hydroxylase (CYP11B1) reside on chromosome 8. In affected individuals, a chimeric gene consisting of the promotor-regulatory region of CYP11B1 and the structural portion of CYP11B2 is located between CYP11B2 and CYP11B1. The protein product resulting from this gene performs all reactions required for aldosterone production, thus, causing ACTH-dependent hyperaldosteronism Ectopic expression of the chimeric protein in the inner cortical zones, which also express CYP17, permits the formation of 18-hydroxy and 18-oxocortisol, the biochemical hallmarks of GRA. Finally, suppressing steroidogenesis in the zona fasciculata and reticularis with exogenous glucocorticoids, alleviates the hypertension. The chimeric gene results from a miotic mismatch and unequal crossing over. In all instances, the crossover is located 5' to intron 4 of the CYP11B genes.

Apparent mineralocorticoid excess

Genetic apparent mineralocorticoid excess (AME) resembles the syndrome observed in persons ingesting large amounts of licorice. Licorice gluttony and treatment with carbenoxalone both cause a volume expansion, low renin, low aldosterone, salt-sensitive form of hypertension, which may also feature metabolic alkalosis and hypokalemia. Interestingly, the hypertension responds to both thiazide and spironolactone, but no abnormal steroid products are present in the urine. Both licorice and carbenoxolone contain glycyrrhetinic acid, which was found to inhibit the enzyme 11 β-hydroxysteroid dehydrogenase. 11 β-hydroxysteroid dehydrogenase is responsible for converting cortisol to cortisone. In the distal renal tubule, this step is crucial for protecting the mineralocorticoid receptor, which has the same affinity for cortisol as it does for aldosterone. This step protects us all from developing AME. Inhibition of 11 β-hydroxysteroid dehydrogenase results in AME. Interestingly, AME may also occur as a rare, autosomal recessive form of monogenic hypertension. Needless to say, the 11 β-hydroxysteroid dehydrogenase gene, which has a renal-specific renal isoform, was a hot candidate gene for this condition. The clinical clues helpful in resolving this condition were volume dependent salt sensitive hypertension, tendency to hypokalemia and metabolic alkalosis, low renin and low aldosterone values, responsiveness to both thiazides and spironolactone despite absence of aldosterone or any abnormal mineralocorticoid products, and resemblance to licorice gluttony. Mune et al. (29) solved the mystery. In 8 of 9 families, mutations in the renal-specific isoform gene for 11 β-hydroxysteroid dehydrogenase were found which indeed rendered the product incapable of converting cortisol to cortisone. Thus, the mineralocorticoid receptor is unprotected from cortisol in these patients and cortisol functions to occupy the mineralocorticoid receptor. The facinating possibility that AME might be relevant in the heterozygous state has been raised by Li et al. (22), who observed a patient with apparent mineralocorticoid hypertension at age 38 years, who had a daughter with homozygous AME. The patient had low renin and aldosterone concentrations and was found to have a mutation in the gene for 11 β-hydroxysteroid dehydrogenase.

Liddle syndrome

Liddle described patients with autosomal-dominant monogenic hypertension who also tended to metabolic alkalosis with hypokalemia. His patients had low renin and low aldosterone values; however, they did not respond to spironolactone, while thiazides and triamterene reduced the blood pressure. This observation convinced Liddle that they probably didn´t have a form of mineralocorticoid excess. Liddle speculated that they would show a distal tubular defect of enhanced sodium and chloride reabsorption. A renal transplant performed on a patient with Liddle syndrome who developed renal failure cured the disease, providing strong evidence that the problem resided within the kidneys rather than in a regulatory system (3). Shimkets et al. (37) subsequently localized the responsible gene of a family with Liddle syndrome to chromosome 16 and were able to show that the gene encodes for the ß subunit of the epithelial sodium channel (ENaC). The channel is amiloride and traimterene sensitive, explaining the efficacy of these drugs in the syndrome. The channel remains inappropriately permeable even in the face of high salt intake, thereby explaining the salt sensitive hypertension. Subsequently a mutation in the γ subunit of ENaC has been found, which can also result in Liddle syndrome (12). The molecular mechanisms of Liddle syndrome involves alteration or deletion of a PY motif in the cytoplasmic tails of the b or γ subunits. As a consequence, Nedd4 binding fails to occur, the channels are not internalized, and instead remain activated on the cell surface (32).

Analogous to the presumed existence of "black holes" and "antimatter", one might speculate that the reverse of such a syndrome could also exist. Indeed, mutations in the subunits of ENaC were found to cause relative hypotension and salt wasting with hyperkalemic acidosis (pseudohypoaldosteronism type I). Mutations in either the α or the β subunit result in loss of channel activity, thereby explaining the pathophysiology of the disease (5). Other channel gene mutations can also result in blood pressure and salt and water regulatory diseases. For instance, Gitelman syndrome is a variant of Bartter syndrome and features inherited hypokalemic alkalosis, hypomagnesemia, and hypocalciuria. The syndrome is caused by mutations in the thiazide-sensitive Na-Cl cotransporter (43). Clinically, the patients look like individuals who surreptitiously are ingesting thiazide diuretics. Bartter syndrome can be caused by several different mutations, including genes for the Na-K-2Cl cotransporter (41), the outwardly directed potassium channel ROMK (42), and the chloride channel gene CLCNKB, on the basolateral cell surface (40). The above syndromes are examples of monogenic "hypotension"; however, they are relevant to hypertension nonetheless.

The gene(s) responsible for pseudohypoaldosteronism type II have recently been mapped, albeit not yet cloned. Pseudohypoaldosteronism type II features familial hyperkalemia and was first described by Gordon. Thiazide diuretics are highly effective in this syndrome, commensurate with salt-sensitivity. A multilocus linkage analysis yielded a lod score of 8.1 for linkage to chromosomes 1q31–q42 and 17p11-q21 (26). Interestingly, the chromosome-17 locus overlaps a syntenic interval in the rat that contains a blood pressure quantitative trait locus. Pseudohypoaldosteronism type II provides promise in leading to cloning of two additional as yet not appreciated genes leading to hypertension.

Autosomal-dominant hypertension with brachydactyly

An additional promising monogenic syndrome is autosomal-dominant hypertension with brachydactyly. We mapped a gene for hypertension to the short arm of chromosome 12 (12p) in a large Turkish kindred with hypertension and type E brachydactyly. In this family, the phenotypes hypertension and brachydactyly always are inherited together; they cosegregate 100 % (35). Affected persons are shorter than nonaffected individuals and do not have volume expansion-induced hypertension as determined by a volume expansion and contraction protocol, but instead resemble patients with essential hypertension (36). The mechanism of the hypertension is unknown. Thus far, this syndrome has only been described in this Turkish kindred and a similar family in Canada. Recently, we encountered another such family in the United States. In these three families, the hypertension also follows an autosomal-dominant mode of inheritance and cosegregates 100 % with short stature and type E brachydactyly. A deletion syndrome in a Japanese child with type E brachydactyly, as well as the additional families, has enabled us to sharply decrease the area on 12p containing the gene (1); however, a 4 million base-pair segment remains and we have not yet cloned the gene.

Primary hypertension

Over a thousand papers were published on this topic since the society last met and only the highlights will be mentioned here. A brief overview of papers in 1997 and 1998 on patients with primary hypertension revealed research on the following genes: angiotensin converting enzyme (ACE), angiotensinogen, β-2 adrenergic receptor, α-adducin, angiotensinase C, renin binding protein, G-protein beta3 subunit, atrial natriuretic peptide, insulin receptor, eNOS in hypertension of pregnancy, angiotensin converting enzyme. Angiotensin converting enzyme has generally not been shown to be associated with hypertension. Even telomere length has been raised as being important to primary hypertension. Despite their interest, discussion of all these genes is beyond the scope of this commentary; however, in my view six genes, ACE, angiotensinogen, α-adducin, the β-2 adrenergic receptor, G-protein beta3 subunit, and the T594M mutation in the β subunit of the epithelial sodium channel, are of particular relevance.

Angiotensin converting enzyme

The ACE gene locus was linked to blood pressure in spontaneously hypertensive rats in 1991, and although the ACE gene insertion/deletion allelic variant has been implicated in arteriosclerotic cardiovascular disease, cardiac hypertrophy, restenosis, progression of diabetic renal disease, and progression of IgA nephropathy, hanging a guilty verdict in terms of hypertension onto the ACE gene has been difficult (44). O'Donnell et al. found evidence for association and genetic linkage of the ACE gene with hypertension and blood pressure in men, but not in women, when they analyzed over 3000 participants from the Framingham Heart Study (31). The data were significant, but not robust. Fornage et al. studied 583 three-generation pedigrees from Rochester, MN, USA, and were able to show that variations in a microsatellite marker within the growth hormone gene, which is close to the ACE gene locus, influenced interindividual blood pressure differences in young white men, but not in women (10).

Angiotensinogen

Jeunemaitre et al. (15) first reported linkage of the angiotensinogen (AGT) gene locus to hypertension in hyptertensive siblings from France and Utah. Subsequent screening identified the so-called AGT 235T variant in hypertensive cases, as being more frequent than in controls. The variant is associated with higher AGT levels and appears to be in tight linkage dysequilibrium with a promoter mutation -6 bp (G-6A) upstream of the initiation site of transcription (13). This mutation may result in a higher basal transcription rate. The haplotype combining the AGT 235T and G-6A polymorphisms appears as the ancestral allele of the human AGT gene and as the one associated with hypertension (14).

Caufield et al. (4) have investigated AGT extensively and reported linkage of the AGT locus to blood pressure in 77 European families (p < 0.000 003). Their studies in African Caribbeans supported the notion that the AGT locus is linked to hypertension. Since the initial reports, many studies have been published on the association between allelic variants in AGT and hypertension. Kunz et al. (20) have recently reviewed the evidence on AGT 235T from 11 studies of 14 populations. Data on 5493 patients showed that the AGT 235T allele was significantly associated with hypertension (OR 1.2 CI 1.11–1.29). These data were significant statistically; however, their clinical significance is another matter. The authors concluded that much more than AGT 235T was responsible for primary hypertension. The AGT gene has been the most scrutinized and the most promising finding of the primary hypertension genes thus far; however, the AGT 235T variant explains only a relatively small part of blood pressure variance.

α-Adducin

To my knowledge, a-adducin is the only example of rat molecular genetic research contributing pertinent information to the molecular genetics of human hypertension. A mutation in rat a-adducin was found to be responsible for 50 % of the hypertension in the Milan hypertensive rat. The mutation was shown to be responsible for an increase in Na-K pump activity in renal cell transfection experiments. Linkage and association studies were subsequently performed in hypertensive patients and controls and a point mutation (G460W) was found in the human a-adducin gene. The 460W variant was shown to be more frequent in hypertensive patients than in controls. The pressure-natriuresis relationship was subsequently studied in 108 hypertensive patients. The relationships suggested a shifted, reduced-slope, salt-sensitive pressure-natriuresis curve in persons bearing the W variant. The a-adducin studies combine molecular genetics and physiology in rats and patients and present a truly remarkable story of careful observations, patience, and scholarship, which has been summarized elsewhere (27). The importance of a-adducin to other hypertensive populations and to salt-sensitive hypertension must await additional studies. Recently, a Japanese group (17) was unable to find an association between α-adducin allelic variants and essential hypertension.

β-2 adrenergic receptor

A restriction fragment length polymorphism in the β-2 adrenergic receptor gene was associated with and linked to salt sensitive hypertensive persons of African origin in earlier studies (47). An amino terminal variant in the β-2 adrenoceptor, which encodes glycine instead of arginine at basepair position 46 (Arg16- >Gly), has been described which appears to have functional significance (50). The variants showed equal affinity for epinephrine or isoproterenol; however, the Gly16 variant exhibited increased down regulation in response to isoproterenol, compared to the Arg16 variant (11). Such a down regulation pattern could lead to impaired vasodilatory responses to circulating β-2 adrenergic agonists. This hypothesis is supported by in vivo studies showing that pulmonary β-2 adrenoceptors with the Gly16 variant also exhibit increased down regulation in response to salbutamol, compared to the Arg16 variant. Furthermore, a recent report indicating that the Gly16 variant in the β-2 adrenoceptor is associated with nocturnal asthma renders further support to the notion that this polymorphism may have major functional importance (49). Finally, increased β-2 adrenoceptor down regulation might serve to explain the decreased β-2 adrenoreceptor expression on the fibroblasts of salt-sensitive, compared to salt-resistant normotensive Europeans (19). Recently, Kotanko et al. (18) performed an association study in 136 African Caribbeans with hypertension and 81 unrelated control persons from the island of St. Vincent. They found significant support for the pro-downregulatory Gly variant with hypertension. These hypertensive persons of African origin would be expected to be salt sensitive, although they were not tested. Data from the Bergen Blood Pressure study support the idea that the Arg16- > Gly allelic variant is important to increased blood pressure (48). However, in that study, the Gly variant was associated with lower blood pressures in a dose-dependent fashion. Obviously, much remains to be done to elucidate the role of the β-2 adrenergic receptor gene in primary hypertension.

G-protein beta3 subunit

The notion that G-proteins might be involved in primary hypertension stems from observations that pertussis toxin sensitive G proteins in lymphoblasts and fibroblasts from selected patients with primary hypertension engaged in enhanced signal transduction (38). Siffert et al. (39) detected a novel polymorphism (C825T) in exon 19 of the gene encoding the G-protein beta3 subunit (GNB3). The T allele is associated with the occurrence of a splice variant, which causes a loss of 41 amino acids and one WD repeat domain of the G beta subunit. The splice variant was shown to be active in expression studies. A genotype analysis of 427 normotensive and 426 hypertensive subjects suggested a signfiicant association of the T allele with essential hypertension. The relevance of these findings will require confirmatory studies.

T594M mutation in the β subunit of the epithelial sodium channel

A variant of the β-subunit of the amiloride-sensitive sodium channel was described by Su et al. (46), who also observed increased channel activity in lymphocytes in African Americans. Baker et al. (2) recently studied 206 hypertensive black patients and 142 normotensive black control subjects in London, UK. Seventeen (8 %) of the hypertensive blacks had the T594M mutation, compared to 2% of normotensive blacks. Persons with the mutation had lower plasma renin activity, supporting the notion of increased sodium reabsorption. Thus, the T594M mutation may serve to explain some degree of salt-sensitivity and hypertension in blacks. The elucidation of Liddle syndrome led to the discovery of this allelic variant. The finding underscores the potential relevance of rare monogenic diseases to complex genetic disease.

Challenge and conundrum

Although major efforts have been expended, excellent experiments have been performed, and exciting stories have been told, the results in the area of human molecular genetics of hypertension are modest. In terms of genetically explaining blood pressure variance for specific genes, we have a long way to go. The above six genes and their allelic variants are worthy of special discussion, in my view, because of the thought processes involved in their evaluation. Linkage analysis was employed in the case of three of the gene variants, namely for the AGT, α-adducin and β-2 adrenergic receptor genes. However, we cannot conclude that these genetic variants were found by linkage analysis. These genes were candidate genes which were selected by investigators and then subjected to a linkage analysis. That the genes of the renin-angiotensin system and the genes for catecholamine receptors, and genes for the enzymes involved in their production and degradation might be involved in hypertension, would have occurred to students of hypertension 50 years ago. α-Adducin and the G-protein beta3 subunit were identified as candidates by whole animal and cell physiology approaches, which resulted in their being selected as candidate gene. A linkage analysis was subsequently performed in hypertensive sibling pairs and the α-adducin gene locus was indeed linked to hypertension. To my knowledge, thus far no gene for a complex disease has been discovered and cloned on the basis of a linkage analysis. One possible explanation for this result is that the genes we seek have relatively small effects. If there are many genes with small effects (such as the gene variants above), the sample size necessary for linkage studies will be prohibitive. Perhaps the right linkage studies have not been done and indeed cohorts of hypertensive sibling pairs exceeding 1000 pairs are being subject to total genome scans in the United States and Europe; however, I am not optimistic.

A review of Pickering's work is enlightening in my view (reviewed in 33). His group obtained a sample of the population at large believed to be representative; first degree relatives of patients with essential hypertension; and first degree relatives of patients without essential hypertension. The data acquisition and data analysis took four years. Pickering found that the frequency distribution curves for blood pressure in the relatives of subjects without hypertension were indistinguishable from those of the population sample. Those for relatives of subjects with essential hypertension were similar in shape but were shifted upwards, by about the same amount at all ages. The increase in blood pressure with age was the same in the relatives of subjects with hypertension as in the rest of the population, but the relatives tended to have higher pressures at all ages. Miall and Oldham performed a similar study in a Welsh mining valley and measured blood pressure in a sample of the population and their first degree relatives (28). The regression coefficient of blood pressure of relatives and propositi was about 0.2, similar to that observed by Pickering's group. Thus, blood pressure appeared to be inherited as a graded characteristic over the whole range of blood pressure, irrespective of the classification: hypotension, normotension, or hypertension. Pickering concluded that the inheritance of blood pressure was quite analagous to the inheritance of height. Were we to consider heights in excess of 170 cm as abnormal, we might as well be looking for "tallness" genes. In all likelihood, we are facing many genes with small effects.

What are our options? The relative power of linkage and association studies for the detection of genes involved in hypertension have been reviewed by Jones (16). He performed power calculations according the methods developed by Risch and Merikangas (34) and showed that if a single major locus causing susceptibility to hypertension were present, nonparametric linkage strategies using affected sibling pairs may prove effective. However, if as suggested by the experiences of the last decade the number of genes is large and their effect is small, the sample size for such linkage analyses will be massive. In that case, a systematic search for allelic association may be more appropriate because of the dramatic reduction in the excess allele sharing for genes of small effect. The transmission disequilibrium test is an example (9). This test requires the collection of trios of two parents and an affected child. The frequency at which alleles are transmitted and not-transmitted to the affected offspring is compared to the Mendelian expectation of 50:50. Importantly, this test determines allelic association requiring the presence of both linkage and linkage disequilibrium in order to yield a significant result. By using non-transmitted alleles as the control population, problems of population admixture and mismatched controls are avoided. Spielman and Ewens (45) have recently expanded the transmission disequilibrium test to permit accruing information from units in which the parents are already dead, as is often the case in cardiovascular diseases. They describe a method termed the sib transmission disequilibrium test that overcomes this problem by using marker data from unaffected siblings instead of from parents, thus, allowing application of the transmission dysequilibrium test to sibships without parental data.

Identifying trios and nuclear families with hypertension is no mean trick. However, perhaps we should take Pickering´s example and concentrate on blood pressure per se, rather than classification. An alternative approach might be to identify quantitative trait loci (QTLs) for blood pressure in normotensive individuals. That such QTLs might be relevant to primary hypertension is highly likely. We have employed studies in monozygotic and dizygotic twins and the parents of the latter. An analysis of monozygotic and dizygotic twins allows heritability estimates to be made. The dizygotic twins and their parents then lend themselves to a linkage analysis. We have linked the insulin-like growth factor (IGF)-1 gene locus to systolic blood pressure and heart size with this approach (30). Recruiting families with multiple children is an alternative approach. The children can then be studied in terms of concordance and discordance for blood pressure and other variables. Excellent cohorts are available for such analyses in the United States. The Rochester Family Heart Study and the San Antonio Heart Study are two examples (24).

We should perhaps reconsider our approach. A powerful tool for the fine structure localization of disease genes in a complex condition, such as hypertension, is linkage dysequilibrium mapping in isolated populations. This novel approach adapts Luria and Delbrück's classical methods for analyzing bacterial cultures to the study of human isolated founder populations with several goals in mind, namely, the estimation of the recombination fraction between a disease locus and a marker, the determination of the expected degree of allelic homogeneity in a population, and the mutation rate of marker loci. Linkage disequilibrium mapping is based on the observation that affected chromosomes descended from a common ancestral mutation should show a distinctive haplotype of the ancestral chromosome. The technique offers increased resolution because it exploits recombination events occurring over the entire history of a population. The best setting in which to apply the method would be a population in which there is a single disease-causing allele with a high frequency, so that the excess of an ancestral haplotype can be detected easily. Furthermore, this allele should have been introduced into the population sufficiently long ago that recombination has made the region of strongest linkage disequilibrium confined, but not too small. The theoretical basis for this "haplotype sharing" method are described in detail elsewhere (7, 8, 21). The combination of focused sampling and the method of mass parallel genotyping (genome scanning) represent a new strategy to identify new genes for complex diseases. Isolated populations are available for study. Finland represents an ideal population for linkage disequilibrium mapping (50). However, there are other relatively isolated populations in many countries on the north American continent, other countries in Europe, the middle east, and elsewhere.

In summary, while our successes with monogenic diseases have been phenomenal, our search for genes causing primary hypertension have been more modest. Interesting finds have been made; however, the surface has barely been scratched. Novel approaches in terms of study design, analyses, and populations will be necessary. Future success will depend less on molecular genetic technology and more on investigator inginuity.

References

1. Bähring S, Nagai T, Toka HR, Nitz C, Toka O, Aydin A, Wienker T, Schuster H, Luft FC (1997) Deletion at 12p in a Japanese child with brachydactyly overlaps the assigned locus of brachydactyly with hypertension in a Turkish family. Am J Human Genet 60: 732–735
2. Baker EH, Dong YB, Sagnella GA, Rothwell M, Onipinia AK, Markandu ND, Cappuccio FP, Cook DG, Persu A, Corvol P, Jeunemaitre X, Carter ND, MacGregor GA (1998) Association of hypertension with T594M mutation in β subunit of epithelial sodium channels in black people resident in London. Lancet 351: 1388–92
3. Botero-Velez M, Curtis JJ, Warnock DG (1994) Liddle's syndrome revisited. N Engl J Med 330: 178–181
4. Caulfield M, Lavender P, Newell-Price J, Kamdar S, Farrall M, Clark AJL (1996) Angiotensinogen in human essential hypertension. Hypertension 28: 1123–1125
5. Chang SS, Grunder S, Hanukoglu A, Rösler A, Mathew PM, Hanukoglu I, Shild L, Lu Y, Shimkets RA, Nelson-Williams C, Rossier BC, Lifton RP (1996) Mutations in subunits of the epithelial sodium channel cause salt wasting with hyperkalaemic acidosis, pseudohypoaldosteronism type I. Nat Genet 12: 248–253
6. de la Chapelle A (1993) Disease gene mapping in isolated human populations: The example of Finland. J Med Genet 30: 857–865
7. de Vries H, van der Meulen MA, Rozen R, Halley JJD, Scheffer H, ten Kate LP, Buys CHCM, te Meerman GJ (1996) Haplotype identity between individuals who share a CFTR mutation allele "identical by descent": Demonstration of the usefulness of the haplotype-sharing concept for gene mapping in real populations. Hum Genet 98: 304–309
8. Donelly KP (1983) The probability that related individuals share some section of genome identical by descent. Theor Pop Biol 23: 43–63
9. Ewens WJ, Spielman RS (1995) The transmission/disequilibrium test: history, subdivision, and admixture. Am J Hum Genet 57: 455–464
10. Fornage M, Amos CI, Kardia S, Sing CF, Turner ST, Boerwinkle E (1998) Variation in the region of the angiotensin-converting enzyme gene influences interindividual differences in blood pressure levels in young white males. Circulation 97: 1773–1779
11. Green SA, Turki J, Innis M, Liggett SB (1994) Amino-terminal polymorphisms of the human β-2 adrenergic receptor impart distinct agonist-promoted regulatory properties. Biochemistry 33: 9414–9419
12. Hansson JH, Nelson-Williams C, Suzuki H, Schild L, Shimkets R, Lu Y, Canessa C, Iwasaki T, Rossier B, Lifton RP (1995) Hypertension caused by a truncated epithelial sodium channel γ subunit: Genetic heterogeneity of Liddle syndrome. Nat Genet 11: 76–82
13. Inoue I, Nakajima T, Williams CS, Quackenbush J, Puryear R, Powers M, Cheng T, Ludwig EH, Sharma AM, Hata A, Jeunemaitre X, Lalouel JM (1997) A nucleotide substitution in the promoter of human angiotensinogen is associated with essential hypertenson and affects basal transcription. J Clin Invest 99: 1786–1797
14. Jeunemaitre X, Inoue I, Williams C, Charru A, Tichet J, Powers M, Sharma AM, Gimenez-Roqueplo, Hata A, Corvol P, Lalouel JM (1997) Haplotypes of angiotensin in essential hypertension. Am J Hum Genet 60: 1448–60
15. Jeunmaitre X, Soubrier F, Kotelevtsev YV, Lifton RP, Williams CS, Charru A, Hunt SC, Hopkins PN, Williams RR, Lalouel JM, Corvol P (1992) Molecular basis of human yhpertension: Role of angiotensinogen. Cell 71: 169–180
16. Jones HB (1998) The relative power of linkage and asscociation studies for the detection of genes involved in hypertension. Kidney Int 53: 1446–1448
17. Kato N, Sugiyama T, Nabika T, Morita H, Kurihara H, Yazaki Y, Yamori Y (1998) Lack of association between the α-adducin locus and essential hypertension in the Japanese population. Hypertension 31: 730–733
18. Kotanko P, Binder A, Tasker J, DeFreitas P, Kamdar S, Clark AJL, Skrabal F, Caulfield M (1997) Essential hypertension in African Caribbeans associates with a variant of the β2-adrenoceptor. Hypertension 30: 773–776
19. Kotanko P, Höglinger O, Skrabal F (1992) β-2 adrenoceptor density in fibroblast culture correlates with human NaCl sensitivity. Am J Physiol 263: C623–C627
20. Kunz R, Kreutz R, Beige J, Distler A, Sharma AM (1997) Association between the angiotensinogen 235T-variant and essential hypertension in whites: A systematic review and methodological appraisal. Hypertension 30: 1331–1337
21. Lander ES, Botstein D (1986) Mapping complex geentic traits in humans: new methods using a complete RFLP linkage map. Cold Spring Harb Symp Quant Biol 51: 49–62
22. Li A, Li KX, Marui S, Krozowski ZS, Batista MC, Whorwood CB, Arnhold IJ, Shackleton CH, Mendonca BB, Stewart PM (1997) Apparent mineralocorticoid excess in a Brazilian kindred: Hypertension in the heterozygous state. J Hypertens 15: 1397–402
23. Lifton RP, Dluhy RG, Powers M, Rich GM, Cook S, Ulick S, Lalouel JM (1992) A chimaeric 11β-hydroxylase/aldosterone synthase gene causes glucocorticoid-remediable aldosteronism and human hypertension. Nature 355: 262–265

24. Luft FC (1998) Scientific conference on the genome: Applications to cardiovascular biology (editorial). J Mol Med 76: 369–371

25. Luft FC, Schuster H, Bilginturan N, Wienker T (1995) "Treasure your exceptions": What we can learn from autosomal dominant inherited forms of hypertension. J Hypertens 13: 1535–1538

26. Mansfield TA, Simon DB, Farfel Z, Bia M, Tucci JR, Lebel M, Gutkin M, Vialettes B, Christofilis MA, Kauppinen-Makelin R, Mayan H, Risch N, Lifton RP (1997) Multilocus linkage of familial hyperkalaemia and hypertension, pseudohypoaldosteronism type II, to chromosomes 1q13-42 and 17p11-q21. Nat Genet 16: 202–5

27. Manunta P, Cusi D, Barlassina C, Righetti M, Lanzani C, D'Amico M, Buzzi L, Stella P, Rivera R, Bianchi G (1998) α-Adducin polymorphisms and renal sodium handling in essential hypertensive patients. Kidney Int 53: 1471–1478

28. Miall WE, Oldham PD (1995) A study of arterial pressure and its inheritance in a sample of the general population. Clin Sci 14: 459–461

29. Mune T, Roberson FM, Nikkilä H, Agarwal AK, White PC (1995) Human hypertension caused by mutations in the kidney isozyme of 11 β-hydroxysteroid dehydrogenase. Nature Genet 10: 394–399

30. Nagy Z, Busjahn A, Bähring S, Faulhaber H-D, Gohlke H-R, Knoblauch H, Schuster H, Luft FC (1997) Quantitative trait loci for blood pressure exist near the IGF-1, the Liddle syndrome, and the angiotensin II-receptor gene loci in man. Hypertension 30: 494A

31. O'Donnell CJ, Lindpaintner K, Larson MG, Rao VS, Ordovas JM, Schaefer EJ, Myers RH, Levy D (1998) Evidence for association and genetic linkage of the angiotensin-converting enzyme locus with hypertension and blood pressure in men but not women in the Framingham Heart Study. Circulation 97: 1766–1772

32. Palmer BF, Alpern RJ (1998) Liddle's syndrome. Am J Med 104: 301 — 309

33. Pickering GW (1982) Systemic artierial hypertension. In: Fishman AP, Richards DW (eds) Circulation Of The Blood, Men and Ideas. American Physiological Society, Bethesda, MD, pp 487–541

34. Risch N, Merikangas K (1996) The future of genetic studies of complex diseases. Science 273: 1516–1517

35. Schuster H, Wienker TF, Bähring S, Bilginturan N, Toka HR, Neitzel H, Jeschke E, Toka O, Gilbert H, Lowe A, Ott J, Haller H, Luft FC (1996) Severe autosomal dominant hypertension and brachydactyly in a unique Turkish kindred maps to human chromosome 12. Nat Genet 4: 98–100

36. Schuster H, Wienker TF, Toka HR, Bähring S, Jeschke E, Toka O, Busjahn A, Hempel A, Tahlhammer C, Oelkers W, Kunze J, Bilginturan N, Haller H, Luft FC (1996) Autosomal dominant hypertension and brachydactyly in a Turkish kindred resembles essential hypertension. Hypertension 28: 1085–1092

37. Shimkets RA, Warnock DG, Bositis CM, Nelson-Williams C, Hansson JH, Schambelan M, Gill JR, Ulick S, Milora RV, Findling JW, Canessa CM, Rossier BC, Lifton RP (1994) Liddle's syndrome: Heritable human hypertension caused by mutations in the β subunit of the epithelial sodium channel. Cell 79: 407–414

38. Siffert W (1998) G proteins and hypertension: an alternative candidate gene approach. Kidney Int 53: 1466–1470.

39. Siffernt W, Rosskopf D, Siffert G, Busch S, Moritz A, Erbel R, Sharma AM, Ritz E, Wichmann HE, Jakobs KH, Horsthemke B (1998) Association of a human G-protein beta3 subunit variant with hypertension. Nat Genet 18: 8–10

40. Simon DB, Bindra RS, Mansfield TA, Nelson-Williams C, Mendonca E, Stone R, Schurman S, Nayir A, Palpay H, Bakkaloglu A, Rodriguez-Soriano J, Morales MN, Sanjad SA, Taylor CM, Pilz D, Brem A, Trachtman H, Griswold W, Richard GA, John E, Lifton RP (1997) Mutations in the chloride channel gene, CLCNKB, cause Bartter's syndrome type III. Nat Genet 17: 171–8

41. Simon DB, Karet FE, Hamdan JM, DiPietro A, Sanjad SA, Lifton RP (1996) Bartter's syndrome, hypokalaemic alkalosis with hypercalciuria, is caused by mutations in the Na-K-2Cl cotransporter NKCC2. Nat Genet 13: 183–8

42. Simon DB, Karet FE, Rodriguez-Soriano J, Hamdan JH, Dipietro A, Trachtman H, Sanjad SA, Lifton RP (1996) Genetic heterogeneity of Bartter's syndrome revealed by mutations in the K+ channel, ROMK. Nat Genet 14: 152–6

43. Simon DB, Nelson-Williams C, Johnson Bia M, Ellison D, Karet FE, Molina AM, Vaara I, Iwata F, Cushner HM, Koolen M, Gainza FJ, Gitelman HJ, Lifton RP (1996) Gitelman's variant of Bartter´s syndrome, in-herited hypokalaemic alkalosis, is caused by mutations in the thiazide-sensitive Na-Cl cotransporter. Nat Genet 12: 24–30

44. Soubrier F (1998) Blood pressure gene at the angiotensin I-converting enzyme locus: Chronicle of a gene foretold. Circulation 97: 1763–1765

45. Spielman RS, Ewsens WJ (1998) A sibship test for linkage in the presence of association: the sib transmission/disequilibrium test. Am J Hum Genet 62: 450–458

46. Su YR, Rutkowski MP, Klanke CA, Wu X, Cui Y, Pun RV, Carter V, Reif M, Menon AG (1996) A novel variant of the β-subunit of the amiloride-sensitive sodium channel in African Americans. J Am Soc Nephrol 7: 2543–49

47. Svetkey LP, Chen Y-T, Mckeown SP, Preis L, Wilson AF (1997) Preliminary evidence of linkage of salt sensitivity in black Americans at the β2-adrenergic receptor locus. Hypertension 29: 918–922
48. Timmermann B, Mo R, Luft FC, Gerdts E, Busjahn A, Omvik P, Li G-H, Schuster H, Wienker TF, Hoehe M, Lund-Johansen P (1998) β-2 Adrenoceptor genetic variation is associated with genetic propensity to essential hypertension: The Bergen Blood Pressure Study. Kidney Int 53: 1455–1460
49. Turki J, Pak J, Green SA, Martin RJ, Ligget SB (1995) Genetic polymorphisms of the β-2 adrenergic receptor in nocturnal and nonnocturnal asthma: Evidence that Gy16 correlates with the nocturnal phenotype. J Clin Invest 95: 1635–1641
50 Yang-Feng TL, Xue FY, Zhong WW, Cotecchia S, Frielle T, Caron MG, Lefkowitz RJ, Francke U (1990) Chromosomal organization of adrenergic receptor genes. Proc Natl Acad Sci USA 87: 1516–1520

Author's address:
Friedrich C. Luft, M.D.
Franz Volhard Clinic
Wiltbergstr. 50
D-13122 Berlin, Germany
E-mail: luft@fvk-berlin.de

Renin-angiotensin system and coronary artery disease – Interaction of angiotensin II with pro-inflammatory cytokines in human stable and unstable coronary plaques

B. Schieffer, H. Drexler

Abteilung Kardiologie und Angiologie, Medizinische Hochschule Hannover, Hannover, Germany

Abstract

Elevated inflammatory markers, such as cytokines (e.g., interleukin 6) and acute phase reactants (C-reactive protein and serum amyloid A) are one of the characteristics of patients with acute coronary syndromes (ACS). In addition, patients with genetically determined elevated serum levels of components of the renin angiotensin system (RAS) have a higher risk of myocardial infarction (MI). Inhibition of angiotensin II formation by angiotensin converting enzyme (ACE) inhibitors reduces the risk of re-infarction in patients after MI as shown in large scale clinical trials, such as SAVE, SOLVD, and AIRE.

Angiotensin II, the effector peptide of the RAS activates via its G-protein coupled type 1 receptor (AT_1) the cascade of Jak kinases and transcription factors of the STAT family (signal transducers and activators of transcription) which is traditionally involved in cytokine induction. *In-vitro* experiments demonstrated that an activated RAS, via the JAK/STAT cascade, interacts with proinflammatory cytokines, e.g., Il-6, which in turn induces the release of prothromobotic factors, such as plasminogen activator 1 and the synthesis of acute phase reactant C-RP and α2-macroglobulin. Blockade of the either the AT_1 receptor or the tyrosine kinase JAK2 abolished this effect. Moreover, *in-vivo* findings obtained by immunhistochemistry in explanted human coronary arteries revealed that ACE, AII, AT_1 receptor, and IL-6 are co-localized with macrophages (CD68 positive cells) at the shoulder region of the plaque. Similarly, co-localization of ACE, AII, AT_1 receptor and Il-6 was documented in atherectomy samples obtained from patients with unstable angina and AII was localized in close proximity to the presumed rupture site of human coronary arteries in acute MI. Thus, these results emphasize that the renin angiotensin system may contribute to inflammatory processes within the vascular wall and thereby may amplify the development of an acute coronary syndrome.

The renin-angiotensin system

In 1898 Robert Tigerstedt first documented that humoral substances can influence blood pressure when he reported that a saline extract of rabbit kidney contained a vasoactive substance. He named this substance "renin" (83). Tigerstedt's observations were further expanded in the 1930s by Harry Goldblatt who reported on different types of renovascular hypertension. Goldblatt and his colleagues developed a renal artery clamp, which they used to produce three different types of experimental hypertension closely resembling human disease (34). In his two kidney-one clip hypertension model, Goldblatt noted that the nervous system is not involved in the development of hypertension. He also noted that following obliteration of the renal vein, previously hypertensive experimental animals became normotensive before eventually dying of uremia, indicating that the kidney secretes a vasoactive substance (78). This observation established the humoral nature of hypertension and refocused attention on renin. It was soon discovered that renin itself had no intrinsic vasoconstrictor effect. Two laboratories working independently reported that renin acted on a substrate found in plasma to produce a heat stable, dialyzable substance that had both vasoconstrictor and pressor effects. Page and Helmer in the United States named their pressor substance angiotonin, while the Braun-Menedez group in Argentina dubbed their substance hypertensin (13, 61). Eventually, the term angiotensin was agreed on, with the propeptide renin substrate being named angiotensinogen. Further research demonstrated that angiotensin exists in multiple forms and lead to the discovery by Skeggs of the dipeptidase, angiotensin converting enzyme (ACE) (14, 79). This enzyme cleaves the carboxyl His-Leu residues from angiotensin I (Ang I) to form the vasoactive octapeptide angiotensin II (Ang II).

The currently accepted model of the renin-angiotensin system (RAS) is shown in Fig. 1. Briefly, the juxtaglomerular cells of the kidney release renin into circulation. Renin acts on angiotensinogen produced in the liver to form the inactive decapeptide Ang I. ACE, produced at many sites including lung and vascular endothelium, cleaves Ang I into the vasoconstrictor Ang II. The heptapeptide Ang III is formed by the actions of an aminopeptidase on Ang II and is a potent inducer of aldosterone secretion by the adrenal gland

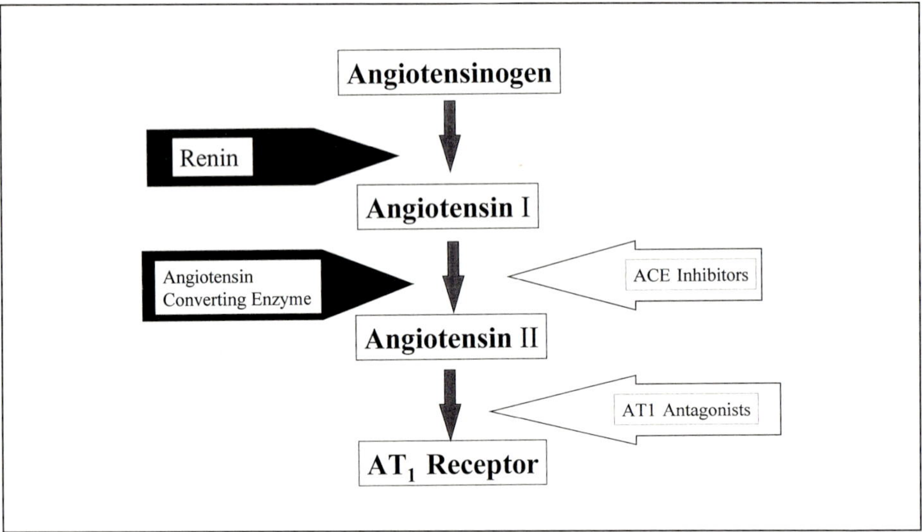

Fig. 1. Classical cascade of angiotensin II generation. Angiotensinogen is synthesized in hepatocytes and released. Cleavage of angiotensiogen to angiotensin I is generated by renin, which in turn is synthetized by juxtaglomerular cells. The octapeptide angiotensin II is predominantly generated by the angiotensin converting enzyme, which is located at the luminal site of endothelial cells in the pulmonary vasculature. Therapeutical interventions interact at the level of the type 1 angiotensin II receptor, which is responsible for basically all hemodynamic function of angiotensin II and at the level of the converting enzyme.

(35). Both Ang II and Ang III are rapidly and nonspecifically inactivated by a number of peptidases.

The effects of Ang II are not limited to vascoconstriction. Ang II has a number of effects on a variety of target tissues. In addition to vasoconstriction, Ang II stimulates the release of aldosterone from the adrenal gland, stimulates both glycogenolysis and gluconeogenesis in the liver, decreases glomerular filtration rate and increases Na^+/H^+ antiporter activity in the kidney, and stimulates the release of arginine vasopressin within the brain (11, 35, 38, 47, 67). In behavioral studies with rats, Ang II has been shown to increase water seeking behavior (67). All of these effects allow Ang II to raise blood pressure and, as a part of the RAS, to achieve fluid homeostasis in the face of constantly changing environmental conditions.

The angiotensin receptors

Since the development of captopril in 1977, ACE inhibitors have become one of the most widely prescribed classes of drugs (20). The clinical efficacy of the ACE inhibitors demonstrates the importance of the RAS in maintaining blood pressure. To better understand the cellular effects of the RAS, the Ang II receptor has to be examined. A number of early studies provided evidence for the existence of multiple Ang receptors. Early physiologic studies showed that Ang III was a more potent stimulator of aldosterone secretion than Ang II, yet Ang II had a greater pressor effect (27, 28). During the 1980s, many studies were undertaken to characterize the Ang II receptor using pharmacological, physiological, and biochemical means. For example, Gunther measured the ^{125}I-angiotensin II binding to liver membranes and found two distinct binding coefficients (37). Gunther reported a high affinity binding site with dissociation constant (K_d) of 0.35 nM and a second lower affinity binding site with $K_d = 3.1$ nM. Furthermore, only binding at the high affinity site could be abolished by treatment with the reducing agent dithiothreitol. In another study, Carson et al. used a photoaffinity analog of Ang II to label adrenal Ang II receptors and found a glycosylated protein of M_r 64,000 (17). Although Ang II and its peptide analogs proved useful in studies of the Ang II receptor, the development of the nonpeptidic Ang II receptor antagonists allowed for a more precise pharmacologic classification. The original report of ACE inhibition by benzyl-substituted imidazoles was published by Furukawa and associates in 1982 (29, 30). Subsequent work led to the development of the compounds DuPont 753 (DuP753, losartan) and Warner Lambert PD 123177 (PD123177) (10, 84). The availability of these pure Ang II antagonists has definitively shown that there are at least two distinct classes of Ang II receptor. The first class blocked by DuP753 is known as the AT_1 receptor subtype; the second receptor class blocked by PD123177 is known as the AT_2 receptor subtype. The subtype-specific receptor antagonists proved useful in functional studies. A large body of work by Wong, Timmermans, and others has established that all of the Ang II-mediated cardiovascular effects, including pressor and tachycardic response are mediated throught the AT_1 receptor subtype (25, 89). The AT_1 receptor subtype also mediates effects, such as aldosterone secretion, water seeking behavior, and hypertension secondary to renal artery stenosis. A physiologic role for the AT_2 receptor subtype has yet not been defined. However, the AT_2 receptor is found in high abundance in fetal and neonatal tissues in the rat and in the failing myocardium, leading to speculation that it may play a role in development (52). Recent work has shown that this receptor subtype is linked to a decrease in intracellular tyrosine phosphorylation in cultured cells, so a better understanding of a physiologic role may soon be revealed (44, 58).

The next major advance was the cloning of the gene for the AT_1 receptor. Because the Ang II receptor loses ligand binding capabilities when it is removed from the cell membrane, isolation of the receptor proved impractical. Therefore, traditional peptide sequencing and library screening with degenerated oligonucleotide primers could not be done. Instead, expression cloning was used to isolate the AT_1 gene by the method of Aruffo and Seed (4, 77). The mRNA used in the cloning procedure was isolated from rat aortic smooth muscle (RASM) cells, which are known to express very high levels of the AT_1 receptor in culture (80). The report of the rat vascular AT_1 receptor by Murphy was concurrent with a report of the bovine adrenal AT_1 receptor sequence (56, 71). These receptors show 92 % amino acid identity. A second rat AT_1 receptor, now known as AT_{1B}, was reported in 1992 by several groups (42, 70). It shows 94 % homology to AT_{1A} but it is the product of a separate gene. Although both rat and mouse have been shown to have two separate AT_1 receptors, there is only a single AT_1 receptor reported in cow, pig, hamster, and human (7, 90). The AT_2 receptor has also recently been cloned (43, 55) and shows 32–35 % amino acid sequence homolgy to the rat AT_1 receptor.

Angiotensin II receptors and Angiotensin II signal transduction

Cell growth, differentiation, and cell-to-cell communication is regulated by the paracrine or autocrine release of extracellular signalling proteins. These molecules stimulate cells via transmembraneous spanning cell surface receptor proteins that initiate intracellular signalling cascades. Several different classes of cell surface receptors have been characterized, including receptors for cytokines, growth factors, and seven transmembrane reaching G-protein coupled receptors (GPCR). Despite their structural diversity, all these receptor types have been shown to induce cell growth, normal and abnormal cell development (72).

Heterotrimeric G proteins

Since AT_1 receptors are members of the GPCR class, they are thought to signal through heterotrimeric G proteins. Heterotrimeric G proteins are made up of three distinct protein subunits known as $G\alpha$, $G\beta$, and $G\gamma$. There are currently 18 distinct $G\alpha$ subunits which can be divided into four classes based on amino acid sequence similarity and effector molecule targets. The $G\alpha_s$ family includes $G\alpha_s$ and $G\alpha_{olf}$ which mediate intracellular change by stimulating adenylyl cyclase and closing Ca^{2+} channels. The $G\alpha_i$ family includes $G\alpha_i$, $G\alpha_o$, $G\alpha_\tau$, $G\alpha_{gust}$, and $G\alpha_z$. This class inhibits adenylate cyclase, opens K^+ channels, stimulates cGMP phosphodiesterase, mediates Ca^{2+} channel closure and inhibits phosphatidylinositol turnover. The third class is the $G\alpha_q$ class and is made up of $G\alpha_q$, $G\alpha_{11}$, $G\alpha_{14}$, $G\alpha_{15}$, and $G\alpha_{16}$.

This class has been shown to couple to phospholipase C-β (PLC-β) and stimulate phosphoinositol-4,5-bisphosphate (PIP$_2$) breakdown to inositol-1,4,5-trisphosphate (IP$_3$) and diacylglycerol (DAG). The fourth class is composed of Gα$_{12}$ and Gα$_{13}$. The effector coupling of this class is unclear at this time.

The Gα subunits range in size from 39–52 kDa and display a similarity of 45–88 % at their amino acid level with approximately 20 % of the amino acids being invariantly conserved. Further diversity is generated by post-translational processing, which can include myristoylation, laurylation, and palmitoylation. The Gα subunits are involved in many of the functions of G proteins including receptor binding, guanine nucleotide binding, and GTP hydrolysis. The intrinsic rate of GTP hydrolysis for the heterotrimeric G proteins is significantly higher than the small G proteins, such as p21ras, which probably accounts for the need of GTPase activating proteins (GAPs) in the small G protein system.

In addition to the wide array of Gα subunits, there are also multiple Gβ and Gγ proteins. Currently there are five known Gβ subunits and seven known Gγ subunits. The Gβ subunits are approximately 36 kDa and display a 50–83 % identity. The Gγ subunits are much smaller (6–9 kDa) and show a wide range of sequence diversity. The Gβ and Gγ subunits form a tightly complexed dimer by interaction of the Gγ with the amino terminal region of the Gβ. This interaction can only be disrupted under denaturing conditions. Some of the Gγ proteins undergo post-translational modification, including isoprenylation, farnesylation or geranylgeranylation of a Cys four residues from the carboxyl terminus. This modification is followed by removal of the three carboxyl amino acid residues and methylation of the new carboxyl terminus. Blocking of these post-translational modifications will still allow dimerization of the Gβγ complex but prevents appropriate interaction of the complex with the lipid membrane (for a review see 63).

Hundreds of receptors have been cloned which display the seven transmembrane helical topology common to G protein-coupled receptors. Ligand binding to a receptor leads to a

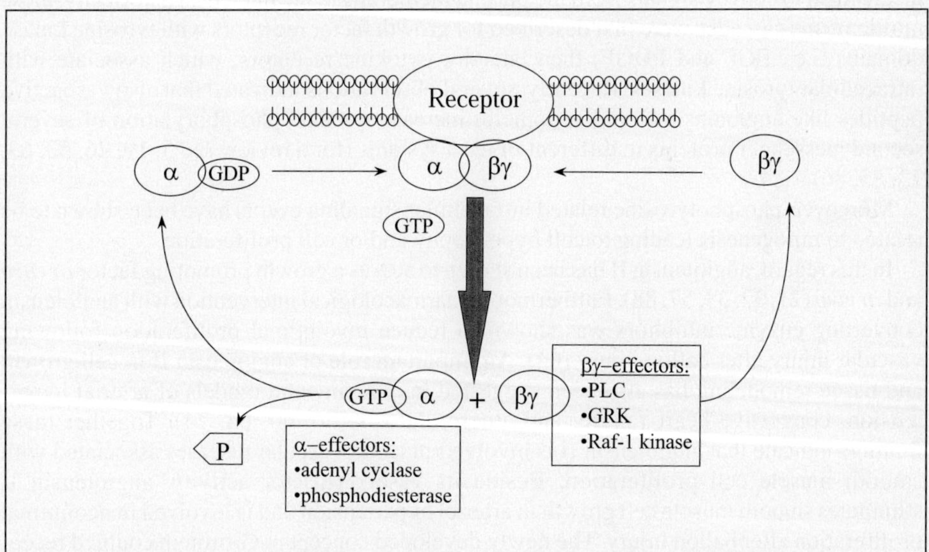

Fig. 2. Modified model of the activation-cascade of heterotrimenic G-protein coupled receptors. Upon receptor ligand binding, the α-subunit couples to GTP which leads to the activation of its down-stream signaling molecules, e.g. adenylate cyclase and phosphodiesterase. The βγ-subunit, in contrast binds to its down-stream signaling molecules and thereby activates them potentially via tyrosine phosphorylation (Schieffer et al., Circulation 1997).

conformational change. This change results in exposure of a high affinity binding site on the receptor for a heterotrimeric G protein in its GDP-bound form. Following interaction with the activated receptor, the Gα subunit undergoes a conformational change leading to a release of GDP and a subsequent binding of GTP. Binding of GTP results in the dissociation of the Gα-GTP from the Gβγ. Due to its hydrolytic activity Gα will hydrolyze the g-phosphate of GTP, releasing free phosphate and returning the Gα to its inactive Gα-GDP state. The Gα-GDP may then reassociate with Gβγ and return the system to its resting state, ready to interact with another receptor.

The active Gα-GTP, formed by interaction with activated receptor, interacts with and activates effector molecules such as adenylyl cyclase or ion channels. The Gβγ has been shown to have signaling effects as well. Probably the most significant effect of Gβγ is in receptor desensitization. The Gβγ can mediate translocation of the b-adrenergic receptor kinase (bARK) from the cytoplasm to the plasma membrane. Once at the plasma membrane, Gβγ anchors bARK to the membrane via isoprenylation of the Gγ subunit and works synergistically with the active receptor to stimulate kinase activity.

A model of traditional G-protein activation by G-protein coupled receptors such as the angiotensin II type 1 receptor is summarized in Fig. 2.

Tyrosine phosphorylation – a common signaling event

Recently, major progress has been achieved in understanding intracellular signaling cascades. Reversible protein phosphorylation has been shown to be a common mechanism by which many cell types regulate growth and differentiation. Protein phosphorylation is regulated by the balanced activation of protein kinases and phosphatases within the cell. The phosphorylation and dephosphorylation of second messenger proteins serves as a mechanism to convey signals from the plasma membrane to the nucleus. Historically, these multienzyme cascades were first described for growth factor receptors with tyrosine kinase domains (i.e., EGF and PDGF) then later for cytokine receptors, which associate with intracellular tyrosine kinases. Recently, several observations indicated that also vasoactive peptides like angiotensin II and endothelin increase tyrosine phosphorylation of several second messenger proteins in different *in vitro* systems (for a review see 5, 19, 26, 53, 63, 73, 85, 86).

Moreover, phosphotyrosine related intracellular signaling events have been shown to be related to mitogenesis leading to cell hypertrophy and/or cell proliferation.

In this regard, angiotensin II has been shown to acts as a growth promoting factor *in vitro* and *in vivo* (21, 32, 33, 57, 88). Furthermore, pharmacological intervention with angiotensin converting enzyme inhibitors was shown to reduce myointimal proliferation following vascular injury after ballon injury (64). An important role of angiotensin II in cell growth and tissue remodeling has also been suggested in experimental models of arterial hypertension, congestive heart failure, and atherosclerosis (36, 60, 64, 74). Together these findings indicate that angiotensin II is involved in cardiovascular diseases associated with smooth muscle cell proliferation. Beside its vasoconstrictor activity, angiotensin II stimulates smooth muscle cell growth in arterial hypertension and is involved in neointimal proliferation after ballon injury. The newly developed concept in G-protein coupled receptors involves the activation of second messenger proteins by tyrosine phosphorylation. Understanding the importance of tyrosine phosphorylation in the signaling cascade of the AT$_1$ receptor may lead to the development of new therapeutical interventions in cardiovascular diseases associated with smooth muscle cell proliferation.

Angiotensin II and the JAK-STAT pathway

In many ways, the AT_1 receptor resembles cytokine receptors such as the interleukin 2 and interferon α receptors, which lack intrinsic tyrosine kinase activity, yet induce tyrosine phosphorylation and mediate cell growth. Activation of both AT_1 receptors and cytokine receptors leads to a rapid increase of *c-fos* mRNA an early growth response gene (68, 69). Although not yet conclusively demonstrated, the induction of *c-fos* is likely to represent an important initial step that participates in a series of molecular events ultimately leading to angiotensin II-induced cell proliferation.

The signaling events whereby angiotensin II induces *c-fos* in VSMC are not completely explored. However, the angiotensin II induction of *c-fos* in general does not require protein *de-novo* synthesis and appears to be regulated by post-translational modifications of transcription factors (68, 69). We hypothized, therefore, that the angiotensin II induced expression of the early growth response gene *c-fos* is under direct regulation of cytoplasmic second messenger pathways.

In this regard, two intracellular pathways have recently been well-defined. The first is a multiple kinase pathway used by a number of growth factors, e.g., PDGF and EGF. In this pathway a ligand activates a cell surface receptor containing intrinsic kinase activity which in turn activates a cascade linking protein tyrosine kinases to serine/threonine kinases such as the p42 mitogen activated protein (MAP) kinase. A second, more direct, signaling pathway is stimulated by cytokines like interferons α and γ. Here, ligand binding to a cell surface receptor activates the JAK family of intracellular tyrosine kinases. Five members

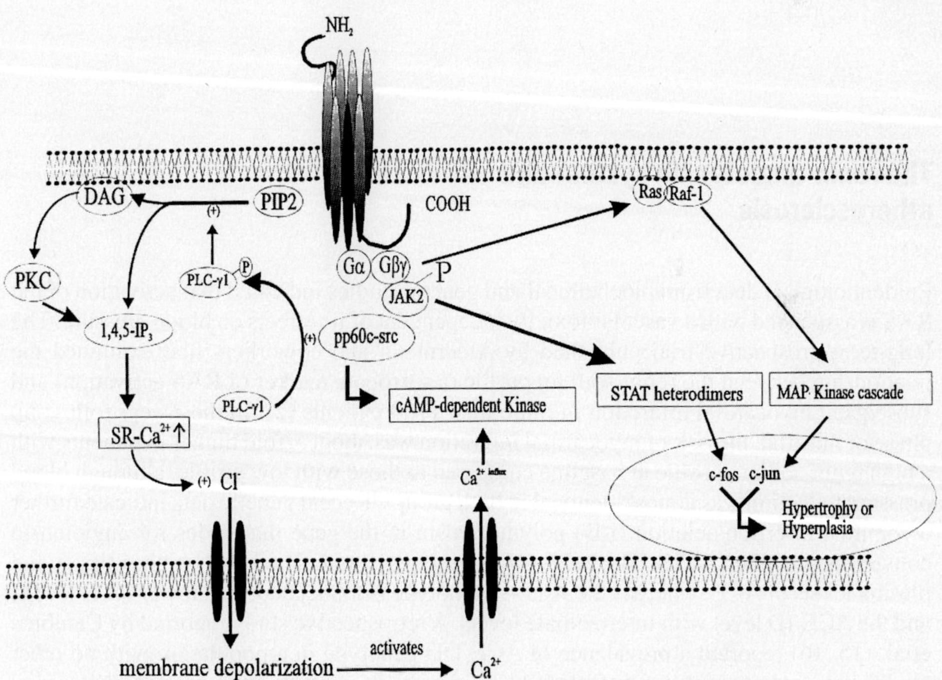

Fig. 3. Summary of signal transduction events mediated by tyrosine phosphorylation initiated by angiotensin II AT_1 receptor activation.

of this family were identified and characterized so far (JAK1, JAK2, JAK3, TYK2, and hopscotch) (22, 75). In response to ligand binding these tyrosine kinases associate with the dimerized cytokine receptor, autophosphorylate, and then activate through phosphorylation other downstream signaling molecules. Well described as JAK substrates are STAT proteins (Signal Transducers and Activators of Transcription) family of transcription factors. When activated by tyrosine phosphorylation, STAT1 (p91) associates with STAT2 (p113) and p48 to form the ISGF3 complex (Interferon Stimulated Growth Factor Complex 3). This complex then translocates to the nucleus where it binds to specific DNA motifs and stimulates early growth response genes, such as *c-fos*. Thus, the JAK-STAT pathway acts as a direct link between a cell surface receptor and transcriptional events.

We demonstrated that angiotensin II stimulates the activation of JAK2 and TYK2 and that these phosphorylations are associated with increased enzyme activity of JAK2. We could further demonstrate that the substrates of the JAK family, STAT1, and STAT2 are rapidly phosphorylated in response to angiotensin II (50). Finally, we were able to demonstrate that this complex then translocates to the nucleus were its binds to specific promotor regions at the serum response element. In addition to our observations, Bhat et al. demonstrated in cultured neonatal fibroblasts stimulated with angiotensin II that the activated STAT1 and STAT3 proteins bind to specific DNA-binding sites previously demonstrated for cytokines (8). These results together suggest that the G protein-coupled AT_1 receptors can signal directly via tyrosine phosphorylation to the nucleus and that angiotensin II stimulates signaling cascades which were previously identified exclusively for cytokines and their receptors.

A hypothetical model of how the G-protein coupled AT_1 receptor may interact with its downstream signaling molecules via tyrosine kinases and G-proteins is summarized in Fig. 3.

The renin-angiotensin system and atherosclerosis

Epidemiological data from biochemical and genetic studies indicated that activation of the RAS is associated with a vascular toxicity independent of its effects on blood pressure. The long-term prospective trial published by Aldermann and coworkers first examined the relationship between the renin-sodium profile (a surrogate marker of RAS activation) and subsequent myocardial infarction in more than 1700 patients (2). In the 8 year follow-up phase of this trial, the risk of myocardial infarction was about 5-fold higher in patients with a high renin-sodium profile at baseline compared to those with low profile, although blood pressure reduction was almost identical in both groups. Recent genetic data indicate further a common insertion/deletion (I/D) polymorphism in the gene that codes for angiotensin converting enzyme (ACE). The ACE-DD genotype is associated with higher tissue and plasma levels of ACE, whereas the ACE-II genotype is associated with lower ACE levels, and the ACE-ID level with intermediate levels. A retrospective study reported by Cambien et al. (15, 16) reported a prevalence of ACE-DD genotype in a population with no other significant cardiovascular risk factors to be greater in subjects with a prior myocardial infarction than in those with no previous infarction. In contrast, Ludwig and coworkers reported no difference in the distribution of ACE genotypes between individuals with and without coronary artery disease, defined as coronary artery stenosis > 60 %. These observations suggest that genetically defined polymorphisms of components of the renin-angiotensin system are associated with an increased risk of myocardial infarction.

Potential mechanisms by which the RAS may enhance the development of artherosclerosis involve the initiation of vasoconstriction and the activation of thrombosis pathways via PAI-1 (62, 81). If triggering of any or all of these mechanisms in vivo, interruption of the RAS by chronic ACE inhibition could theoretically reduce the risk of myocardial infarction. In fact, numerous studies in patients with left ventricular dysfunction including, AIRE, SOLVD, SAVE, and TRACE have consistently demonstrated a reduction of 7–9 % per year in the rate of myocardial infarction during long-term ACE inhibition. Nevertheless, it is not known whether ACE inhibitors will prevent ischemic events in patients with normal ventricular function. However, there is evidence that ACE inhibition can retard the development of experimental artherosclerosis. In a variety of animal models including apoE deficient mice, Watanabe rabbits, and cholesterol fed-monkeys, ACE inhibition has been shown to reduce the extent of vascular lesions (for a review see 12).

Inflammation in coronary artery disease

Laboratory and clinical evidence strongly suggested that focal inflammation in the coronary arteries at the culprit lesion may be involved in the genesis of unstable coronary syndromes. Liuzzo and coworkers reported that the acute-phase reactants, C-reactive protein and serum amyloid A are increased in patients with unstable angina, including those who subsequently had a myocardial infarction (66, 76). The authors further raised the question of the source of the inflammatory stimulus in two contexts: (A) that of the evidence of increased infiltration of coronray arteries by inflammatory cells in patients with unstable angina and (B) that of the possibility that repeated episodes of ischemia may induce inflammatory responses in the myocardium or its microvasculature (3).

Morphological and molecular bases of coronary inflammation

Morphology of human artherosclerotic plaques ranges from a solid fibrous structure to those with substantial lipid cores, covered by only a thin fibrous cap on its luminal aspect (23, 48). Pathological studies demonstrated that rupture of these coronary artheromas precipitates the formation of the occluding thrombus that causes myocardial infarctions. Plaque rupture predominantly occurs on the edges of the plaque's fibrous cap, the shoulder region, areas frequently associated with accumulations of monocyte-derived macrophages and mast cells in close proximity to vascular smooth muscle cells (23, 41, 46). Moreover, biomechanical analysis revealed that at the shoulder region maximal circumferential stress occurs (49), predisposing this plaque region to rupture. Vascular smooth muscle cells by synthesizing and releasing macromolecules, such as collagen and elastin, contribute to the stability of the plaque's fibrous cap. In contrast, macrophages and T-Lymphocytes via the release of proteases and cytokines, such as chymase, tryptase, and interleukin 6, stimulate their neighboring cells (smooth muscle cells and fibroblasts) to erode the collagen and elastin resulting in a decay of the framework which forms the plaque's cap (31). Thus, the interaction of vascular smooth muscle cells with macrophages seems to be crucial for the stability of the artheromatous plaque. Although these mechanisms may probably play a prominent role in an advanced stage of plaque rupture, other factors may trigger earlier crucial steps responsible for the development of an unstable coronary syndrome.

Recent studies demonstrated that the sites of artheromatous plaque rupture contain a strong inflammatory component (87). Interleukin 6, a powerful mediator of inflammation, was shown to be elevated in patients with unstable angina (51) and in acute myocardial infarctions (9). Multifunctional cytokines, such as IL-6, stimulate a variety of intracellular signaling mechanisms including the traditional cytokine signaling cascade of the JAK kinases and STAT transcription factors (45). Via this signaling cascade, IL-6 mediates a variety of physiological functions including macrophage differentiation, B-cell maturation, acute phase protein synthesis, and smooth muscle cell proliferation. Moreover, it was shown that cytokine-stimulated smooth muscle cells synthesize and release enzymes required for extracellular matrix digestion (matrix metalloproteinases), thereby potentially destabilizing the plaques's fibrous cap (31). This latter emphasizes the importance of pro-inflammatory cytokines, such as interleukin 6, in the development of an acute coronary syndrome. Biomechanical analysis by Loree and coworkers demonstrated that the shoulder region of the fibrous cap is the predilection site for plaque rupture, since maximal circumferential stress occurs at this location (49). An increase in circumferrential stress appears, when the vessel diameter is reduced, e.g., induced by vasoconstrictors.

The angiotensin II forming enzyme ACE was shown to be expressed in human coronary artheromatous lesions at the shoulder region of plaques in areas of clustered macrophages

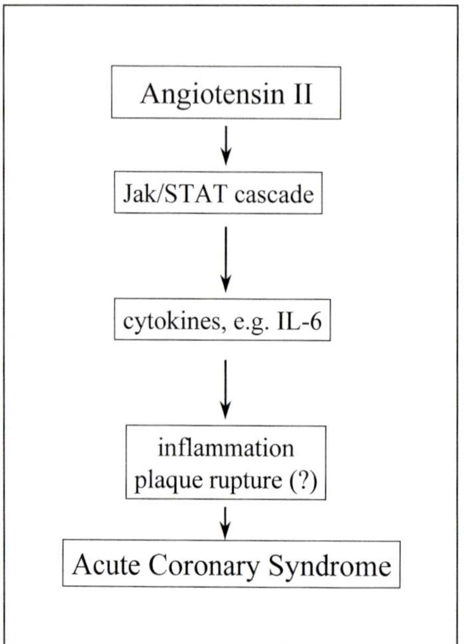

Fig. 4. Hypothetical model describing potential effects of angiotensin II via the JAK/STAT cascade in human stable and unstable coronary plaques.

(40). Moreover, as indicated above, recent studies demonstrated evidence that the RAS may be involved in the development of an acute coronary syndrome. Studies in patients with left ventricular dysfunction have suggested that blockade of the angiotensin II formation by ACE inhibitors reduces the incidence of recurrent myocardial infarctions and angina. Interestingly, the results of several of these studies have demonstrated that the beneficial effects of ACE inhibition occurs via a mechanism that is, in part, independent of its blood pressure regulating action. Although there is additional experimental evidence that ACE inhibition can retard the development of artherosclerosis in a variety of experimental models, the underlying mechanism still remains unknown (1, 18, 59). These data suggest a role for the renin-angiotensin system and its effector peptide angiotenisn II in the development of an acute coronary syndrome.

Since experimental data suggested that angiotensin II, similarly to IL-6, activates the JAK/STAT cascade, we speculated that angiotensin II may via this pathway generate similar physiological effects as reported for IL-6 (50). We tested the hypothesis whether angiotensin II via Jak/STAT cascade induces the synthesis and release of IL-6. As shown in Fig. 4 the results revealed that blockade of Jak2 by selective tyrosine kinase inhibitors, such as AG490, abolished angiotensin II induced IL-6 release (54). Moreover, since IL-6 is involved in fibrinolysis and acute-phase reactions, the hypothesis was tested, whether angiotensin II, via IL-6 induces the synthesis and release of the acute-phase reactant C-RP and the pro-thrombotic factor PAI-1. In vitro data showed that angiotensin I induces the release of PAI-1 and C-RP via an autocrine-paracrine mechanisms, since neutralizing IL-6 receptor antisera blunted the angiotensin II effects (24). *In vitro* findings are summarized in Fig. 5, suggesting a model in which angiotensin II via IL-6 may amplify the development of an acute coronary syndrome via the induction of PAI-1, CR-P, and other potential artherogenic factors, such as macrophage chemoatractant protein 1 [MCP-1] and nitric oxide.

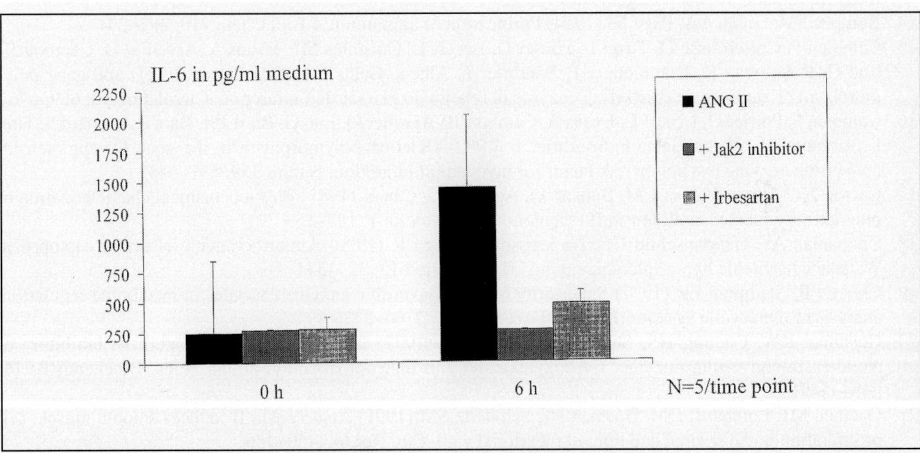

Fig. 5. Angiotensin II induces the release of interleukin-6 in human coronary smooth muscle cells. Summary of results obtained by enzyme linked immune absorbance assay (ELISA) from smooth muscle cells stimulated with angiotensin II. Results demonstrate that interleukin 6 is synthestized and released following angiotensin II-AT$_1$ receptor stimulation. Blockade of the AT$_1$-receptor by Irbesartan abolished IL-6 release. Moreover, selective blockade of the tyrosine kinase JAK2 (by AG690 10 μM, Meydan et al., Nature 1996) prevented IL-6 release, indicating that the JAK/STAT cascade is particularly involved in the inflammatory respsone in angiotensin II stimulated smooth muscle cells.

Based on these findings, we suggest the hypothesis that an activated renin angiotensin system, via its effector peptide angiotensin II, may interact with proinflammatory cytokines, such as interleukin 6, to amplify or boost the development of an acute coronary syndrome.

Acknowledgment The authors are indebt to Elisabeth Schieffer, M.D., Denis Hilfiker-Kleiner, Ph.D., and Res Hilfiker, Ph.D., for their excellent technical assistance and helpful discussions. Results presented in this manuscript were supported by DFG grants Dre 486/6-1 and Schie 386/3-1.

References

1. Aberg G, Ferrer P (1990) Effects of Captopril on artherosclerosis in cynomoglus monkeys. J Cardiovasc Pharmacol 15 (Suppl I): S65–S72
2. Aldermann MH, Madhavan S, Ooi WL, Cohen H, Sealy JE, Laragh JH (1991) Association of the renin-sodium profile with the risk of myocardial infarction in patients with hypertension. N Engl J Med 324: 1098–1104
3. Alexander RW (1994) Inflammation and Coronary Artery Disease. N Engl J Med 331 (7): 468–469
4. Aruffo A, Seed B (1987) Molecular cloning of a CD28 cDNA by a high-efficiency COS cell expression system. Proc Nat Acad Sci USA 84: 8573–8577
5. Barford D (1991) Molecular mechanisms for the control of enzymatic activity by protein phosphorylation. Biochem Biophys Acta 1133: 55–62
6. Bernstein KE, Alexander RW (1992) Counterpoint: Molecular analysis of the angiotensin II receptor. Endocr Rev 13: 381–386
7. Bernstein KE, Berk BC (1993) The biology of angiotensin II receptors. Am J Kid Dis 22: 745–754
8. Bhat CJ, Thekkumara TJ, Thomas WG, Conrad KM, Baker KM (1994) Angiotensin II stimulates sis-inducing factor-like DNA binding activity. Evidence that the AT_{1A} receptor activates transription factor stat91 and/or a related protein. J Biol Chem 269: 31443–31449
9. Biassuci L, Vitelli A, Liuzzo G, Altamura S, Caliguri G, Monaco C, Rebuzzi A, Ciliberto G, Maseri A (1996) Elevated levels of interleukin-6 in unstable angina. Circulation 94: 874–877
10. Blankley CJ, Hodges JC, Kelly JS, Klutchko SR (1988) European Patent No. 0 245 637
11. Boer P, Mamet R, Sperling O (1991) Acceleration of purine synthesis in mouse liver by glycogenolytic hormones. Biochem Med Metabol Biol 46: 185–195
12. Brown N, Vaughan D (1998) Angiotensin converting enzyme inhibitors. Circulation 97: 1411–1420
13. Braun-Menendez E, Fasciola JC, Leloir JF, Munoz JM (1939) La substancia hipertensora de la sangre del rinon isquimiado. Rev Soc Argent Biol 15: 420
14. Bumpus FM, Green AA, Page IH (1954) Purification of angiotonin. J Biol Chem 210: 287–294
15. Cambien F, Costerousse O, Tirret L, Poirier O, Lecerf L, Gonzales MF, Evans A, Arveilier D, Cambou JP, Luc G, Rakotovao R, Ducimetiere P, Sourbrier F, Alhenc-Gelas F (1994) Plasma levels and gene polymorphism of angiotensin converting enzyme in relation to myocardial infarction. Circulation 90: 669–676
16. Cambien F, Poirier O, Lecerf L, Evans A, Cambou JP, Arvelier D, Luc G, Bard JM, Bara R, Richard S, Tiret L, Amouyel P, Alhenc-Gelas F, Sourbrier F (1992) Deletion polymorphism in the gene for angiotensin-converting enzyme is a potent risk factor for myocardial infarction. Nature 359: 641–644
17. Carson MC, Leach Harper CM, Baukal AJ, Aguilera G, Catt K (1987) Physicochemical characterization of photoaffinity-labeled angiotensin II receptors. Mol Endocrin 1: 147–153
18. Chobanian AV, Haudenschild CC, Nickerosn C, Drago R (1990) Antiartherogenic effect of captopril in Watanabe herritable hyperlipidemic rabbits. Hypertension 15: 327–331
19. Chock PB, Stadtman ER (1977) Superiority of interconvertible enzyme cascades in metabolite regulation: analysis of metacyclic systems. Proc Natl Acad Sci 74: 2766–2770
20. Cushman DW, Cheung HS, Sabo EF, Ondetti MA (1977) Design of potent competitive inhibitors of angiotensin-converting enzyme. Carboxyalkanoyl and mercaptoalkanoyl amino acids. Biochemistry 16: 5484–5491
21. Daemen MJ, Lombardi DM, Bosman FT, Schwartz SM (1991) Angiotensin II induces smooth muscle cell proliferation in the normal and injured rat arterial wall. Circ Res 68: 450–456
22. Darnell JE, Kerr IM, Stark GR (1994) JAK-Stat pathways and transcriptional activation in response to IFNs and other extracellular signaling proteins. Science 264: 1415–1421
23. Davies MJ, Thomas AC (1985) Plaque fissuring: the cause of acute myocardial infarction, sudden ischemic death, and crescendo angina. Br Heart J 53: 363–373
24. Diet F, Pratt R, Berry GJ, Momose N, Gibbons G, Dzau VJ (1996) Increased accumulation of tissue ACE in human artherosclerotic coronary artery disease. Circulation 94: 2576–2767
25. Dudley DT, Panek RL, Major TC, Lu GH, Bruns RF, Klinkefus BA, Hodges JC, Weishaar RE (1990) Subclasses of angiotensin II binding sites and their functional significance. Mol Pharmacol 38: 370–377

26. Fantl WJ, Johnson DE, Williams LT (1993) Signalling by receptor tyrosine kinases. Annu Rev Biochem 62: 453–481

27. Freeman RH, Davis JO, Lohmeier TE (1975) Des-asp1 angiotensin II: Possible intrarenal role in homeostasis in the dog. Circ Res 37: 30

28. Freeman RH, Davis JO, Lohmeier TE, Spielman WS (1977) (Des-asp1)angiotensin II: Mediator of the renin-angiotensin system? Fed Proc 36: 1766

29. Furukawa Y, Kishimoto S, Nishikawa K (1982) US Patent No. 4 340 598

30. Furukawa Y, Kishimoto S, Nishikawa K (1982) US Patent No. 4 355 040

31. Galis ZS, Muszynski M, Sukhova GK, Simon-Morrissey E, Unemori EN, Lark M, Amento E, Libby P (1994) Cytokine-stimulated human vascular smooth muscle cells synthesize a complement of enzymes required for extracellular matrix digestion. Circ Res 75: 181–189

32. Geisterfer AA, Peach MJ, Owens GK (1988) Angiotensin II induces hypertrophy, not hyperplasia, of cultured rat aortic smooth muscle cells. Circ Res 62: 749–756

33. Gibbons GH, Pratt RE, Dzau VJ (1992) Vascular smooth muscle cell hypertrophy versus hyperplasia. Autocrine transforming growth factor-beta 1 expression determines growth response to angiotensin II. J Clin Invest 90 (2): 456–461

34. Goldblatt H, Lynch J, Hanzal RF, Summerville WW (1934) Studies on experimental hypertension. I. The production of persistent elevationof systolic blood pressure by means of renal ischemia. J Exp Med 59: 347–380

35. Goodfriend TL, Peach MJ (1975) Angiotensin III: (des-aspartic acid)-angiotensin II, evidence and speculation for its role as an important agonist in the renin-angiotensin system. Circ Res 36 (suppl): I38–I48

36. Gottlieb SS, Dickstein K, Fleck E, Kostis J, Levine TB, LeJemtel T, DeKock M (1993) Hemodynamic and neurohormonal effects of the angiotensin II antagonist losartan in patients with congestive heart failure. Circulation 88 (4): 1602–1609

37. Gunther S (1984) Characterization of angiotensin II subtypes in the rat liver. J Biol Chem 259: 7622–7629

38. Harris PJ (1992) Regulation of proximal tubule function by angiotensin. Clin Exp Pharmacol Physiol 19: 213–222

39. Hausdorff WP, Caron MG, Lefkowitz RJ (1990) Turning off the signal: desensitization of β-adrenergic receptor function. FASEB J 4: 2881–2889

40. Hayek T, Keidar S, Mei-Yi, Oikine J, Breslow J (1995) Effect of angiotensin converting enzyme inhibitors on LDL lipid peroxidation and artherosclerosis progression in apoE deficient mice. Circulation 92 (Suppl I): I-625

41. Kaartinen M, Pentilä A, Kovanan P (1994) Accumulation of activated mast cells in the shoulder region of human coronary artheroma, the predilection site of of artheromatous rupture. Circulation 90: 1669–1678

42. Kakar SS, Sellers JC, Devor DC, Musgrove LC, Neill JD (1992) Angiotensin II type-1 receptor subtype cDNAs: differential tissue expression and hormonal regulation. Biochem Biophys Res Comm 183: 1090–1096

43. Kambayashi Y, Bardhan S, Takahashi K, Tsuzuki S, Inui H, Hamakubo T, Inagami T (1993) Molecular cloning of a novel angiotensin II receptor isoform involved in phosphotyrosine phosphatase inhibition. J Biol Chem 268: 24543–24546

44. Kambayashi Y, Takahashi K, Bardhan S, Inagami T (1994) Molecular structure and function of angiotensin type 2 receptor. Kid Intern 46: 1502–1504

45. Kishimoto T, Akira S, Narazaki M, Taga T (1995) Interleukin 6 family of cytokines and gp130. Blood 86: 1243–1254

46. Kovanen PT, Kaartinen M, Paavonen T (1995) Infiltrates of activated mast cells at the site of coronary arthero-matous erosion or rupture in myocardial infarction. Circulation 92: 1084–1088

47. Laragh JH, Angers M, Kelly WG, Lieberman D (1960) Induction of arginine-vasopressin in the central-nervous system of hypertensive rats. J Am Med Assoc 174: 234–242

48. Libby P (1995) Molecular Bases of the acute coronary syndrome. Circulation 21: 2844–2850

49. Loree HM, Kamm RD, Stringfellow RG, Lee RT (1992) Effects of fibrous cap thickness on peak circum-ferential stress in model artherosclerotic vessels. Circ Res 71: 850–858

50. Marrero MB, Schieffer B, Paxton WG, Heerdt L, Berk BC, Delafontaine P, Bernstein KE (1995) Direct stimulation of JAK/STAT pathway by the angiotensin II AT_1 receptor. Nature 375: 247–250

51. Marx N, Neumann FJ, Ott I, Gawaz M, Koch W, Pikau T, Schömig A (1997) Induction of cytokine expression in leucocytes in acute myocardial infarction. J Am Coll Cardiol 30: 165–170

52. Millan MA, Carvallo P, Izumi S-I, Zemel S, Catt KJ, Aguliera G (1989) Novel site of expression of functional angiotensin II receptors in the late gestation fetus. Science 244: 1340–1342

53. Molloy CJ, Taylor DS, Weber H (1993) Angiotensin II stimulation of rapid tyrosine phosphorylation and protein kinase activation in rat aortic smooth muscle cells. J Biol Chem 268: 7338–7345

54. Moreno PR, Falk E, Palaicos IF, Newell JB, Fuster V, Fallon JT (1994) Macrophage infiltration in acute coronary syndromes. Implications for plaque rupture. Circulation 90: 775–778

55. Mukoyama M, Nakajima M, Horiuchi M, Sasamura H, Pratt RE, Dzau VJ (1993) Expression cloning of type 2 angiotensin receptor reveals a unique class. of seven-transmembrane receptors. J Biol Chem 268: 24539–24542

56. Murphy TJ, Alexander RW, Griendling KK, Runge MS, Bernstein KE (1991) Isolation of a cDNA encoding the vascular type-1 angiotensin II receptor. Nature 351: 233–236

57. Naftilan AJ, Pratt RE, Dzau VJ (1989) Induction of platelet-derived growth factor A-chain and c-myc gene expression by angiotensin II in cultured rat vascular smooth muscle cells. J Clin Invest 83: 1419–1424

58. Nahmias C, Cazaubon SM, Briend-Sutren MM, Lazard D, Villageois P, Strosberg AD (1995) Angiotensin II AT$_2$ receptors are functionally coupled to protein tyrosine dephosphorylation in N1E-115 neuroblastoma cells. Biochem J 306: 87–92

59. Northemann W, Braciak TA, Hattori M, Lee F, Fey GH (1989) Structure of the rat interleukin 6 gene and its expression in macrophage-derived cells. J Biol Chem 264: 16072–16082

60. Owens GK, Schwartz SM (1982) Alterations in smooth muscle cell mass in spontaneously hypertensive rats. Role of cellular hypertrophy, hyperploidy and hyperplasia. Circ Res 51: 280–289

61. Page IH, Helmer OM (1940) A crystalline pressor substance (angiotonin) resulting from the reaction between renin and renin activator. J Exp Med 71: 29–42

62. Pfeffer M, Braunwald E, Moye L, Basta L, Brown EJ, Cuddy TE, Davis BR, Geltmann EM, Goldman S, Flaker GC, Klein M, Lamas G, Packer M, Rouleau J, Rutherford J, Wertheimer JH, Hawkins CM (1992) Effect of captopril on martality and morbidity in patients with left ventricular dysfunction after myocardial infarction: Results of the survival and ventricular enlargement trial. N Engl J Med 327: 669–677

63. Pouyssegur J (1990) In: Birnbaumer L, Iyengar R (eds) G-proteins. Academic Press, Orlando, FL, pp 550–570

64. Powell JS, Clozel JP, Muller RKM, Kuhn H, Hefti F, Hosang M, Baumgartner HR (1989) Inhibitors of angiotensin-converting enzyme prevent myointimal proliferation after vascualr injury. Science 245: 186–188

65. Ridker PM, Gaboury CJL, Conlin PR, Seely EW, Williams GH, Vaughan DE (1993) Stimulation of plasminogen activator inhibitor in vivo by infusion of angiotensin II: evidence of a potential interaction between the renin-angiotensin system and fibrinolytic function. Circulation 87: 1969–1973

66. Ross R (1993) Pathogenesis of artherosclerosis: A perspective for the 1990s. Nature 362: 801–809

67. Saavedra J (1992) Brain and pituitary angiotensin. Endocr Rev 13: 329–380

68. Sadoshima J, Izumo S (1993) Molecular characterization of angiotensin II-induced hypertrophy of cardiac myocytes and hyperplasia of cardiac fibroblasts: Critical role of the AT$_1$ receptor subtype. Circ Res 73: 413–423

69. Sadoshima J, Izumo S (1993) Signal transduction pathways of angiotensin II induced *c-fos* gene expression in cardiac myocytes in vitro. Circ Res 73: 424–438

70. Sandberg K, Hong J, Clark AJ, Shapira H, Catt KJ (1992) Cloning and expression of a novel angiotensin II receptor subtype. J Biol Chem 267: 9455–9458

71. Sasaki K, Yamano Y, Bardham S, Iwai N, Murray JJ, Hasegawa M, Matsuda Y, Inagami T (1991) Cloning and expression of a complementary DNA encoding a bovine adrenal angiotensin II type-1 receptor. Nature 351: 230–233

72. Schieffer B, Paxton WG, Marrero MB, Bernstein KE (1996) Importance of tyrosine phosphorylation in Angiotensin II Type 1 Receptor mediated signalling. Hypertension 27: 476–480

73. Schieffer B, Paxton WG, Marrero MB, Bernstein KE (1996) Importance of tyrosine phosphorylation in Angiotensin II AT$_1$ receptor mediated signalling. Hypertension 27: 476–480

74. Schieffer B, Wirger A, Meybrunn M, Seitz S, Holtz J, Riede UN, Drexler H (1994) Comparative effects of chronic angiotensin-converting enzyme inhibition and angiotensin II type 1 receptor blockade on cardiac remodeling after myocardial infarction. Circulation 89 (5): 2273–2282

75. Schindler C, Darnell JE (1995) Transcriptional responses to polypeptide ligands: the Jak-Stat pathway. Annu Rev Biochem 64: 621–651

76. Schwartz SM, Heimark RL, Majesky MW (1990) Developmental mechanisms underlying pathology of arteries. Physiol Rev 70 (4): 1177–1209

77. Seed B, Aruffo A (1987) Molecular cloning of the CD2 antigen, the T-cell erythrocyte receptor, by a rapid immunoselection procedure. Proc Nat Acad Sci USA 84: 3365–3369

78. Skeggs LT, Dorer FE, Kahn JR, Lentz KE, Levin M (1981) Experimental renal hypertension: The discovery of the renin-angiotensin system. In: Soffer RL (ed) Biochemical Regulation of Blood Pressure. Wiley, New York, NY, pp 3–38

79. Skeggs LT, Marsh WH, Kahn JR, Shumway NP (1954) The existence of two forms of hypertensin. J Exp Med 99: 275

80. Smith JB (1986) Angiotensin-receptor signaling in cultured vascular smooth muscle cells. Am J Physiol 250 (Renal Fluid Electrolyte Physiol 19): F759–F769

81. The SOLVD Investigators (1992) Effect of enalapril on moratlity and the development of heart failure in asymptomatik patients with reduced left ventricular ejection fraction. N Engl J Med 327: 568–574

82. Stouffer GA, Owens GK (1982) Angiotensin II-induced mitogenesis of spontaneously hypertensive rat-derived cultured smooth muscle cells is dependent on autocrine production of transforming growth factor-beta. Circ Res 70: 820–828
83. Tigerstedt R, Bergman PG (1898) Niere und Kreislauf. Scand Arch Physiol 8: 223
84. Timmermans PBMWM, Wong PC, Chiu AT, Herblin WF (1991) Nonpeptide angiotensin II receptor antagonists. Trends Pharmacol Sci 12: 55–62
85. Tsuda T, Kawahara Y, Shii K, Koide M, Ishida Y, Yokoyama M (1991) Vasoconstrictor induced protein-tyrosine phosphorylation in cultured rat vascular smooth muscle cells. FEBS Lett 285: 44–48
86. Van Der Geer, Hunter T, Lindberg RA (1994) Receptor protein tyrosine kinases and their signal transduction. Annu Rev Cell Biol 10: 251–338
87. Van der Waal AC, Becker AE, Loos CM, Das PK (1994) Site of intimal rupture or erosion of thrombosed coronary artherosclerotic plaques is characterized by an inflammatory process irrespective of the dominant plaque morphology. Circulation 89: 34–44
88. Weber H, Taylor DS, Molloy CJ (1994) Angiotensin II induces delayed mitogenesis and cellular proliferation in rat aortic smooth muscle cells. Correlation with the expression of specific growth factors and reversal by suramin. J Clin Invest 93 (2): 788–798
89. Wong PC, Hart SD, Zaspel AM, Chiu AT, Ardecky RJ, Smith RD, Timmermans PBMWM (1990) Functional studies of nonpeptide angiotensin II receptor subtype-specific ligands: DuP753 (AII-1) and PD123177 (AII-2). J Pharm Exp Therap 255: 584–592
90. Yoshida H, Kakuchi J, Guo D, Furuta H, Iwai N, van der Meer de Jong R, Inagami T, Ichikawa I (1992) Analysis of the evolution of angiotensin II type 1 receptor gene in mammals (mouse, rat, bovine and human). Biochem Biophys Res Commun 186: 1042–1049

Author's address:
Helmut Drexler, M.D.
Abteilung Kardiologie und Angiologie
Medizinische Hochschule Hannover
Carl Neuberg Strasse 1
30625 Hannover, Germany
e-mail: Drexler.Helmut@MH-Hannover.de

Genetics of Lipoprotein(a)

H. G. Kraft

Institute for Medical Biology and Human Genetics, Innsbruck, Austria

Abstract

Lipoprotein(a) [Lp(a)] is a complex in human plasma consisting of an LDL particle to which a glycoprotein designated apolipoprotein(a) [apo(a)] is bound via a disulfide bridge. High levels of lipoprotein(a) are considered as genetic risk factor for premature atherosclerosis. Lp(a) plasma levels vary over 1000-fold between individuals. Sib-pair and twin studies have revealed that in Caucasians this variation of Lp(a) concentrations is almost completely determined by the gene locus of one of its protein constituents, namely apo(a). Here we describe the effect of 4 polymorphisms in the apo(a) gene on Lp(a) levels in 4 populations from Africa, and Europe and their relation with coronary heart disease (CHD).

The distribution of Lp(a) levels differs significantly between populations. In each population the Kringle-IV-2 polymorphism (K-IV-2 VNTR) exerts the major effect on Lp(a) levels and the type of the association is the same in all populations (i.e., alleles with low numbers of K-IV repeats are associated with high Lp(a) levels and vice versa). However, differences in K-IV-2 allele frequencies do not explain differences in Lp(a) concentration between populations. Therefore, other polymorphisms in the apo(a) gene were studied.

Two polymorphisms in the promoter region of the apo(a) gene were studied regarding their effect on Lp(a) levels. Between 6 and 11 TTTTA repeats can be detected at – 1.3 kb from the transcription start in individual apo(a) alleles. The effect of this polymorphism on Lp(a) concentrations is much smaller than the effect of the size polymorphism and only present in Caucasian populations.

Secondly, a C/T polymorphism that creates an additional start codon and thereby reduces apo(a) translation *in vitro* was studied. In all populations, mean and median Lp(a) concentrations were lower in CT heterozygotes compared to CC homozygotes. This difference was significant only in the African populations (Blacks and KhoiSan). In all but in the KhoiSan, strong linkage disequilibria were detected between the C/T polymorphism and the two other polymorphisms which likely explain the lack of a significant effect in some populations.

Finally, a mutation that causes an aminoacid (Met/Thr) polymorphism in Kringle IV-10 was analyzed. This mutation was not present in the KhoiSan and had a significant lower frequency in Blacks compared to Caucasians. In contrast to the other polymorphisms, this mutation showed no effect whatsoever on Lp(a) levels.

Since the size polymorphism in the apo(a) gene has such a strong effect on Lp(a) levels, we studied if it is also associated with risk for CHD. We determined Lp(a) levels and apo(a) alleles in 69 patients with CHD and age and sex matched controls. The patients had not only higher Lp(a) levels but also a higher frequency of small sized apo(a) alleles that are associated with high Lp(a) levels. Thus, the size of the apo(a) alleles turned out to be a better risk factor than Lp(a) levels.

Introduction

Lipoprotein(a) [Lp(a)] is a complex consisting of an LDL (low density lipoprotein) particle to which a glycoprotein designated apolipoprotein(a) [apo(a)] is bound via a disulfide bridge. Hence the physico-chemical properties of Lp(a) resemble very much those of LDL and the differences (e.g., higher density, larger size) can be attributed to the presence of the additional apolipoprotein. In a given individual, Lp(a) plasma levels are genetically determined and remain very constant throughout life but vary over 1000-fold between individuals. High levels of lipoprotein(a) are generally accepted as risk factor for premature atherosclerosis leading to coronary heart disease or stroke. Twin and Sib-pair studies have revealed that the apo(a) gene is the major gene determining Lp(a) concentrations in plasma. The apo(a) gene has been located on chromosome 6q2.7 in close vicinity to the gene for plasminogen from which it is thought to have evolved. Like plasminogen, apo(a) contains a signal peptide, Kringle (K) domains, and a protease domain. In contrast to plasminogen, which possesses 5 types of Kringles, apo(a) has lost K-I, K-II, and K-III but instead has accumulated a high number of identical and almost identical K-IV repeats. Within the apo(a) locus, several types of variations have been identified which potentially influence Lp(a) levels (Fig. 1).

Kringle-IV repeat polymorphism
and Lp(a) levels

The strongest effect on Lp(a) levels has been attributed to the size polymorphism of the apo(a) glycoprotein which is caused by a variable number of Kringle IV repeats [K-IV VNTR], which are encoded by 5.6 kb units in the apo(a) gene. This size polymorphism can be demonstrated on the protein level by SDS agarose gel electrophoresis followed by immunoblotting but also on the DNA level by pulsed field gel electrophoresis of restriction enzyme fractionated genomic DNA and Southern blotting (Fig. 2). Although the two methods have a comparable resolution leading to similar patterns, different information is gained. The DNA analysis gives information about the size of the apo(a) alleles present in an individual (usually expressed as the number of K-IV repeats); the protein analysis

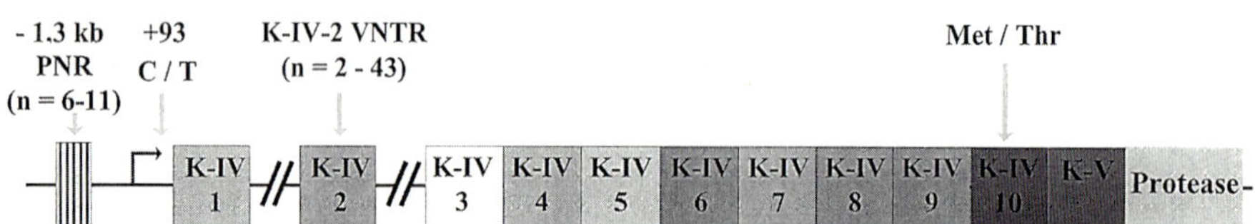

Fig. 1. The sketch shows the genomic structure of the apo(a) gene together with the position of the 4 polymorphisms analyzed

Fig. 2. Presentation of the apo(a) size polymorphism as analyzed on the DNA (upper panel) and protein (lower panel) level. Genomic DNA and plasma of 11 individuals were size separated by electrophoretic procedures, and apo(a) (DNA fragment or isoform, respectively) was visualized by chemoilluminescence. At the bottom, the apo(a) genotype of each individual is presented where individuals 1–10 are heterozygous for 2 different sized alleles and individual 11 is homozygous for an apo(a) allele with 32 K-IV repeats. Both procedures give the same result with 2 exceptions. In the immunoblot, individuals 5 and 8 also show only 1 isoform because of the low expression of the second isoform.

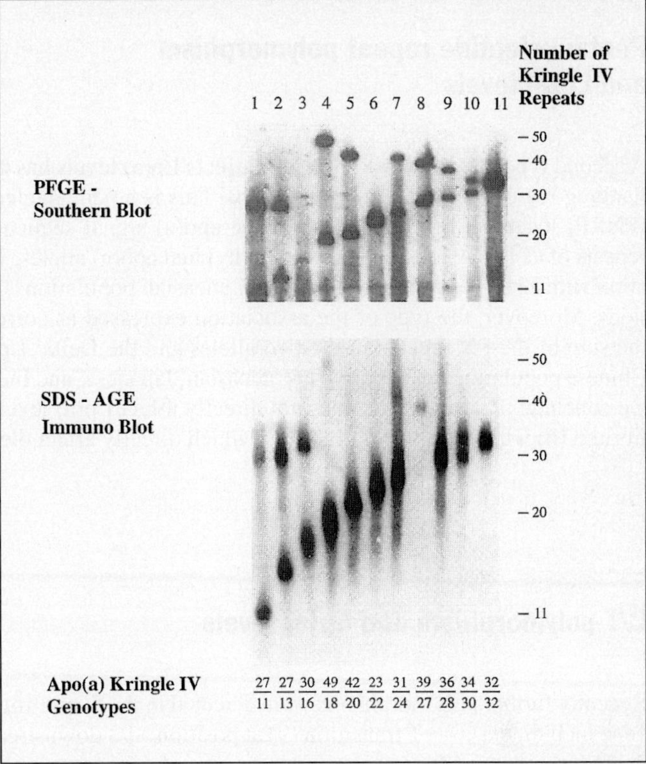

depicts if this allele is expressed and at which level. Hence, due to the allele frequencies and in agreement with expectations based on Hardy-Weinberg equilibrium, > 90 % of all individuals are heterozygous on the DNA level, i.e., they have two apo(a) alleles with a different number of K-IV repeats. The protein analysis on the other hand results in a high number of individuals with a single apo(a) isoform. The majority of them are not true homozygotes but heterozygotes with a second apo(a) allele with a very low expression.

The total number of K-IV repeats ranges between 11 and 52. In every population studied to date, an inverse association has been detected between the number of K-IV repeats and the Lp(a) concentration in plasma. Thus, the size polymorphism explains a significant part of the variation of Lp(a) levels in the population. The magnitude of this effect is, however, different in respective populations. The strongest effect was detected in a Chinese population (4). The K-IV VNTR explains 70 % of the Lp(a) level variation in this sample. The smallest effect was present in Blacks from South Africa (30 %). The homogeneity of the K-IV effect in various populations suggests a basic and causal mechanism that has been explained *in vitro* by different retention times of the apo(a) glycoprotein in the endoplasmic reticulum (1, 8).

Since the size polymorphism does not explain completely the effect of the apo(a) gene on Lp(a) variation and since the size of this effect differs between ethnicities, we conclude that other types of genetic variation in the apo(a) gene which differ among ethnic groups must also operate.

Pentanucleotide repeat polymorphism and Lp(a) levels

A second type of variation which also affects Lp(a) levels has been identified within the 5' flanking region of the apo(a) gene (5, 6). This is a pentanucleotide repeat polymorphism [PNRP] located 1.3 kb upstream of the apo(a) signal sequence (Fig. 1). Between 6–11 repeats of (TTTTA) were detected in individual apo(a) alleles. The association of this variation with Lp(a) levels is significant in Caucasian populations – but not in African populations. Moreover, the type of the association expressed as correlation coefficient between the sum of the PN repeats in the two alleles and the Delta[1] Lp(a) value is positive in the Chinese population but negative in Caucasian, Japanese, and Indian populations. From this, we conclude that the PNRP does not directly affect Lp(a) levels but is in linkage disequilibrium (6) with unknown variation(s) which directly affect the Lp(a) concentrations.

C/T polymorphism and Lp(a) levels

Recently further polymorphisms were detected in the 5' non-translated region of the apo(a) gene including a C → T transition (9) at position +93 downstream of the transcription start that creates a new ATG translation start codon. *In vitro* assays showed that this base change reduced apo(a) translation by 58 % (9) because the ATG is followed by stop codons soon thereafter. We have analyzed the *in vivo* effect of this polymorphism by population studies. Lp(a) levels, apo(a) size alleles, and the C/T genotype were determined in 4 populations, 2 from Europe (Austrians and Danes) and 2 from Africa (Blacks and Khoi San from the Republic of South Africa).

C/T allele frequencies

The allele frequencies were determined by "gene counting" and are shown in Table 1. The allele frequencies in the individual populations were in agreement with expectations based on Hardy-Weinberg equilibrium.

---

[1] The Delta Lp(a) value was calculated to account for the influence of the K-IV polymorphism. In each population a linear regression was calculated with Lp(a) as depending variable and the number of K-IV repeats in the two alleles as independent variables. Using the resulting equations, the expected Lp(a) level was calculated for every individual. The Delta value is the difference between the measured Lp(a) level and this expected value.

Table 1. Allele frequencies (%) of the C and T allele in 4 populations

Population (N)	KhoiSan (58)	Blacks (127)	Austrians (133)	Danes (96)
C	85.0	92.5	88.0	85.4
T	15.0	7.5	12.0	14.6

C/T polymorphism and Lp(a) concentration

Mean and median Lp(a) levels for CC and TT homozygotes and CT heterozygotes in the 4 populations are shown in Table 2. The number of TT homozygotes was very small; therefore, they were not considered in the statistical analysis. In all populations, the CT heterozygotes had lower mean Lp(a) levels compared with the CC homozygotes. The difference in Lp(a) levels between the genotypes was significant in the two African populations, of borderline significance in the Austrian population, but not significant in the Danish population. In the 2 Caucasian populations the difference was completely explained by the size polymorphism (see expected mean in Table 2).

The presence of lower mean Lp(a) levels in CT heterozygotes in all populations is most likely explained by a direct *in vivo* effect of this base change, which has been shown to a reduce apo(a) translation *in vitro* by 58 %. The lack of a statistical significance of this effect in a Caucasian population may be explained by the linkage disequilibria in this population described below. CT heterozygosity was associated with apo(a) alleles which have intermediate numbers of K-IV repeats and 9 PNRs in Caucasians. In these populations such apo(a) alleles are associated with low and very low Lp(a) plasma concentrations. It is, therefore, likely that the effect of the CT polymorphism on Lp(a) levels is masked by the confounding effect of the 2 other polymorphisms.

No such masking was present in the two African populations. In the KhoiSan there was no linkage disequilibrium of the K-IV VNTR and/ or PNRP with C/T alleles. In the Blacks there was linkage disequilibrium but here apo(a) alleles with a "T" had allele sizes associated with high Lp(a) levels.

Table 2. Lp(a) concentrations [mg/dl] and C/T polymorphism

	KhoiSan				Black South Africans				Austrians				Danes			
Genotype	CC	CT	TT	p	CC	CT	TT	p	CC	CT	TT	p	CC	CT	TT	p
mean	38.5	22.9	23.9		30.9	16.5	–		18.3	11.7	0.5		16.9	13.7	–	
SD	28.8	24.3	12.5		27.2	15.8	–		22.9	15.2	–		20.5	24.6	–	
median	32.2	14.2	23.9	0.033	21.0	12.4	–	0.007	8.9	5.8	0.5	0.0465	6.5	10.0	–	0.843
expected mean	33.5	38.1	42.8		28.3	30.0	–		18.1	13.1	3.0		17.0	12.5	–	

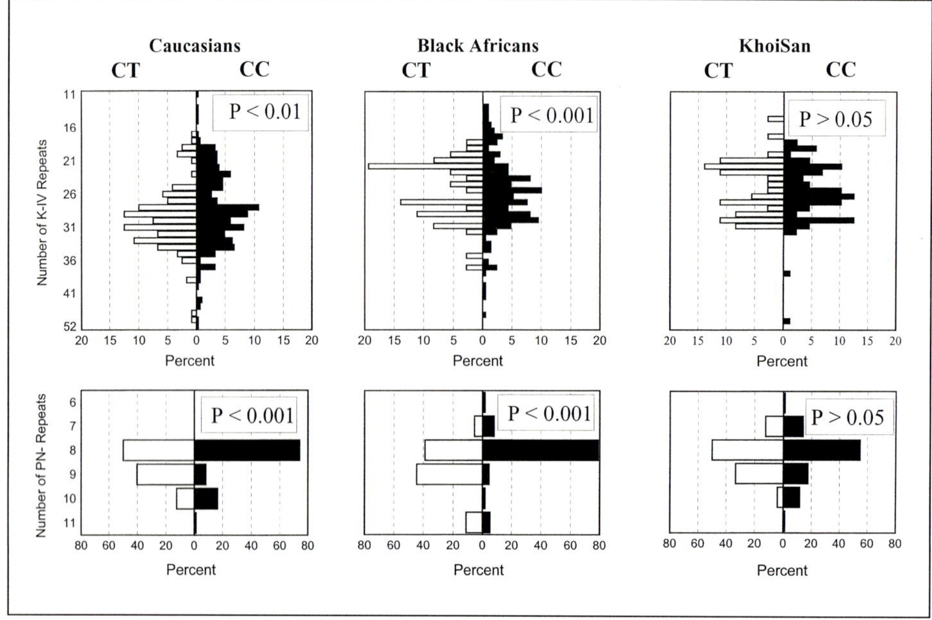

Fig. 3. Graphical presentation of linkage disequilibria in the apo(a) gene between the C/T polymorphism and the size polymorphism (upper panel) and the PNRP (lower panel), respectively. In Caucasians CT heterozygotes are associated more frequently with apo(a) alleles of intermediate size (K-IV 28–32) and less frequently with "small" apo(a) alleles (K-IV < 23) than CC homozygotes. In Black Africans just the opposite was true. Regarding the PNRP significant linkage disequilibria were detected in Caucasians and Blacks with "T" alleles having predominantly 9 PN repeats in both populations. In the KhoiSan there was no linkage disequilibrium detectable for both polymorphisms.

Linkage disequilibrium between C/T polymorphism and Kringle IV polymorphism and the pentanucleotiderepeat polymorphism

The relation between the apo(a) C/T polymorphism and the K-IV VNTR and PNRP, respectively is illustrated in Fig. 3. A statistically significant difference in the distribution of PNRP alleles was detected between CC homozygotes and CT heterozygotes in Caucasians and in Blacks but not in the KhoiSan population. In all populations, where a linkage disequilibrium was detected, the T alleles were found almost exclusively on alleles with 9 (TTTTA) repeats.

The relation between the C/T polymorphism and the K-IV alleles was inhomogeneous. Significant linkage disequilibria (employing the Estimating Haplotypes program) were detected in Blacks and Caucasians but the situation was opposite in Blacks versus Caucasians. C alleles were overrepresented on alleles with 21-25 K-IV repeats (associated with high Lp(a) levels) in Caucasians but the opposite was true in Blacks.

Met/Thr polymorphism and Lp(a) levels

Finally a polymorphism in the coding region of the apo(a) gene was analyzed (2). It is a T→C substitution leading to an aminoacid (Met→Thr) change at position 66 in K-IV type 10. This Kringle is thought to be important for the lysine binding activity of Lp(a) or apo(a). Genotypes for this polymorphism were analyzed by a PCR based method and the mean and expected mean Lp(a) levels were compared for the 3 genotypes as described above. In contrast to the 3 other polymorphisms, this variation showed no effect on Lp(a) levels in any population that was not completely explained by linkage disequilibria with the size polymorphism.

Apo(a) alleles and risk for CHD

In every case-control and prospective study Lp(a) levels were found to be higher in patients with CHD than in controls (for review see (7)). In a few studies, however, the difference was not statistical significant. Nevertheless, increased Lp(a) levels (above 30 mg/dl) are generally accepted as an independent risk factor for CHD and stroke. Since the apo(a) size polymorphism explains ca. 50 % of the variation of Lp(a) concentration in Caucasians, we wanted to study if apo(a) alleles alone can be also regarded as risk factors for CHD. Sixty-nine patients with CHD were analyzed for Lp(a) levels and apo(a) size together with the same number of age and sex matched controls from the same geographic region. The patients had significantly higher mean (p = 0.002) Lp(a) levels than controls (39.2 mg/dl vs. 19.0 mg/dl). The relative risk (expressed as odds ratio) associated with quintiles of Lp(a) levels are shown in Table 3. Only the highest quintile (> 33.6 mg/dl) had a significantly increased risk for CHD. Apo(a) alleles with a low number of K-IV repeats (< 23) were significantly more frequent in the patients group whereas large alleles (> 25 K-IV repeats) were more frequent within the controls. The calculation of relative risk for CHD dependent on the presence of specific apo(a) alleles resulted in a significantly increased risk (OR = 4.63) for individuals with small apo(a) alleles (16 < K-IV < 20) and in a significantly decreased risk (OR = 0.314) for individuals possessing only large sized apo(a) alleles (K-IV > 25).

Table 3. Relative risk (odds ratio) for CHD depending on Lp(a) levels or K-IV number in apo(a) alleles

Lp(a) concentration range (mg/dl)	CHD risk (Odds Ratio)	Apo(a) allele Number of K-IV repeats	CHD risk (Odds Ratio)
0– 2.5	0.472	17–19	4.63*
2.5– 6.0	0.805	20–22	2.08
6.0–11.4	0.805	23–25	1.09
11.4–33.6	0.666	> 25	0.314**
> 33.6	2.55*		

* P < 0.05; ** P < 0.001

Although the difference in size allele frequencies did not completely explain the increased Lp(a) level in the patients group (3), this result clearly documents that apo(a) alleles must be regarded as significant risk factors for CHD.

References

1. Brunner C, Lobentanz EM, Pethö-Schramm A, Ernst A, Kang C, Dieplinger H, Müller HJ, Utermann G (1996) The number of identical kringle IV repeats in apolipoprotein(a) affects its processing and secretion by HepG2 cells. J Biol Chem 271: 32403–32410
2. Kraft HG, Haibach C, Lingenhel A, Brunner C, Trommsdorff M, Kronenberg F, Müller HJ, Utermann G (1995) Sequence polymorphism in kringle IV 37 in linkage disequilibrium with the apolipoprotein (a) size polymorphism. Hum Genet 95: 275–282
3. Kraft HG, Lingenhel A, Köchl S, Hoppichler F, Kronenberg F, Abe A, Mühlberger V, Schönitzer D, Utermann G (1996) Apolipoprotein(a) kringle IV repeat number predicts risk for coronary heart disease. Arterioscler Thromb Vasc Biol 16: 713–719
4. Kraft HG, Lingenhel A, Pang RWC, Delport R, Trommsdorff M, Vermaak H, Janus ED, Utermann G (1996) Frequency distributions of apolipoprotein(a) Kringle IV repeat alleles and their effects on lipoprotein(a) levels in Caucasian, Asian, and African populations: The distribution of null alleles is non-random. EJHG 4: 74–87
5. Mooser V, Mancini FP, Bopp S, Pethö-Schramm A, Guerra R, Boerwinkle E, Müller HJ, Hobbs HH (1995) Sequence polymorphisms in the apo(a) gene associated with specific levels of Lp(a) in plasma. Hum Mol Gen 4: 173–181
6. Trommsdorff M, Köchl S, Lingenhel A, Kronenberg F, Delport R, Vermaak H, Lemming L, Klausen IC, Faergeman O, Utermann G, Kraft HG (1995) A pentanucleotide repeat polymorphism in the 5' control region of the apolipoprotein(a) gene is associated with lipoprotein(a) plasma concentrations in Caucasians. J Clin Invest 96: 150–157
7. Utermann G (1995) Lipoprotein(a). In: Scriver CR, Beaudet AL, Sly WS, Stanbury JB, Wyngaarden JB, Fredrickson DS (eds) The Metabolic and Molecular Bases of Inherited Disease. New York:McGraw-Hill, Inc. p 1887–1912
8. White AL, Guerra B, Lanford RE (1977) Influence of allelic variation on apolipoprotein(a) folding in the endoplasmic reticulum. J Biol Chem 272: 5048–5055
9. Zysow BR, Lindahl GE, Wade DP, Knight BL, Lawn RM (1995) C/T Polymorphism in the 5í untranslated region of the apolipoprotein(a) gene introduces an upstream ATG and reduces in vitro translation. Arterioscler Thromb Vasc Biol.15: 58–64

Author's address:
H. G. Kraft
Institute for Medical Biology and Human Genetics
Schöpfstr. 41
A-6020 Innsbruck, Austria

The molecular mechanisms of inherited hypercholesterolemia

W. März[1], M. S. Nauck[1], E. Fisher[2], M. M. Hoffmann[1], H. Wieland[1]

[1]Division of Clinical Chemistry, Department of Medicine, Albert Ludwigs-University, Freiburg im Breisgau, Germany, [2]Gustav Embden Center of Biological Chemistry, University Hospital, Johann Wolfgang Goethe-University, Frankfurt am Main, Germany

Abstract

Both observational and intervention studies have proven that hypercholesterolemia is a major risk factor for cardiovascular disease. Genetic factors are significant determinants of cholesterol and LDL cholesterol. Among the sources of genetic variation are monogenetic disorders resulting in severe clinical phenotypes and genetic polymorphisms affecting the metabolism of plasma lipoproteins. The best characterized monogenetic disorders of lipoprotein metabolism are familial hypercholesterolemia and familial defective apo B-100. In familial hypercholesterolemia (FH), the primary defect is a mutation in the gene encoding the LDL receptor. More than 300 mutant allels distorting receptor function are known to date. This genetic heterogeneity has to be accounted in the diagnosis of familial hypercholesterolemia at the molecular level. Familial defective apo B-100 has for a long time been considered to result from one point mutation changing codon 3500 from arginine to glutamine. Recent work, however, shows that this disorder is heterogeneous at the genetic level as well and that approaches to diagnose familial defective apo B-100 by probing for the arg$^{3500}\rightarrow$gln substitution will fail to detect other, more rare variants of apo B-100 also associated with decreased binding of LDL to LDL receptors. The most extensively studied genetic polymorphism affecting LDL cholesterol is the polymorphism of apolipoprotein E. Three common alleles exist at the apo E gene locus, namely apo E2, apo E3, and apo E4. Apo E3 represents the wild type allele. Compared to apo E3 homozygotes, carriers of one or two alleles of apo E4 have slightly higher LDL cholesterol concentrations whereas carriers of apo E2 tend to have lower LDL cholesterol. A small proportion of apo E2 homozygotes, however, develope type III hyperlipoproteinemia, a highly atherogenic form disorder of lipoprotein metabolism characterized by the accumulation of remnant particles derived from the incomplete catabolism of triglyceride-rich lipoproteins. In very rare cases, type III hyperlipoproteinemia may be transmitted in an autosomal dominant fashion. The common feature of mutations underlying this form of type III hyperlipoproteinemia appears to be that they severly impair the interaction of apo E with heparin sulfate proteoglycans rather than with lipoprotein receptors.

Introduction

High concentrations of cholesterol, in particular those of LDL cholesterol, are among the principal risk factors of atherosclerosis. However, despite changes in lifestyle and the availability of effective pharmacological approaches to lower plasma cholesterol concentrations, cardiovascular disease continues to be the major cause of death in North America, Europe, and much of Asia. The plasma levels of LDL vary widely within the population. They are affected by common factors such as sex, age, diet, exercise, and ethnic background. It is, however, also clear that genetic factors significantly influence LDL concentrations. Thus, the overall inter-individual variation of LDL levels results from a hereditary and an environmental component. Among the genetic factors affecting LDL metabolism are monogenetic disorders producing severe clinical phenotypes such as familial hypercholesterolemia (due to mutations in the LDL receptor gene) and familial defective apo B-100. Although these two disorders belong to the most frequent inborn errors of metabolism in humans, they are too rare to make significant contributions to the variance of LDL cholesterol concentrations observed in the general population.

On the other hand, polymorphisms of genes involved in lipoprotein metabolism have been implicated in determining LDL cholesterol. Genetic polymorphisms occur at frequencies high enough to explain a substantial fraction of the population variance of LDL concentrations although they may have a small effect on LDL cholesterol in a single individual. This article will discuss recent progress made in the study of two forms of inborn errors of LDL metabolism, namely familial hypercholesterolemia (FH) and familial defective apo B-100. Finally, it will attempt to explain how the interplay of frequent and rare variants of apo E with non-genetic factors may affect the metabolism of lipoproteins and, ultimately, the risk of atherosclerosis.

A glance at the metabolism of plasma lipoproteins

Lipoproteins are macromolecular complexes involved in the intercellular transport of lipids. All lipoproteins have a common structure of a neutral lipid core (triglycerides and cholesteryl esters) surrounded by a surface monolayer of amphipathic lipids (phospholipids and unesterified cholesterol). The protein moiety of lipoproteins, the apolipoproteins, are amphipathic in nature as well in that they possess hydrophobic and hydrophilic domains, thus, being able to interact with the lipid core and the aqueous environment of the lipoproteins. Beyond this detergent-like function, apolipoproteins serve as effectors of enzymes of lipid metabolism and as ligands for cell surface lipoprotein receptors.

Lipoproteins are classified according to their hydrated densities. Chylomicrons are large triglyceride-rich particles produced by the intestine. They transport triglycerides and cholesterol to the liver. Very low density lipoproteins (VLDL) are triglyceride-rich particles synthesized in the liver. Intermediate density lipoproteins (IDL) represent a transitory pool of lipoproteins originating from hepatic VLDL. Low density lipoproteins (LDL) transport the bulk of cholesterol in the blood. LDL possess one molecule of apoB-100 per particle. Apo B-100 is a ligand of the LDL receptor (LDL-r) and mediates the transfer of LDL cholesterol from the blood into peripheral cells or hepatocytes. The lipid moiety of high density lipoproteins (HDL) mainly consists of cholesteryl esters and phospholipds.

There are three major routes of lipid transport in plasma: the exogenous, the endogenous and the reverse cholesterol transport pathway (Fig. 1). The exogenous pathway is initiated by the secretion of chylomicrons into the intestinal lymph. These particles enter the bloodstream via the thoracic duct, thus, by-passing the liver. Their triglyceride moiety (as much

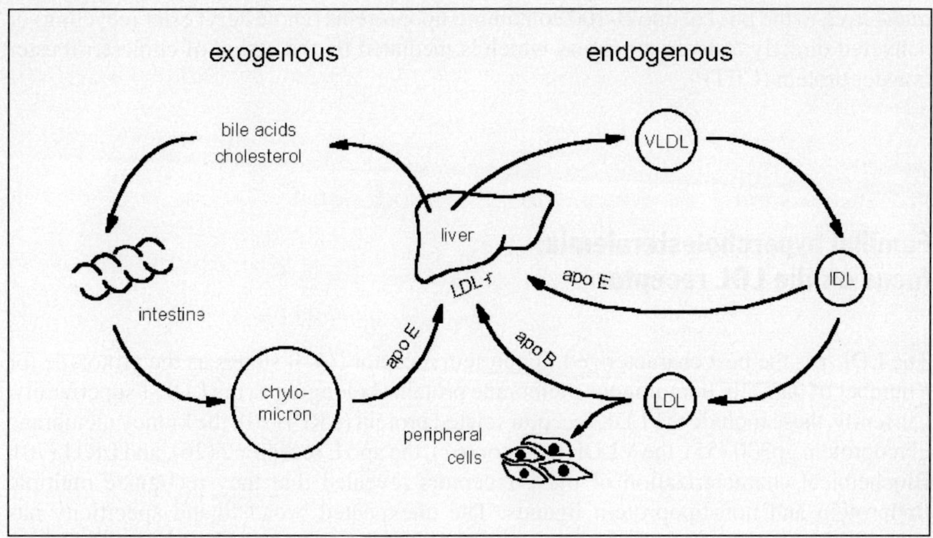

Fig. 1. The metabolism of plasma lipoproteins. For details see text.

as 150 g/d) is hydrolyzed by the enzyme lipoprotein lipase, which resides on the lumenal surface of the capillary endothelium. The free fatty acids generated in this reaction are taken up by the tissues such as adipose, for storage, and muscle, for oxidation. As a consequence of the hydrolysis of triglycerides, chylomicrons are converted to smaller remnant particles. During this transformation, excess surface components (phospholipids and apolipoproteins) are transferred to HDL. The remnant particles become enriched in cholesterol and acquire apo E from HDL. Since their apo B-48 residue lacks the receptor binding domain of apo B-100, apo E is needed to mediate the uptake of remnant particles into the liver through specific cell surface receptors including the low density lipoprotein receptor (LDL-r) and the LDL receptor-related protein (LRP). In summary, there are, thus, two major steps in the catabolism of chylomicrons: hydrolysis of triglycerides in the circulation and receptor-mediated catabolism of cholesterol in the liver.

Essentially, the same principles apply to the endogenous pathway. Triglycerides and cholesterol synthesized by the liver are packaged and secreted as VLDL. Similar to chylomicrons, VLDL are rich in triglycerides. Their major apolipoproteins are apo B-100, apo C, and apo E. VLDL undergo lipolysis in the circulation to give rise to IDL. A significant fraction of the IDL is rapidly taken up by the liver; the remainder undergoes further lipolysis to produce LDL. This conversion probably depends on the action of another lipolytic enzyme, hepatic triglyceride lipase (HTGL). LDL particles contain most of the cholesterol in blood. Their only protein constituent is apo B-100. LDL are taken up into peripheral cells by the LDL-r. This provides cholesterol which is utilized in the synthesis of cell membranes and steroid hormones. However, roughly two thirds of the LDL are catabolized by the liver, again via the LDL receptor pathway.

HDL are formed from precursor particles released from the intestine and from the liver. In addition, surface material derived from the catabolism of chylomicrons is a source of HDL particles. Such nascent HDL particles mobilize free cholesterol from peripheral cells which is then immediately esterified by the enzyme lecithin:cholesterol acyltransferase. During this process, mature HDL particles are generated. Esterified cholesterol is then transferred to the pool of apo B-100 containing lipoproteins (cholesteryl ester recycling) or delivered directly to liver, a process which is mediated by the action of cholesterol ester transfer protein (CETP).

Familial hypercholesterolemia: focus on the LDL receptor

The LDL-r is the best characterized lipoprotein receptor (6). It stands as the prototype for a number of partially homologous membrane proteins belonging to the LDL-r superfamily. Currently, these include the LDL receptor related protein (LRP) (20), the kidney membrane glycoprotein gp330 (55), the VLDL receptor (61), the apo E receptor 2 (26), and LR11 (70). Biochemical characterization of these receptors revealed that they recognize multiple lipoprotein and non-lipoprotein ligands. The unexpected broad ligand specificity has extended lipoprotein research far into previously unrelated areas such as neurobiology or developmental biology. However, as members of the LDL-r superfamily other than the LDL-r have not been unequivocally been implicated in the development of genetic disease in humans, these molecules will not be treated here.

The major function of the LDL-r is to mediate the cellular uptake of LDL. The LDL-r, thus, has key role in regulating cellular and systemic cholesterol homeostasis. The LDL-r recognizes apo B-100, the only protein constituent of LDL particles, apo E (6), and LPL (41). Apo B-48, the intestinal isoform of apo B, is not recognized by the LDL-r since it lacks the receptor binding domain present in apo B-100 (see below).

The LDL-r is a cell membrane-spanning glycoprotein consisting of the five structural domains: the ligand binding domain, the epidermal growth factor homology region, the O-linked carbohydrate domain, the transmembrane region and the cytoplasmic tail (Fig. 2). LDL-r are expressed at varying levels in almost every type of cell or tissue (liver paren-chymal cells, intestine, adipocytes, lymphocytes, ovaries, adrenal, monocytes and macrophages, endothelial cells, and smooth muscle cells). LDL-r on the surface of liver cells are responsible for approximately more than two thirds of the catabolism of LDL in the body (6).

Cellular cholesterol originates from two sources, the de novo synthesis from activated acetic acid and the receptor mediated uptake of cholesterol containing lipoproteins. As the cell must balance internal and external sources of cholesterol while avoiding shortage or over-accumulation, cholesterol needs to be balanced by feedback-control. In the absence of extracellular sources of cholesterol, cells enhance the production of LDL-r, together with coordinate increases in the rate-limiting enzymes of the sterol biosynthesis pathway (6, 17). In contrast, when cells are cultured in the presence of LDL, cholesterol biosynthesis declines by more than 90 % and the number of LDL-r decreases.

Exogenous cholesterol is delivered to the cells by receptor-mediated endocytosis of LDL. The lipoprotein particle first binds to LDL-r. LDL-r are clustered in specialized regions of the cell surface, the clathrin-coated pits. Once ligand particles have bound to LDL-r, the entire coated pit undergoes internalization and is converted into an endocytotic coated vesicle. Subsequently, the vesicles' coat is removed and their contents are acidified. The receptor molecule undergoes a pH dependent conformational transition which results in the dissociation of the ligand from the LDL-r. The latter is recycled to the cell surface while the lipoprotein is forwarded to the lysosomes where the protein and lipid moiety are

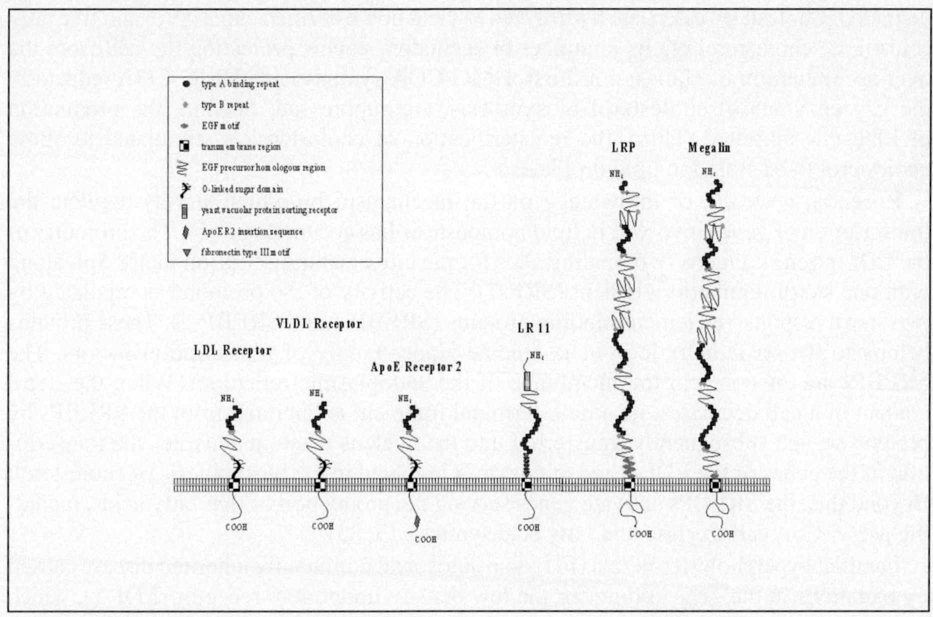

Fig. 2. Members of the LDL-r gene superfamily expressed in humans. **The LDL-r** is a membrane protein consisting of five domains. The aminoterminal domain is responsible for the binding of ligands; it is rich in cysteine residues and consists of seven homologous type A binding repeats in which the positions of six cysteine residues are highly conserved. Each of these cysteine residues is involved in the formation of disulfide bonds. The binding of apo B-100 and apo E to the type A repeats is mediated by clusters of negatively charged amino acids residues (glutamate and aspartate) between the fourth and the sixth cysteine residue. When these residues are protonized in the endosomes, ligand molecules are released from its binding to the receptor. The second domain of the LDL-R shares a high degree of homology with the epidermal growth factor precursor. This domain includes two cysteine-rich type B repeats, a spacer region, and a third type B repeat. The third domain contains 18 threonine or serine residues and O-linked carbohydrate residues. The transmembrane region consists of 22 hydrophobic amino acids. The cytoplasmic domain mediates the clustering of receptor molecules in coated-pits and the sorting of receptors to the basolateral cell surface in polarized cells. The **VLDL receptor** is highly homologous to the LDL-r, but contains eight type A binding repeats, in contrast to seven in the LDL-r. The VLDL-r is abundantly expressed on the lumenal surface of endothelial cells of the heart, the muscle, the adipose tissue and the brain. The **apo E receptor 2** consists of five functional domains resembling the LDL-r and the VLDL-r. This receptor has seven type A repeats. The primary structure of these repeats is more closely related to those in the VLDL-r than to those in the LDL-r. The cytoplasmic tail of the apo E-r2 contains a unique insertion of 59 amino acids; the function of this domain is not known. These apo E-r2 is most highly expressed in human brain and placenta, but hardly in any other tissue. **LR11** is a 250 kDa membrane protein. Its extracellular portion contains one cluster of 11 type A binding repeats, one spacer region, six tandemly arranged fibronectin type III repeats reminiscent of neural adhesion molecules, and a domain with similarity to a yeast receptor for vacuolar protein sorting. The cytoplasmic domain has features characteristic of endocytosis-competent receptors. LR11 is expressed abundantly in the central nervous system. The **LDL receptor related protein** contains 31 type A repeats, arranged in four clusters of 2, 8, 10, and 11 repeats. There are 22 type B repeats compared to three in the LDL-r. The type B repeats are constituents of four complete and four truncated EGF precursor homology regions. The cytoplasmic domain of LRP contains 100 amino acids and is, thus, twice as long as the cytoplasmic domain of the LDL-r. It contains two NPYX motifs which serve as internalization signals. Mature LRP is a heterodimer of two non-covalently linked subunits with apparent molecular masses of 515 and 85 kDa, respectively. They arise from a monomeric 600 kDa precursor which is endoproteolytically cleaved by furin in the trans-Golgi complex. **Megalin** is the autoantigen of Heymann's nephritis, an autoimmune glomerulonephritis in rats. In humans, megalin consists of 4655 amino acid residues. In the extracellular region, there are 36 type A binding repeats, clustering in four distinct domains, 16 type B repeats separated by eight spacer regions, and one epidermal growth factor motif. There is one single transmembrane region and an intracellular C-terminal region of 209 amino acids. The latter contains two copies of the NPXY internalization signal and, interestingly, several Src-homology 3 recognition motifs, one Src-homology 2 recognition motif for the p85 regulatory subunit of phosphatidylinositol 3-kinase, and additional sites for protein kinase C, casein kinase II, and cAMP-/cGMP-dependent protein kinase.

degraded. Cholesteryl esters are hydrolyzed to yield non-esterified cholesterol and free fatty acids. Free cholesterol elicits a number of regulatory events protecting the cell from the over-accumulation of cholesterol. First, HMG-COA synthase and HMG-COA reductase, the key enzymes of cholesterol biosynthesis, are suppressed. Second, the production of LDL-r is inhibited. Third, the re-esterification of cholesterol is stimulated to allow cholesterol to be stored in lipid droplets.

Recently, a wealth of knowledge on the mechanism by which sterols regulate the transcription of genes involved in lipid homoestasis has accumulated (5). The promoter of the LDL-r gene contains two binding sites for the universal transcription factor Spl, along with one sterol regulatory element (SRE-1). The activity of the promoter is regulated by two sterol responsive element binding proteins (SREBP-1 and SREBP-2). These proteins belong to the basic-helix-loop-helix-leucine zipper family of transcription factors. The SREBPs are anchored in the membrane of the endoplasmic reticulum. When the sterol content of a cell decreases, an amino-terminal fragment is liberated from the SREBPs by proteolysis and subsequently transferred into the nucleus where it activates the transcription of the genes of the LDL-r and of enzymes involved in the biosynthesis of cholesterol. Beyond this, the SREBPs activate genes serving the production of free fatty acids, including acetyl-CoA carboxylase and fatty acid synthase (3, 33).

Familial hypercholesterolemia (FH) is an autosomal dominantly inherited disease caused by mutations in the gene coding for the low density lipoprotein receptor (LDL-r), which mediates the specific uptake and catabolism of plasma LDL (18). Heterozygous FH individuals with express only half the number of functional LDL-r and have a markedly raised plasma cholesterol. These patients may present with tendon xanthomas, accelerated atherosclerosis, and premature coronary artery disease. Homozygous FH individuals are more severely affected and, without intensive cholesterol-lowering treatment, may succumb before the age of maturity.

The prevalence of heterozygous FH is approximately 1 in 500 in Europe and North America (18). In some areas with culturally and geographically isolated populations, however, the frequency of this disease and of specific mutations is much higher, presumably as a result of a founder effect; examples include the French Canadians (32), Sephardic Jews (31), Lebanese Christian Arabs (29), South African Afrikaners (30), and the Finns (1).

So far, more than 300 different mutant alleles of the LDL-r gene have been reported (21), and except for the few populations in which founder mutations prevail, each family is, a priori, expected to have a unique LDL-r mutation. For a number of mutations identified so far, the mutant gene product has functionally been characterized, either in cultured cells derived from the patient or by mutagenesis and expression of the mutant allele in heterologous cells *in vitro*.

Since the LDL receptor is a multifunctional protein consisting of distinct structural domains, different mutations result in mutant proteins; the structure and function of which are impaired in different ways and to a different extent. Defining mutations at the protein level allowed the identification of five classes of functional defects of the receptor. These classes include defects in synthesis, intracellular transport, ligand binding, internalization, and recycling of the receptor. Consequently, the characterization of the specific mutation in the LDL-r gene of a FH patient not only provides insights in the way the LDL-r functions *in vivo*, but also allows an accurate diagnosis to be made on which treatment and counseling can be based. It has long been recognized that there is considerable variation in the severity of the disease in FH patients, regarding both the degree of hypercholesterolemia and the age of onset of clinical symptoms of coronary heart disease. Comparing groups of patients with either the same or different mutations in the LDL-r gene may, in the future, allow better assessment of the underlying genetic or environmental causes of this variation.

In addition, the first reports comparing the results of medical treatment in individuals with different LDL-r gene mutations indicate that knowledge of the molecular defect may be a tool allowing better predictions of clinical response to treatment.

Our strategy to identify mutations in the LDL-r gene is based on the amplification of the 18 exons of LDL-r gene including the splice site consensus sequences and the known regulatory elements of the promoter, followed by denaturing gradient gel electrophoresis (44) and direct sequencing (Fig. 3). Using this approach we characterized 100 unrelated patients in whom we diagnosed FH according to clinical criteria (sex-adjusted cholesterol levels above the 90th percentile of the German population, tendon xanthomas, and/or premature coronary artery disease in the patient or a first degree relative) (Table 1). Eight of these individuals were heterozygous for apo B-100 (arg^{3500}→gln) (see below). Mutations in the LDL-r gene were detected in 57 out of the 100 subjects; among these were two true homozygotes, while one individual was a compound heterozygote, carrying two mutations on different alleles. One patient was heterozygous for both apo B-100 (arg^{3500}→gln) and a point mutation in the LDL-r (asp^{108}→asn). Only seven out of 45 different mutations occurred more than once. To our knowledge 19 of these mutations have been described previously whereas the remaining 26 mutations were encountered for the first time. It is very likely that these novel mutations represent the causes of hypercholesterolemia in the affected individuals since these were the only molecular defects identified in the entire coding and splice-site consensus sequences of the LDL-r gene. In addition, most of these mutations affected amino acid residues that have already been shown to be crucial to the function of the LDL-r in previous investigations. Together, these results confirm the genetically heterogeneous nature of FH and emphasize the need to screen for mutations in each newly identified index patient.

Ligand defective apo B-100: a frequent monogenetic disorder of LDL metabolism

Apo B-100 is a glycoprotein of approximately 550 kDa; it is an integral constituent of VLDL, IDL, and LDL. The apo B gene on the short arm of chromosome 2 is 43 kb in length and consists of 29 exons (27). Exon 26 is one of the longest contiguous exons of the human genome. In humans, apo B-100 is exclusively expressed in the liver. Apo B-48, the intestinal isoform of apo B, contains the aminoterminal part of apo B-100. Apo B-48 is the major protein component of chylomicrons. Both apo B isoforms are products of a single gene. Apo B-48 mRNA is derived from apo B-100 mRNA through RNA editing. The editing of apo B mRNA is an intranuclear event that occurs post-transcriptionally, coincident with splicing and polyadenylation (58, 62). The interaction of apo B-100 with LDL-r is responsible for the transfer of LDL cholesterol from blood into the liver and most other cells in the body. The receptor-binding domain of apo B-100 resides in the carboxyterminal half of apo B-100 (4). As apo B-48 is lacking this part of the molecule, it is not able to bind to lipoprotein receptors. The clearance of intestinal lipoproteins, therefore, crucially depends on apo E.

Familial defective apo B-100 (FDB) is a group of autosomal dominantly inherited disorders, in which the cellular uptake of LDL from the blood is diminished due to mutations within the of apo B-100 receptor binding domain. The biochemical and clinical character-

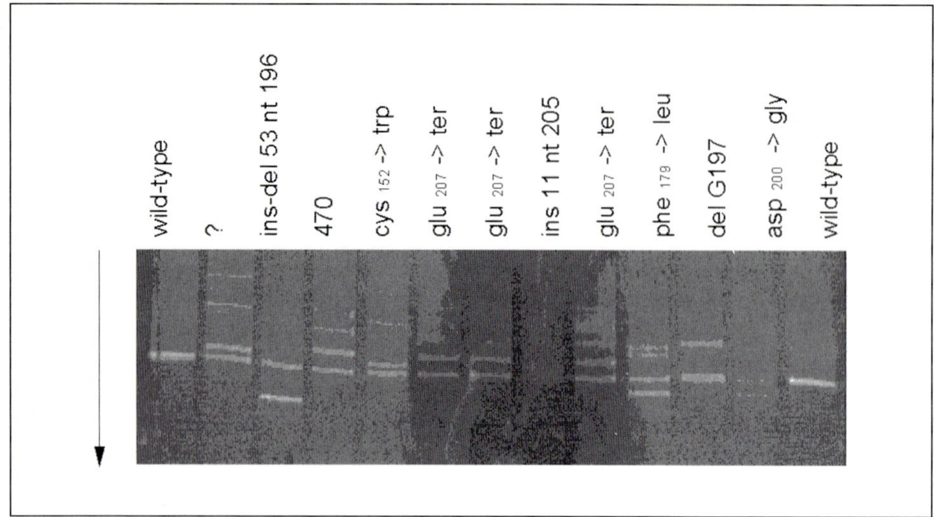

Fig. 3. Screening for mutations in the gene of the LDL-r using denaturing gradient gel electrophoresis. The 18 exons of LDL-r gene including the splice site consensus sequences and the known regulatory elements of the promoter were amplified by polymerase chain reaction. The amplification products were then analyzed by denaturing gradient gel electrophoresis (44). As an example, the electrophoretic behavior of mutations within the fourth exon of the LDL-r gene is shown. Those samples revealing an abnormal pattern were directly sequenced in both directions using fluorescence-labeled primers and the thermo sequenase cycle sequencing. Sequencing results are indicated on top of the respective lanes.

istics of FDB are moderately to severely elevated LDL cholesterol, tendon xanthoma, arcus lipoides, and premature coronary artery disease. A number of point mutations of the putative receptor binding domain of apo B-100 have been identified (59). Only three of these mutations have so far been proven to produce binding-defective apo B-100 by appropriate genetic and functional investigations (15, 48, 59). The first one to be discovered and, apparently the most frequent one, is apo B-100 (arg^{3500}→gln) (59). The other two substitutions, apo B-100 (arg^{3500}→trp) 15 and apo B-100 (arg^{3531}→cys) 48, are generally considered to occur less frequently. The arg^{3531}→cys mutation has been identified in two families of different ethnic origin (48), in four CAD patients from the Great Salt Lake Basin area, all of Caucasian origin (34), in two families in the United Kingdom (68), and two French individuals (49). Compared to apo B-100 (arg^{3500}→gln), the mutation at codon 3531 is associated with a lesser increase in LDL cholesterol (48, 68). Consistently, apo B-100 (arg^{3531}→cys) containing LDL exhibited less reduction of LDL receptor binding in vitro than LDL endowed with apo B-100 (arg^{3500}→gln) (48, 68). Apo B-100 (arg^{3500}→trp) has been described in just one family of European origin (15) so far, twice in a mixed Chinese and Malayan hypercholesterolemic cohort (7), and in the originally reported family of Asian descent living in the Glasgow region (15). The receptor binding of apo B-100 (arg^{3500}→trp) has been claimed to be similar to apo B-100 (arg^{3500}→gln) (15).

In an attempt to search for new genetic variants affecting the receptor binding of apo B-100, we examined a 2121 base pair (codons 3131–3837) portion of the apo B gene, including the putative receptor binding region, using polymerase chain reaction and temperature gradient gel electrophoresis in 297 unrelated individuals with primary hypercholesterolemia (LDL cholesterol greater than 1.55 g/L and triglycerides less than 2.0 g/L) recruited in the Rhein-Main area. We identified three unrelated carriers (1 %) of a silent

Table 1. Mutations of the gene of the LDL-r identified in 100 individuals clinically diagnosed as familial hypercholesterolemia in Germany

no.	exon	codon change	nucleotide change	type	origin	status[1]	number of patients
1	1	met^{-21}→val	ATG→GTG	missense	Netherlands	het	2
2	Intron 1	nt 67+1	G→A	splice site	new	het	2
3	3	211 del 1	– G	frameshift	North Ireland	het	1
4	3	trp^{66}→gly	TGG→GGG	missense	French-Canadian 4	het	1
5	Intron 3	nt 313+1	G→A	splice site	Elverum	het	3
6	Intron 3	nt 313+2	T→C	splice site	Netherlands	het	4
7	4	nt 93 del 5	–TTTCG	frameshift	new	het	1
8	4	nt 310 del 5	–GTCGT	frameshift	new	het	1
9	4	asp^{108}→asn	GAC→AAC	missense	new	com FDB	1
10	4	cys^{113}→arg	TGC→CGC	missense	new	het	1
11	4	glu^{119}→asn	GAG→GAC	missense	new	het	1
12	4	cys^{122}→arg	TGC→CGC	missense	new	het	1
13	4	cys^{152}→trp	TGC→TGG	missense	new	het	1
14	4	phe^{179}→leu	TTC→CTC	missense	new	het	1
15	4	nt 570 del 1	–G	frameshift	Lithuania	het	1
16	4	196 del 37		frameshift	new	het	1
17	4	asp^{200}→gly	GAC→GGC	missense	Padua	het	1
18	4	asp^{203}→val	GAC→GTC	missense	Germany	het	1
19	4	gln^{207}→stop	GAG→TAG	nonsense	Marocco	het/com	4/1
20	4	nt 615 ins 11	ACGGTATGGAC	frameshift	new	het	1
21	5	arg^{232}→trp	CGG→TGG	missense	new	het	1
22	5	asp^{245}→glu	GAT→GAA	missense	Cincinatti 1	het	1
23	6	ser^{265}→arg	AGC→AGA	missense	Greece	het	1
24	6	ser^{285}→leu	TCA→TTA	missense	Amsterdam	het	1
25	7	gly^{302}→ser	GGC→AGC	missense	new	het	1
26	7	cys^{317}→tyr	TGC→TAC	missense	new	hom	1
27	7	arg^{329}→stop	CGA→TGA	nonsense	United Kingdom	het	1
28	8	cys^{371}→trp	TGC→TGG	missense	new	het	1
29	9	val^{408}→met	GTG→ATG	missense	Africaner 2	het	2
30	9	trp^{422}→cys	TGG→TGC	missense	North Platt	het	1
31	Intron 9	nt 1358+2	T→A	splice site	new	het	2
32	10	pro^{505}→ser	CCT→TCT	missense	Cincinatti 3	het	1
33	11	gly^{528}→asn	GGT→GAT	missense	Genua	het	1
34	11	asn^{543}→his	AAT→CAT	missense	Denmark	het	1
35	12	arg^{553}→cys	CGG→CAG	missense	new	het	1
36	13	asn^{604}→thr	AAC→ACC	missense	new	het	1
37	13	val^{618}→asp	GTC→GAC	missense	new	het	1
38	14	cys^{646}→trp	TGT→TGG	missense	new	hom	1
39	14	leu^{661}→phe	CTC→TTC	missense	new	het	1
40	14	phe^{664}→leu	CCG→CTG	missense	Gujerat	het	1
41	15	thr^{705}→ile	ACC→ATC	missense	Paris 9	Com	1
42	15	717 ins 1	nukl. 2214 ins C	frameshift	new	het	1
43	15	thr^{721}→ile	ACC→ATC	missense	new	het	1
44	17	val^{785}→asp	GTC→GAC	missense	new	het	1
45	17	nt 2393 del 9	–TCCTCGTCT	deletion	Utah	het	1

[1] het indicates heterozygous; hom, homozygous; com, compound heterozygous

substitution (CTG→CTA) affecting the codon for leucine^{3350}, four carriers of apo B-100 (glu^{3405}→gln) (1.3 %), and two subjects with apo B-100 (arg^{3500}→trp) (0.7 %). Apo B-100 (arg^{3500}→gln) was found in 21 individuals (7.1 %). When extrapolated to the general population, this corresponded to a frequency of 1.4 % (1:71) among healthy individuals in the Rhein-Main area, the highest prevalence of apo B-100 (arg^{3500}→gln) reported so far.

Functional studies revealed that binding, uptake and degradation of apo B-100 (arg^{3500}→trp) was lower than normal, but higher compared to apo B-100 (arg^{3500}→gln). This stands in contrast to results by Gaffney and colleagues (15) who found no difference between the two apo B-100 variants affecting codon 3500. The observation of higher binding and uptake of apo B-100 (arg^{3500}→trp) compared to apo B-100 (arg^{3500}→gln) suggests that the substitution of trp^{3500} for arg may cause less severe reduction in binding than the substitution of gln. Another interesting observation was made in individuals heterozygous for apo B-100 (glu^{3405}→gln). LDL from these subjects bound to LDL receptors normally, but were taken up and degraded at significantly reduced rates, suggesting that domains of apo B-100 involved in binding and uptake do not completely overlap. Together, these data indicate that FDB is more heterogeneous on the molecular level than previously assumed and that diagnostic approaches solely designed for detecting of apo B-100 (arg^{3500}→gln) will clearly underestimate the frequency of this disorder.

We and others identified homozygous FDB patients (14, 37, 40, 43). Hypercholesterolemia was less severe in these subjects as compared to patients homozygous for FH in whom the LDL receptor is defective. We studied the receptor mediated endocytosis of LDL from a homozygous FDB patient in normal cultured human skin fibroblasts (37). Binding, internalization, and degradation of FDB-LDL (1.019 to 1.063 kg/l) was diminished, but not completely abolished. We noticed that this was due to the presence of multiple subfractions of LDL which markedly differed with regard to their receptor binding. The small dense LDL subfractions (densities above 1.040 kg/l) of our homozygous patient were completely defective in binding. In contrast, the cellular uptake of buoyant LDL (1.019 to 1.034 kg/l) was normal, due to the presence apo E on the surface of these particles. Consistently, only the binding-defective small dense LDL, but not the buoyant LDL accumulated in the plasma of this patient (37). Using a stable isotope labeling technique, we studied the turnover *in vivo* of lipoproteins in the fasting state in our FDB homozygous patient and in clinically healthy, normolipidemic individuals not carrying the FDB mutation (56). The

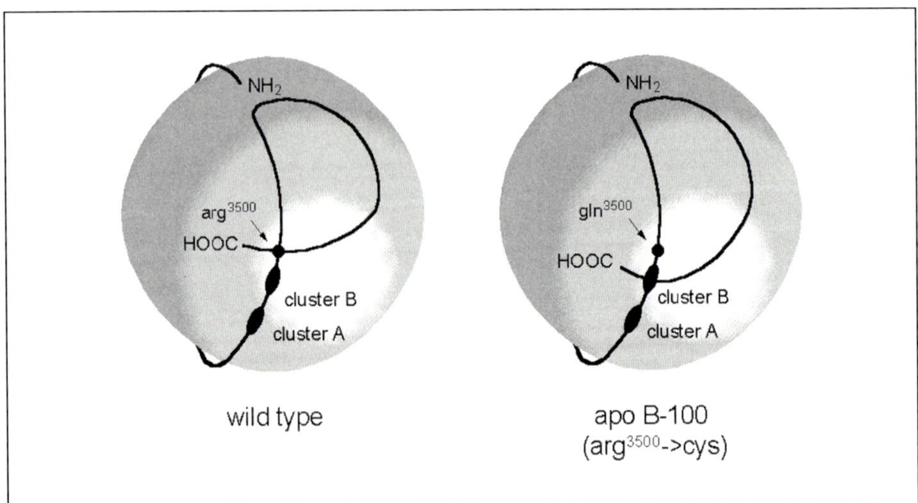

Fig. 4. Proposed model of the role of arg^{3500} in modulating the binding of LDL to LDL-r. The receptor binding domain of apo B-100 contains two clusters, A (3147-3157) and B (3359-3367), of basic amino acid residues. The carboxyterminus of apo B-100 forms a loop which is normally immobilized by interacting with arg^{3500}. If arg^{3500} is replaced by glutamine or tyrosine, the carboxyterminal portion of apo B-100 is detached from residue 3500 and may then mask cluster B, thus hindering it to interact with the LDL-r.

residence time of LDL apo B-100 was prolonged 3.6-fold in homozygous FDB, but the production rate of LDL apo B-100 was decreased compared to normal. These data clearly show that the *in vivo* metabolism of apo B-100 containing lipoproteins in FDB is different from that in FH: In both conditions the residence times of LDL apo B-100 appears increased at approximately the same degree, but LDL production is increased in FH and decreased in FDB. Most likely, the decreased production of LDL apo B-100 in FDB resulted from an enhanced removal of apo E containing LDL precursors by LDL-r which may be up-regulated in response to the decreased flux of LDL derived cholesterol into hepatocytes. Apo E thus partially compensates for the defective binding of apo B-100 in FDB.

The discovery of familial defective apo B-100 (FDB) has significantly enhanced the understanding of the molecular interaction between apo B-100 and the LDL receptor (24, 59). In the current model of the apo B-100 receptor binding domain two clusters A (3147–3157) and B (3359–3367) of basic amino acids, which are linked through a disulfide bond between residues 3167 and 3297, are thought to mediate the binding to the LDL-r. Arg^{3500} is not directly involved in receptor binding. According to very recent work, the carboxyterminus of apo B-100 is able to diminish receptor binding by forming a loop covering cluster B of basic amino acids. By interacting with the carboxyterminal loop, arg^{3500} is able to immobilize the tail of apo B-100, thus, unmasking cluster B. Substitution of arg^{3500} for glutamine or tyrosine disrupts this interaction and allows the apo B-100 carboxyterminus to camouflage cluster B (Fig. 4). It is consistent with this model that apo B-100 ($arg^{3500}{\rightarrow}gln$) still possesses some residual receptor binding which may be mediated by the basic cluster A (37).

Genetic variants of apolipoprotein E affecting LDL and triglyceride metabolism

Apolipoprotein (apo) E is a glycoprotein of 34 kDa. In plasma, it is associated with triglyceride-rich lipoproteins and high density lipoproteins (35). Apo E serves as a ligand of members of the LDL-r gene family including the LDL-r, LRP (2), VLDL-r (61), apo E-r2 (26), and LR11 (70).

More than 90 % of the circulating apo E is derived from the liver (39). Beyond this, apo E is expressed in a variety of other tissues and organs including macrophages and macrophage-like cell lines, in specific cells of the adrenal, in the ovary, keratinocytes, and smooth muscle cells.

The most extensively studied function of apo E is to mediate the uptake of chylomicron and VLDL remnants into the liver. Apo E also promotes the efflux of cholesterol from non-hepatic cells (23) and may mediate the transfer of HDL cholesterol into hepatocytes. Apart from its roles in transporting lipids, apo E has been attributed endocrine or paracrine functions. Among these are the modulation of cellular immune responses, the inhibition of the platelet aggregation and the regulation of the production of steroid hormones.

Apo E is polymorphic in sequence. In humans, there are three common alleles designated ε2, ε3, ε4 at the apo E locus, giving rise to three homozygous and three heterozygous genotypes (Fig. 5). The apo E isoforms differ from one another at positions 112 and 158 of the amino acid sequence (35). Apo E3, the most frequent isoform, has arginine at position 112 and cysteine at position 158. Apo E4 has arginine, and apo E2 has cysteine at both posi-

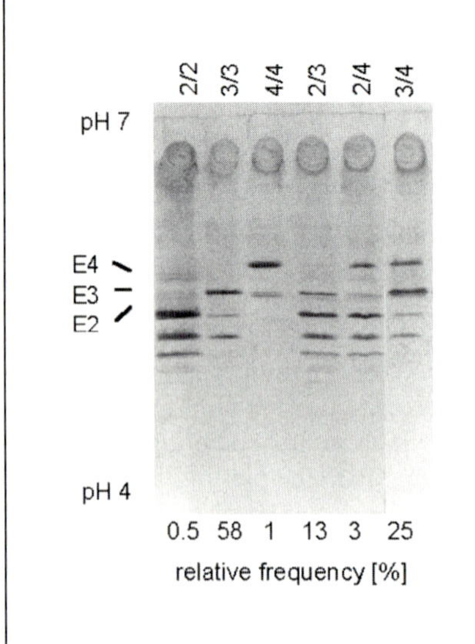

Fig. 5. Demonstration of the apo E polymorphism by iso-electric focusing and immunoblotting. There are three frequent alleles at the apo E locus: $\varepsilon2$, $\varepsilon3$ and $\varepsilon4$ giving rise to three homozgygous (E2/2, E3/3, E4/4) and three heterozygous (E2/3, E2/4, E3/4) phenotypes. The minor bands migrating anodically to the major apo E isoforms are due to post-translational modification of apo E with sialic acid.

tions. Apo E4 is the ancestral allele (19); apo E2 and apo E3 arose after the split of the human and chimpanzee lineages. Thus, evolutionary pressure could have favored apo E3. Consistently, men homozygous for apo E3 appear to be significantly more fertile than those with the other common genotypes (16).

Apo E4 is associated with elevated LDL concentrations. The prevalence of an E4 allele increases both the risk of artherosclerosis and Alzheimer's disease (8, 53). One of the functional differences between apo E4 and apo E3 is that apo E4 (arginine at residue 112) preferentially associates with VLDL, whereas apo E3 (cysteine at 112) associates with HDL. The region of apo E which is responsible for binding to lipids resides in the carboxyterminus of the molecule. How does then the replacement of arginine for cysteine at position 112 modify the lipid binding of apo E? In apo E3, glutamic acid 109 forms a salt bridge with arginine 61. In apo E4, this salt bridge is replaced by a salt bridge between glutamic acid 109 and arginine 112. This enables the arginine 61 side chain to interact with glutamic acid 255 in the carboxyl-terminal lipid-binding domain and is believed to direct the binding of apo E4 to VLDL (11).

The polymorphism of apo E affects the concentration of LDL by modifying the expression of hepatic LDL-r. By virtue of its preferential association with triglyceride-rich lipoproteins, apo E4 enhances the catabolism of remnants. Consequently, hepatic LDL receptors are down-regulated and LDL plasma levels increase.

The $\varepsilon2$ allele exerts an opposite effect on lipoprotein levels. Apo E2 is defective in binding to lipoprotein receptors (28, 57). This is unexpected as the site of the sequence difference between apo E2 and apo E3 (residue 158) is remote from the cluster of positively charged amino acids considered to constitute the LDL-r binding domain of apo E (residues 136 through 150) (28). The replacement of arginine at position 158 by cysteine disrupts a salt bridge between residue 158 and asparagine at position 154. As a consequence, a new salt bridge occurs between asparagine 154 and arginine 150. Ultimately, this shifts arginine 150 out of the receptor binding domain (10).

As mentioned, the clearance of chylomicrons and VLDL remnants depends on functional apo E. As a consequence of the defective binding of apo E2 to lipoprotein receptors, homozygotes for apo E2 accumulate remnant particles in their circulation. This decreases the flux of dietary cholesterol into the liver, up-regulates hepatic LDL-r, and lowers LDL cholesterol. Ultimately, apo E2 may, thus, confer protection against the development of vascular disease.

For yet unknown reasons, however, a small proportion of the apo E2/2 homozygotes develops type III hyperlipoproteinemia, a disorder characterized by the accumulation of excessive amounts of cholesterol-rich remnant lipoproteins derived from the partial catabolism of chylomicrons and very low density lipoproteins (63). Homozygosity for apo E2 is necessary, but not sufficient by itself to precipitate type III hyperlipoproteinemia (HLP). Nine out of ten patients with type III HLP are homozygous for apo E2, but only about one in 20 individuals carrying the E2/2 phenotype finally develops type III HLP. This has led to the suggestion that further factors, genetic, metabolic, or environmental, are required for the phenotypic expression of type III HLP (63).

Rare apo E variants have been identified. Some of these variants have been associated with the dominant expression of type III hyperlipoproteinemia. This form of type III HLP is considered to have a high degree of penetrance. To date, the dominant variants of apo E (Table 2) include apo E3-Leiden, apo E2 (lys^{146}→gln), apo E3 (cys^{112}→arg, arg^{142}→cys),

Table 2. Apolipoprotein E variants

	position	codon change	clinical phenotype	Reference
common variants				
E2	158	arg→cys	Typ III HLP - r	50, 51
E3			wild type	51, 66
E4	112	cys→arg	HC, CAD	46, 66
			Alzheimer's disease	
apo E variants associated with type III HLP				
E0	nt 3592	A→G	type III HLP - r	9
		(donor splice site)		
E0[1]	nt 2919, 2920, 2921	del G	type III HLP - r	9
E0[2]	nt? del 10		type III HLP - r	9
E0	20	trp→stop	type III HLP - r	[3]
E3-Leiden	112	cys→arg	type III HLP - d	9
	121–127	seven amino acids		
		tandem duplication		
E1-Hammersmith	146	lys→asn	type III HLP - d	22
	147	arg→trp		
E1	127	gly→asp	type III HLP - r	9
	158	arg→cys		
E1-Harrisburg	146	lys→glu	type III HLP - d	9
E1	142	arg→leu	type III HLP - u	52
	158	arg→cys		
E2-Christchurch	136	arg→ser	type III HLP - u	9
E2	136	arg→cys	type III HLP - r	38
E2-Fukuoka	224	arg→gln	type III HLP - u	9
E2	145	arg→cys	type III HLP - u	9
E2	146	lys→gln	type III HLP - d	9
E3-Washington	210	trp→stop	type III HLP - r	9
E3	112	cys→arg	type III HLP - d	9
	142	arg→cys		
E3-Kochi	145	arg→his	type III HLP - u	60
E4-Philadelphia	13	glu→lys	type III HLP - d	9
	145	arg→cys		
Apo E4-Fridingen	93–97	*inframe* Deletion	Typ III HLP- d	[3]
			amyloidosis	

Table 2. Continued

	position	codon change	clinical phenotype	Reference
variants associated with other types of hyperlipoproteinemia				
E1	158	arg→cys	hypercholesterolemia	9
	252	leu→glu		
Apo E1-Baden	180	arg→cys	hypertriglyceridemia	3
E2	236	val→glu	hypertriglyceridemia	9
E2-Dunedin	228	arg→cys	hypertriglyceridemia	9
E3	112	cys→arg	hypertriglyceridemia	9
	251	arg→gly		
E4-Freiburg	28	Leu→Pro	low HDL cholesterol	45
E5	3	glu→lys	hypercholesterolemia	9
E5	13	glu→lys	hypercholesterolemia	9
			hypertriglyceridemia	
E5-Frankfurt	81	gln→lys	hypercholesterolemia	54
E5-Heidelberg	212	glu→lys	hypertriglyceridemia?	13
E7-Suita	224	glu→lys	hypercholesterolemia	9
	245	glu→lys	hypertriglyceridemia	
variants not associated with hyperlipidemia				
E2	134	arg→gln	normal	9
E2	213	arg→tyr	normal	4
E3	46	gln→his	normal	4
E3	99	ala→thr	normal	9
	152	ala→pro		
E3-Freiburg	42	thr→ala	normal	69
E3	112	cys→arg	normal	9
	274	arg→his		
E4	296	ser→arg	normal	9
E5-Madgeburg	66	Glu→Lys	normal	3
E5	84	pro→arg	normal	9

[1] the exact position of the G deletion could not be established due to the occurrence of three G as the last nucleotide of codon 30 and the first two nucleotides of codon 31. Codon 30 remains unchanged, codons 31 through 59 all differ from the original sequence due to the frameshift which produces a stop at codon 60.

[2] a 10 bp deletion leads to a loss of codons 209 through 212, the subsequent codons all differ from the wild-type sequence, codon 229 is converted into stop codon.

[3] Hoffmann, M.M, not published

[4] Funke, H, not published

apo E4 (glu[13]→lys, arg[145]→cys), apo E2 (arg[145]→cys), apo E1 (lys[146]→glu), apo E1 (lys[146]→asn, arg[147]→trp), and apo E4-Fridingen, an in frame deletion of amino acid residues 93 through 97 recently identified by our group (Hoffmann M.M. et al., not published). With the exception of apo E3-Leiden and apo E4-Fridingen, the dominant apo E variants involve substitutions of the basic residues at positions 142, 145, 146, and 147. These amino acids are all located within the first heparin binding domain of the apo E molecule which extends from residues 142 through 147 (67). Thus, the apo E variants conferring dominant type III HLP appear to differ from apo E2 in that they exhibit reduced binding to cell surface HSPG (25, 36), whereas apo E2 (Arg[158]→cys) possesses significant residual heparin binding (25, 36).

The importance of impaired binding to heparin to the expression of dominant type III HLP is underscored by a recent investigation of apo E2 (arg[136]→cys) from our laboratory (38). Site-specific mutagenesis studies have implicated arg[136] of wild type apo E in LDL receptor binding; conversion of arg[136] to ser resulted in approximately 60 % decrease in

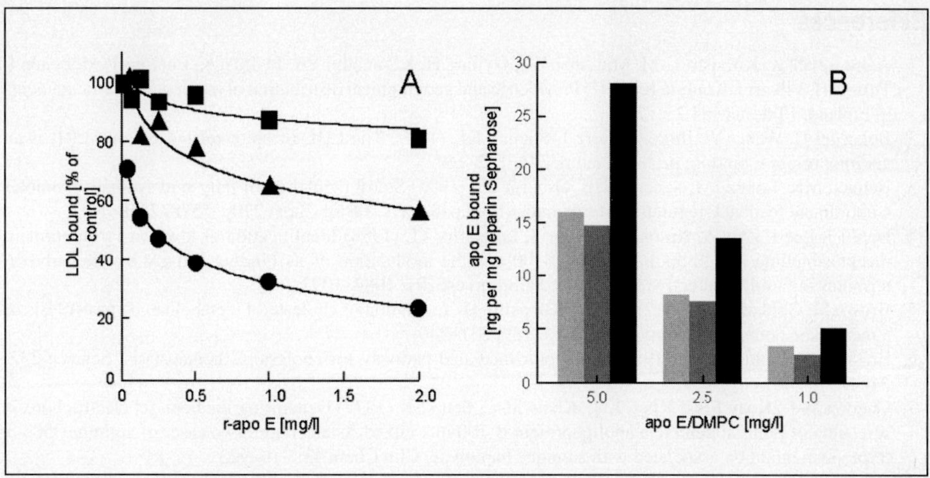

Fig. 6. Receptor (panel A) and heparin (panel B) binding of recombinant apo E2 (Arg[136]→Cys), apo E2 (Arg[158]→Cys), and apo E3 incorporated into DMPC complexes. Panel A: Normal human skin fibroblasts were grown in 24-well polystyrene plates and incubated for 40 hours with medium containing 10 % (v/v) human lipo-protein-deficient serum. The cells then received 5 mg/l ^{125}I-labeled LDL and apo E-DMPC complexes as competitors at apo E concentrations indicated on the abscissa for 1 h at 4 °C. Each data point represents the aver-age of two experiments, each performed in triplicate. Triangles: apo E2 (Arg[136]→Cys); squares: apo E2 (Arg[158]→Cys); circles: apo E3. Panel B: Heparin binding of apoE3 (solid bars), apoE2 (Arg[158]→Cys) (dark grey bars), and apo E2 (Arg[136]→Cys) (light grey bars). Recombinant ^{125}I-labeled apo E was incorporated into DMPC vesicles and incubated at the indicated apo E concentrations with heparin Sepharose or Sepharose, respectively. All incubations were performed in triplicate; results were corrected for binding to Sepharose alone and expressed as ng apo E per mg heparin Sepharose.

LDL receptor binding (28). As arg[136] lies outside the putative heparin binding domain of apo E, point mutations at this site would be supposed to result in recessive apo E variants. However, this has been controversial. Three point mutations affecting codon 136 of mature apo E have been described: apo E2-Christchurch (arg[136]→ser) (65), apo E3 (arg[136]→his) (42), and apo E2 (arg[136]→cys) (64). Apo E3 (arg[136]→his) is apparently not associated with dominant type III HLP (42). Both apo E2-Christchurch (arg[136]→ser) and apo E2 (arg[136]→cys) have been linked to incomplete, late-onset dominance of type III HLP (12, 47). Walden et al. (64), in contrast, identified four carriers of apo E2 (arg[136]→cys), one apo E2 (arg[136]→cys)/3 heterozygote and three apo E2 (arg[136]→cys)/2 (arg[158]→cys) heterozygotes; only one of them, a 39-year-old, obese apo E2 (Arg[136]→cys)/2 (arg[158]→cys) heterozygote, presented with type III HLP. Hence, these investigators concluded that apo E2 (arg[136]→cys) contributed to type III HLP in a recessive rather than in a dominant fashion.

We studied four apo E2 (Arg[136]→Cys)/3 heterozygotes 38. Two of them exhibited type IV hyperlipidemia and two had normal lipid concentrations. LDL receptor binding activities were studied using recombinant apo E loaded to dimyristoylphosphatidylcholine (DMPC) vesicles and to VLDL and from an apo E-deficient individual (Fig. 6). LDL receptor binding of apo E2 (arg[136]→cys) was 14 % of apo E3 and was, thus, higher than that of apo E2 (arg[158]→cys). Both apo E2 (arg[136]→cys) and apo E2 (arg[158]→cys) displayed substantial heparin binding (61 and 53 % of apo E3, respectively) which is in line with the clinical finding that none of the heterozygous carriers of apo E2 (Arg[136]→cys) presented with type III HLP in our study. Our observations further suggest that mutations within the receptor binding domain of apo E will not give rise to dominant type III HLP as long as they do not compromise the interaction of apo E with HSPG of the cell surface.

References

1. Aalto-Setälä K, Koivisto U-M, Miettinen TA, Gylling H, Keseniämi YA, Pyörälä K, Ebeling T, Mononen I, Turtola H, Viikari J, Kontula K (1992) Prevalence and geographical distribution of major gene rearrangements in Finland. J Intern Med 231: 227
2. Beisiegel U, Weber W, Ihrke G, Herz J, Stanley KK (1989) The LDL-receptor-related-protein, LRP, is an apolipoprotein E binding protein. Nature 341: 162–164
3. Bennett MK, Lopez JM, Sanchez HB, Osborne TF (1995) Sterol regulation of fatty acid synthase promoter – coordinate feedback regulation of two major lipid pathways. J Biol Chem 270: 25578–25583
4. Borén J, Lee I, Zhu W, Arnold K, Taylor S, Innerarity TL (1988) Identification of low density lipoprotein receptor-binding site in apolipoprotein B100 and the modulation of its binding activity by the carboxyl terminus in familial defective apo B-100. J Clin Invest 101: 1084–1093
5. Brown M, Goldstein JL (1997) The SREBP pathway: regulation of cholesterol metabolism by proteolysis of a membrane bound transcription factor. Cell 89: 331–340
6. Brown MS, Goldstein JL (1986) A receptor mediated pathway for cholesterol homeostasis. Science 232: 34–47
7. Choong M-L, Koay ESC, Khoo K-L, Khaw M-C, Sethi SK (1997) Denaturing gradient-gel electrophoresis screening of familial defective apolipoprotein B-100 in a mixed Asian cohort: two cases of arginine 3500-> tryptophan mutation associated with a unique haplotype. Clin Chem 43: 916–923
8. Davignon J, Gregg RE, Sing CF (1988) Apolipoprotein E polymorphism and atherosclerosis. Arteriosclerosis 8: 1–21
9. de Knijff P, van den Maagdenberg AMJM, Frants RR, Havekes LM (1994) Genetic heterogeneity of apolipoprotein E and its influence on plasma lipid and lipoprotein levels. Hum Mut 4: 178–194
10. Dong LM, Parkin S, Trakhanov SD, Rupp B, Simmons T, Arnold KS, Newhouse YM, Innerarity TL, Weisgraber KH (1996) Novel mechanism for defective binding of apolipoprotein E2 in type III hyperlipoproteinemia. Nat Struct Biol 3: 718–722
11. Dong LM, Weisgraber KH (1996) Human apolipoprotein E4 domain interaction. Arginine 61 and glutamic acid 255 interact to direct the preference for very low density lipoproteins. J Biol Chem 271: 19053–19057
12. Feussner G, Albanese M, Mann WA, Valencia A, Schuster H (1996) Apolipoprotein E2 (Arg136Cys), a variant of apolipoprotein E associated with late-onset dominance of type III hyperlipoproteinemia. Eur J Clin Invest 1996: 13–23
13. Feussner G, Scharnagl H, Scherbaum C, Acar J, Dobmeyer J, Lohrmann J, Wieland H, März W (1996) Apolipoprotein E5-Heidelberg (Glu212Lys): Increased binding to cell surface proteoglycans, but decreased uptake and degradation in cultured fibroblasts. J Lipid Res 37: 1632–1645
14. Funke H, Rust S, Seedorf U, Brennhausen B, Chirazi A, Motti C, Assmann G (1992) Hozygosity for familial defective apolipoprotein B-100 (FDB) is associated with lower plasma cholesterol concentrations than homozygosity for familial hypercholesterolemia (FH). Circulation 86 (Suppl I): I-691
15. Gaffney D, Reid JM, Cameron IM, Vass K, Caslake MJ, Shepherd J, Packard CJ (1995) Independent mutations at codon 3500 of the apolipoprotein B gene are associated with hyperlipidemia. Arterioscler Thromb Vasc Biol 15: 1025–1029
16. Gerdes LU, Gerdes C, Hansen PS, Klausen IC, Faergeman O (1996) Are men carrying the apolipoprotein epsilon 4- or epsilon 2 allele less fertile than epsilon 3 epsilon 3 genotypes? Hum Genet 98: 239–242
17. Goldstein JL, Brown MS (1990) Regulation of the mevalonate pathway. Nature 343: 425–430
18. Goldstein JL, Hobbs HH, Brown MS (1995) Familial hypercholesterolemia. In: Scriver CR, Beaudet AL, Sly WS, Valle D (eds) The Metabolic Basis and Molecular Basis of Inherited Diasease. Vol. I. McGraw Hill Book Co., Orlando, pp 1981–2030
19. Hanlon CS, Rubinsztein DC (1995) Arginine residues at codons 112 and 158 in the apolipoprotein E gene correspond to the ancestral state in humans. Athersosclerosis 112: 85–90
20. Herz J, Hamann U, Rogne S, Myklebost O, Gausepohl H, Stanley KK (1988) Surface location and high affinity for calcium of a 500 kD liver membrane protein closely related to the LDL-receptor suggest a physiological role as lipoprotein receptor. EMBO J 7: 4119–4127
21. Hobbs HH, Brown MS, Goldstein JL (1992) Molecular genetics of the LDL receptor gene in familial hypercholesterolemia. Hum Mutat 1: 445–466
22. Hoffer MJ, Niththyananthn S, Naoumova RP, Kibirige MS, Frants RR, Havekes LM, Thompson GR (1996) Apolipoprotein E1-Hammersmith (Lys146→Asn, Arg147→Trp), due to a dinucleotide substitution, is associated with early manifestation of dominant type III hyperlipoproteinemia. Atherosclerosis 124: 183–189
23. Huang Y, von Eckardstein A, Wu S, Maeda N, Assmann G (1994) A plasma lipoprotein containing only apo E and with gamma-mobility on electrophoresis releases cholesterol from cells. Proc Natl Acad Sci USA 91: 1834–1838
24. Innerarity TL, Weisgraber KH, Arnold KS, Mahley RW, Krauss RM, Vega GL, Grundy SM (1987) Familial defective apolipoprotein B-100: Low density lipoproteins with abnormal receptor binding. Proc Natl Acad Sci USA 84: 6919–6923

25. Ji Z-S, Fazio S, Mahley RW (1994) Variable heparan sulfate proteoglycan binding of apolipoprotein E variants may modulate the expression of type III hyperlipoproteinemia. J Biol Chem 269: 13421–13428

26. Kim DH, Iijma H, Goto K, Sakai J, Ishii H, Kim HJ, Suzuki H, Kondo H, Saeki S, Yamamoto T (1996) Human apolipoprotein E receptor 2. J Biol Chem 271: 8373–8380

27. Knott T, Rall SC, Innerarity TL, Jacobson SF, Urdea MS, Levy-Wilson B, Powell LM, Pease RJ, Eddy R, Nakai H, Byers M, Priestly LM, Robertson E, Rall LB, Betsholtz C, Shows TB, Mahley RW, Scott J (1985) Human apolipoprotein B: structure of carboxyl-terminal domains, sites of gene expression, and chromosomal localization. Science 230: 37–43

28. Lalazar A, Weisgraber KH, Rall SC, Giladi H, Innerarity TL, Levanon AZ, Boyles JK, Amit B, Gorecki M, Mahley RW, Vogel T (1988) Site-specific mutagenesis of human apolipoprotein E. Receptor binding activity of variants with single amino acid substitutions. J Biol Chem 263: 3542–3545

29. Lehrman MA, Schneider WJ, Brown MS, Davis CG, Elhammer A, Russel DW, Goldstein JL (1987) The Lebanese allele at the low density lipoprotein receptor locus. Nonsense mutation produces truncated receptor that is retained in endoplasmic reticulum. J Biol Chem 262: 401–410

30. Leitersdorf AK, Van Der Westhuyzen DR, Coetzee GA, Hobbs HH (1989) Two common low density lipoprotein receptor gene mutations cause familial hypercholesterolemia in Afrikaners. J Clin Invest 84: 954

31. Leitersdorf E, Reshef A, Meiner V, Dann EJ, Beigel Y, van Roggen FG, van der Westhuyzen DR, Coetzee GA (1993) A missense mutation in the low density lipoprotein receptor gene causes familial hypercholesterolemia in Sephardic Jews. Hum Genet 91: 141

32. Leitersdorf E, Tobin EJ, Davignon J, Hobbs HH (1990) Common low-density lipoprotein receptor mutations in the French Canadian population. J Clin Invest 84: 1014

33. Lopez JM, Bennet MK, Sanchez HB, Rosenfeld JM, Osborne TF (1996) Sterol regulation of acetyl CoA carboxylase: a mechanism for coordinate control of cellular lipid. Proc Natl Acad Sci USA 93: 1049–1053

34. Ludwig EH, Hopkins PN, Allen A, Wu LL, Williams RR, Anderson JL, Ward RH, Lalouel J-M, Innerarity TL (1997) Association of genetic variations in apolipoprotein B with hypercholesterolemia, coronary artery disease, and receptor binding of low density lipoproteins. J Lipid Res 38: 1361–1373

35. Mahley RW (1988) Apolipoprotein E: Cholesterol transport protein with expanding role in cell biology. Science 240: 622–630

36. Mann WA, Meyer N, Weber W, Meyer S, Greten H, Beisiegel U (1995) Apolipoprotein E isoforms and rare mutations: parallel reduction in binding to cells an to heparin reflects severity of associated type III hyperlipoproteinemia. J Lipid Res 36: 517–525

37. März W, Baumstark MW, Scharnagl H, Ruzicka V, Buxbaum S, Herwig J, Pohl T, Russ A, Schaaf L, Berg A, Böhles H-J, Usadel KH, Groß W (1993) Accumulation of "small dense" low density lipoproteins in a homozygous patient with familial defective apolipoprotein B-100 results from heterogenous interaction of LDL-subfractions with the LDL receptor. J Clin Invest 92: 2922–2933

38. März W, Hoffmann MM, Scharnagl H, Fisher E, Chen M, Nauck MS, Feussner G, Wieland H (1998) Apolipoprotein E2 (Arg136→Cys) mutation in the receptor binding domain of apo E is not associated with dominant type III hyperlipoproteinemia. J Lipid Res 39: 658–669

39. März W, Peschke B, Ruzicka V, Siekmeier R, Groß W, Scheuermann E (1993) Type III hyperlipoproteinemia acquired by by liver transplantation. Transplantation 55: 284–288

40. März W, Ruzicka V, Pohl T, Usadel KH, Groß W (1992) Familial defective apolipoprotein B-100: mild hypercholesterolemia without atherosclerosis in a homozygous patient. Lancet 340: 1362

41. Medh JD, Bowen SL, Fry GL, Ruben S, Andracki M, Inoue I, Lalouel JM, Strickland DK, Chappel DA (1996) Lipoprotein lipase binds to low density lipoprotein receptors and induces receptor-mediated catabolism of very low density lipoproteins in vitro. J Biol Chem 271: 17073–17080

42. Minnich A, Weisgraber KH, Newhouse Y, Dong L-M, Fortin L-J, Tremblay M, Davignon J (1995) Identification and characterization of a novel apolipoprotein E variant, apolipoprotein E3' (Arg136→His): Association with mild dyslipidemia and double pre-β very low density lipoproteins. J Lipid Res 36: 57–66

43. Myant NB (1993) Familial defective apolipoprotein B-100: a review, including some comparisons with familial hypercholesterolaemia. Atherosclerosis 104: 1–18

44. Nissen H, Guldberg P, Hansen AB, Petersen NE, Horder M (1996) Clinically applicable mutation screening in familial hypercholesterolemia. Hum Mutat 8: 168–177

45. Orth M, Wei W, Funke H, Steinmetz A, Assmann G, Nauck M, Dierkes J, Ambrosch A, Weisgraber KH, Mahley RW, Wieland H, Luley C (1999) Effects of a frequent apolipoprotein E isoform, apo E4-Freiburg (Leu28→Pro) on lipoproteins and the prevalence of coronary artery disease in Caucasians. Arterioscler Thromb Vasc Biol (in press)

46. Paik YK, Chang DJ, Reardon CA, Davies GE, Mahley RW, Taylor JM (1985) Nucleotide sequence and structure of the human apolipoproteion E gene. Proc Natl Acad Sci USA 82: 3445–3449

47. Pocovi M, Cenarro A, Civeira F, Myers RH, Casao E, Esteban M, Ordovas JM (1996) Incomplete dominance of type III hyperlipoproteinemia is associated with the rare apolipoprotein E2 (Arg136→Ser) variant in multigenerational pedigree studies. Atherosclerosis 122: 33–46

48. Pullinger CR, Hennessy LK, Chatterton JE, Liu W, Love JA, Mendel CM, Frost PH, Malloy MJ, Schumaker VN, Kane JP (1995) Familial ligand-defective apolipoprotein B. Identification of a new mutation that decreases LDL receptor binding affinity. J Clin Invest 95: 1225–1234

49. Rabes JP, Varret M, Saint-Jore B, Erlich D, Jondeau G, Krempf M, Giraudet P, Junien C, Boileau C (1997) Familial ligand-defective apolipoprotein B-100: simultaneous detection of the Arg3500→Gln and Arg3531→Cys mutations in a French population. Hum Mut 10: 160–163

50. Rall SC, Weisgraber KH, Innerarity TL, Mahley RW (1982) Structural basis for receptor binding heterogeneity of apolipoprotein E from type III hyperlipoproteinemic subjects. Proc Natl Acad Sci USA 79: 4696–4700

51. Rall SC, Weisgraber KH, Mahley RW (1982) Human Apolipoprotein E. The complete amino acid sequence. J Biol Chem 257: 4171–4178

52. Richard P, Thomas G, de Zulueta MP, De Gennes J-L, Thomas M, Cassaigne A, Béréziat G, Iron A (1994) Common and rare genotypes of human apolipoprotein Ev determined by specific restriction profiles of polymerase chain reaction-amplified DNA. Clin Chem 40: 24–29

53. Roses AD (1997) Apolipoprotein E, a gene with complex biological interactions in the aging brain. Neurobiol Dis 4: 170–185

54. Ruzicka V, März W, Russ A, Mondorf W, Groß W (1993) Characterization of the gene for apolipoprotein E5-Frankfurt (Gln81→Lys, Cys112→Arg by polymerase chain reaction, restriction isotyping and temperature gradient gel electrophoresis. Electrophoresis, Electrophoresis 14: 1032–1037

55. Saito A, Pietromonaca S, Kwor-chie Loo A, Farquhar M (1994) Complete cloning and sequencing of rat gp330/'megalin', a distinctive member of the low density lipoprotein receptor gene family. Proc Natl Acad Sci USA 91: 9725–9729

56. Schäfer J, Scharnagl H, Baumstark M, Steinmetz A, Schweer H, Zech LA, Seyberth HJ, März W (1997) Homozygous familial defective apolipoprotein B-100: Enhanced removal of apolipoprotein E containing low density lipoprotein precursors and decreased production of low density lipoproteins. Arterioscler Thromb Vasc Biol 17: 348–353

57. Schneider WJ, Kovanen PT, Brown MS, Goldstein JL, Utermann G, Weber W, Havel RJ, Kotite L, Kane JP, Innerarity TL, Mahley RW (1981) Familial dysbetalipoproteinemia: Abnormal binding of mutant apolipoprotein E to low density lipoprotein receptors of human fibroblasts and membranes from liver and adrenals of rats, rabbits and cows. J Clin Invest 68: 1075–1085

58. Scott J (1995) A place in the world for RNA editing. Cell 81: 833–836

59. Soria LF, Ludwig EH, Clarke HRG, Vega GL, Grundy SM, McCarthy BJ (1989) Association between a specific apolipoprotein B mutation and familial defective apolipoprotein B-100. Proc Natl Acad Sci USA 86: 587–591

60. Suehiro T, Yoshida K, Yamano T, Ohno F (1990) Identification and characterization of a new variant of apolipoprotein E (apoE-Kochi). Jpn J Med 29: 587–594

61. Takahashi S, Kawabayasi Y, Nakai T, Sakai J, Yamamoto T (1992) Rabbit very low density lipoprotein receptor; A low density lipoprotein receptor like protein with distinct ligand specificity. Proc Natl Acad Sci USA 89: 9252–9256

62. Teng B, Burant CF, Davidson NO (1993) Molecular cloning of the apolipoprotein B mRNA editing protein. Science 260: 1816–1819

63. Utermann G, Hees M, Steinmetz A (1977) Polymorphism of apolipoprotein E and occurrence of dysbetalipoproteinaemia in man. Nature 269: 604–607

64. Walden CC, Huff MW, Leiter LA, Connelly PW, Hegele RA (1994) Detection of a new apolipoprotein-E mutation in type III hyperlipoproteinemia using deoxyribonucleic acid restriction typing. J Clin Endorinol Metab 78: 699–704

65. Wardell MR, Brennan SO, Janus ED, Fraser R, Carrel RW (1987) Apolipoprotein E2-Christchurch (136Arg→Ser). New variant of human apolipoprotein E in a patient with type III hyperlipoproteinemia. J Clin Invest 80: 483–490

66. Weisgraber KH, Rall SC, Mahley RW (1981) Human E apoprotein heterogeneity. Cysteine arginine interchanges in the amino acid sequence of the apoE isoforms. J Biol Chem 256: 9077–9083

67. Weisgraber KH, Rall SC, Mahley RW, Milne RW, Marcel YL, Sparrow JT (1986) Human apolipoprotein E. Determination of the heparin binding sites of apolipoprotein E3. J Biol Chem 261: 2068–2076

68. Wenham PR, Henderson BG, Penney MD, Ashby JP, Rae PWH, Walker SW (1997) Familial ligand-defective apolipoprotein B-100: detection, biochemical features and haplotype analysis of the R3531C mutation in the UK. Atherosclerosis 129: 185–192

69. Wieland H, Funke H, Krieg J, Luley C (1991) Apo E3-Freiburg and apo E4-Freiburg are two genetic apo E variants which are caused by exchanges of uncharged amino acids and do not appear to be associated with lipid disorders or heart disease. In: Abstract Book of the 9th International Symposium on Atherosclerosis, Rosement IL., p 164
70. Yamazaki H, Bujo H, Kusonoki J, Seimiya K, Kanaki T, Morisaki N, Schneider WJ, Saito Y (1996) Elements of neural adhesion molecules and a yeast vascular protein sorting receptor are present in a novel mammalian low density lipoprotein receptor family member. J Biol Chem 271: 25761–25768

Author's address:
Priv.-Doz. Dr. med. Winfried März
Division of Clinical Chemistry, Department of Medicine
Albert Ludwigs-University
Hugstetter Straße 55
79106 Freiburg im Breisgau (Germany)
E-mail: maerz@mzl200.ukl-freiburg.de

Insulin resistance: A pathogenic link between cardiovascular risk factors and atherosclerosis

D. Müller-Wieland, J. Kotzka, B. Knebel, J. Brüning, W. Krone

Klinik II und Poliklinik für Innere Medizin der Universität zu Köln, Cologne, Germany

Abstract

Patients with insulin resistance and/or type 2 diabetes have a 5-fold increased coronary risk and cardiovascular mortality rate. Therefore, it is a current issue of discussion that arterial hypertension, lipid disorders as well as visceral obesity are coronary risk factors, which might belong to a syndrome that is caused by decreased insulin sensitivity. Insulin resistance is associated with specific alterations of lipid metabolism. Typically there are elevated triglyceride levels and low HDL cholesterol levels. Furthermore, this dyslipoproteinemia is associated with alterations in the composition of LDL particles possibly increasing their atherogenicity. The relation between insulin resistance and arterial hypertension is much more evident in patients with obesity. Recently, a general change in our understanding of the pathogenesis of obesity has emerged, realizing that the fat cell is not only a passive reservoir of triglycerides, but might be active in the synthesis and secretion of endocrine active peptides, e.g., leptin or angiotensinogen. Concerning a possible molecular link between insulin resistance, atherosclerosis and obesity, we focus in our research on questions looking for a molecular link between cholesterol metabolism, insulin action, and obesity.

Sterol regulatory element binding proteins (SREBPs) are transcription factors, which are regulated by the intracellular content of cholesterol. Recently, we could show, that these SREBPs are also modulated by insulin and growth factors like PDGF. Interestingly, one of the SREBPs (SREBP-1c) is identical to the transcription factor called ADD1 (adipocyte differentation determination factor 1). ADD1 plays an essential role in mechanisms linked to adipocyte differentiation. Therefore, these transcription factors might be a gene regulatory convergence point not only for metabolic but also endocrine signals. In an attempt to identify genetic defects of insulin resistance, we have characterized various postreceptor defects of insulin affecting the MAP-kinase cascade. This intracellular signaling cascade couples the insulin receptor to major gene regulatory events including the transcription factors mentioned above. These studies provide evidence that single gene defects in a signaling step affecting various gene regulatory events might be associated with a very complex clinical phenotype.

Introduction

The cardiovascular risk in patients with diabetes mellitus is increased 2- to 5-fold. Haffner et al. (11) have shown recently that diabetic patients without previous myocardial infarction have a similar risk of myocardial infarction as non-diabetic patients with previous myocardial infarction. This study compared the 7-year incidence of fatal and non-fatal myocardial infarction among 1,373 non-diabetic subjects with the incidence among 1,059 diabetic subjects in Finnland. Therefore, it is a current issue of discussion that type 2 diabetes and coronary heart disease have some common predisposing environmental and genetic factors in their pathogenesis. Several recent studies indicate that arterial hypertension, lipid disorders as well as visceral obesity are coronary risk factors, which might belong to a syndrome that is caused by decreased insulin sensitivity with consecutive hyperinsulinaemia. Prospective epidemiological studies in non-diabetic and diabetic patients indicate that hyperinsulinaemia as a marker of insulin resistance is a coronary risk factor. The San Antonio Heart Study (12) has shown prospectively over eight years in more than 1100 non-diabetic, normotensive, non-obese individuals that probands with high plasma insulin levels had a significantly increased incidence of clinical overt hypertension, dyslipidaemia, and diabetes compared to individuals with relatively low plasma insulin levels. These prospective clinical studies support the hypothesis that insulin resistance with hyperinsulinaemia increases the risk of atherosclerosis or macroangiopathy via increased incidence of multiple coronary risk factors. Beside the increased incidence of coronary risk factors associated with decreased insulin sensitivity, other molecular processes with an atherogenic potential might play a role (5), e.g., endothelial dysfunction as well as alterations in the coagulation or fibrinolytic system which might also be directly affected by insulin.

In the following, we will focus first clinical aspects of insulin resistance and dyslipoproteinaemia as well as arterial hypertension and then new molecular mechanisms possibly linking insulin resistance with cellular cholesterol metabolism and obesity.

Dyslipoproteinaemia:
A major feature of insulin resistance

Patients with insulin resistance and/or type 2 diabetes have an 5-fold increased coronary risk and cardiovascular mortality rate. About 60 % of patients with type 2 diabetes have alterations of their plasma lipids, and recently, a subgroup analysis of the 4-S Study (27) showed that treatment of patients with diabetes mellitus and coronary heart disease with a cholesterol synthesis inhibitor can decrease the incidence of severe coronary events over the 5.4 years by more than 50 % (22). In addition the MRFIT Study showed that patients with diabetes mellitus have an increased coronary risk at every plasma cholesterol level (33). One possible explanation for this increased coronary risk is that insulin resistance might aggravate the genetic predisposition for an increased coronary risk and/or be associated with specific plasma lipid alterations. Recently, a Canadian study showed that the extent of coronary stenosis in patients with a genetically defined hypercholesterinaemia, i.e., a heterozygous LDL receptor gene mutation, is increased several fold in patients with additional insulin resistance (10). Furthermore, insulin resistance is associated with specific alterations in lipid metabolism (21). Typically there are elevated plasma triglyceride levels and low HDL cholesterol levels. This dyslipoproteinaemia is associated with alterations in the composition of LDL particles. These LDL particles can be smaller, denser, and are often enriched in triglyceride concentration and can be altered in their apoprotein composition as well as be chemically modified by glycosylation and/or oxidation. These modifications may render the LDL particles with lower affinity for the LDL receptor leading to a prolonged pertinence in the vascular system and being potentially more atherogenic. The alterations in LDL particle composition appear to be associated with already minor increases in plasma triglyceride levels. This means that a LDL cholesterol plasma level might indicate a higher atherogenic risk in a patient with diabetes compared to non-diabetic individuals. Therefore, the American Diabetes Association recommends (1) to aim for LDL cholesterol levels at least below 130 mg/dl in all patients with diabetes mellitus. In patients with clinical overt coronary heart disease and in diabetics with clinical overt coronary heart disease or only one coronary risk factor, LDL values below 100 mg/dl are recommended.

Hypertension and obesity

Ferranini et al. (8) were the first to show that essential hypertension in patients with normal weight is associated with reduced insulin sensitivity. Several other studies have confirmed these findings in about 50 – 70 % of all patients with essential hypertension. The facts that insulin resistance persists despite an effective blood pressure lowering drug treatment and that reduced insulin sensitivity is usually not observed in patients with secondary forms of hypertension indicate that insulin resistance is not only an epiphenomenon but rather an essential pathogenic factor. Some pathophysiological links between insulin resistance and elevated arterial blood pressure might be, for example, an increased sodium and volume retention, an altered peripheral resistance, and an increased activation of the sympathetic nervous system (7, 37).

However, the relation between insulin resistance and arterial hypertension is much more evident in patients with obesity (20, 37). Therefore, the clinical manifestation of arterial hypertension in patients with insulin resistance appears to be greatly affected by additional hemodynamic and pathogenic factors which appear to be related to the extent and especially distribution of adipose tissue. Recently, a general change in our understanding of the pathogenesis of obesity and its clinical relevance was observed. The novel understanding of the fat cell is that these cells are not only a passive reservoir of triglycerides, but might be active in the synthesis and secretion of endocrine active peptides (32). The best example given is the recently identified hormone leptin (9). Alterations in the secretion and action of leptin were observed in various models of obesity with and without diabetes. Leptin appears to act in certain areas of the hypothalamus and stimulates the synthesis of neuropeptide Y. Leptin secretion appears to be elevated in most patients with obesity and is most likely due to leptin resistance and, therefore, associated with increased food intake. There is cumulating speculation that leptin regulates more than only food intake. Several studies are on their way to revealing the relation between leptin resistance and insulin resistance as well as the relation to the activation of the sympathetic adrenergic system, adrenal activity, and hemodynamic vasoregulatory effects. However, leptin appears not to be the only product of fat cells, and other vasogenic peptides are increasingly identified, e.g., tumor necrosis factor α, which can decrease insulin action, and the adipose tissue can generate angiotensinogen which might contribute as a vasoconstrictor to the aterial hypertension observed in obesity and diabetes.

Concerning a possible molecular link between insulin resistance, atherosclerosis and obesity, we focus in our research laboratories on three questions:

▸ Is there a molecular link between cholesterol and insulin affecting gene regulation and thereby cell biology?
▸ Is this molecular link related to obesity?
▸ Are there genetic defects in patients with insulin resistance affecting intracellular signaling cascades coupled to gene regulatory events?

Sterol regulatory element binding proteins (SREBPs) as gene regulatory convergence points of metabolic and endocrine signals

Alterations of cellular cholesterol homeostasis appear to play a major role in the pathogenesis of atherosclerosis. A break through in understanding the cellular cholesterol metabolism was the characterization of the LDL receptor and its mutations in patients with familial hypercholesterolaemia and premature atherosclerosis. In accordance with this, several large prospective clinical trials have shown recently that treatment of patients with (25, 27, 35) and without (6, 28) coronary heart disease with statins to lower plasma cholesterol levels leads to a great reduction of cardiovascular morbidity and mortality. One key question in the understanding of cellular cholesterol homeostasis and statin action is what happens to cell metabolism when intracellular cholesterol concentration is reduced. In this respect a new and broader perspective has been developed by the group of Brown and Goldstein (7). They have identified and characterized a family of cholesterol sensitive transcription factors called SREBPs. These intracellular proteins appear to transmit the signal of membrane-embedded cholesterol level to the nucleus regulating the expression rate of multiple genes. The promoter of the LDL receptor gene contains a sterol regulatory element (sre-1/ATCAC-CCCAC), which is regulated by the intracellular content of sterols. This DNA sequence in the promoter of the LDL receptor gene can bind three transcription factors named SREBP-1a, SREBP-1c, and SREBP-2. These transcription factors are activated by a novel cholesterol regulated proteolytic mechanism that controls the cytosolic release of these proteins and thereby for example the transcription rate of the LDL receptor gene. These transcription factors are localized in the endosplasmatic reticulum. Decrease of intracellular sterol levels can activate protease activity, which cleaves the transcription factors in the endoplasmatic reticulum. The N-terminal domains with the molecular weight of approximately 68 kDa translocate by unknown mechanisms into the nucleus. In the nucleus, the N-terminal activated transcription factors bind to a sterol responsive element not only in the LDL receptor gene but also in many others. Although the sterol sensitive proteolytic processing mechanisms of the SREBPs appear to be unique, some essential features of their structure-function relationship let them belong to the family of basic helix-loop-helix leucine zipper (bHLH-LZ) transcription factors. The basic domain of these proteins regulates DNA binding to a consensus sequence referred to as E-box motif (CANNTG). This latter motif is found in promoters of many genes. Most bHLH-LZ proteins contain an arginine in the basic region restricting protein-DNA interaction to this E-box motif. However, SREBPs uniquely contain a tyrosine at this position instead of an arginine. Thereby, SREBPs have a dual specificity (13), i.e., not only for E-box, but also for sre-1-like elements. Sterol-responsive sre-1-like cis-elements (consensus-sequence: Py-CA-Py; Py: pyrimidine) seem to exist in many more promoters of various genes coding for enzymes involved not only in cholesterol metabolism but also in triglyceride synthesis and possibly others. It has been shown that beside the LDL receptor gene promoter SREBPs can regulate the transcription rate of genes, e.g., coding for the HMG-CoA reductase, HMG-CoA synthase, farnesyl diphosphate synthase, acetyl CoA carboxylase, fatty acid synthase, glycerol-3-phosphate, alcyltransferase (2, 19). Interestingly, the gene of SREBP-2 but not SREBP-1 contains a sterol-responsive regulatory element, so that differential autoregulation of these transcription factors might play a role (26).

The LDL receptor gene is not only regulated by cholesterol, but also by drugs, growth factors, and hormones. It has been shown that insulin and PDGF can induce the number of LDL receptor at the cell surface in hepatic and non-hepatic cells and can elevate the LDL receptor mRNA levels. Recently, we showed that the insulin-induced effect on LDL receptor mRNA levels can even be seen in the presence of LDL cholesterol levels, which completely suppress LDL receptor gene expression (34). This was one indirect evidence that both, intracellular sterol levels and insulin, might have a common convergence point in LDL receptor gene regulation. Further experiments using various 5' deleted and in vitro mutated LDL receptor promoter constructs showed that the insulin sensitive cis-element in the LDL receptor promoter is identical to the sterol sensitive and SREBP-binding cis-element sre-1 (34). Using different pharmacological and cell biological approaches including SREBP-1 and SREBP-2 deficient human hepatoma cell lines, which we generated by antisense techniques as well as recombinant GST fusion proteins, we showed (24) that SREBPs mediate different gene regulatory effects, i.e., not only of cholesterol but also of insulin and that they are coupled to the intracellular MAP-kinase cascade.

SREBP-1c/ADD 1 as a possible link between insulin resistance and obesity

Insulin resistance and obesity are closely related and appear to be associated with glucose intolerance, type 2 diabetes and an increased risk for cardiovascular complications. The major breakthrough in the understanding of the relationship between insulin sensitivity and adipogenesis was the discovery of the peroxisome proliferator-activated receptor (PPAR), a member of the nuclear hormone receptor superfamily (30, 31). PPAR-γ was identified and cloned as a component of an adipocyte differentiation-dependent regulatory factor (ARF6), which binds to the adipose-specific enhancer from the aP2 gene and is an obligate heterodimer with the retinoid X receptor (RXR). PPAR-γ is alternatively spliced at the N-terminus generating two subtypes called PPAR-γ1 and PPAR-γ2. PPAR-γ2 is most abundantly expressed in adipocytes and appears to be a major player in adipocyte differentiation and lipid metabolism. Accordingly, the ectopic expression and activation of PPAR-γ2 leads to a highly significant conversion rate of fibroblastic cell lines to adipocytes (14). Furthermore, PPARs are drug targets for lipid lowering agents like fibrates, and PPAR-γ is the intracellular receptor for the new blood glucose lowering insulin sensitizers called thiazolidinediones (18). We recently identified an inactivating mutation of PPAR-γ2 in unrelated individuals with obesity (23). One essential factor modulating (4, 30) the PPAR activity – also involved in cellular cholesterol metabolism – is the adipocyte determination- and differentiation dependent factor (ADD) 1. ADD-1 was cloned by the group of Spiegelman et al. (36) as an adipogenesis related transcription factor and is the human homologue to the SREBP-1c, involved in cellular cholesterol metabolism as described above. Over-expression of ADD-1/SREBP-1c in fibroblasts (14) of transgenic mice induces lipoprotein lipase and fatty acid synthase. Further studies indicate that ADD-1/SREBP-1c can promote adipocyte differentiation and increase the transcriptional activity of PPAR-γ2. Therefore, ADD-1/SREBP-1c appears to be a key link between cholesterol and lipid metabolism, adipogenesis as well as insulin sensitivity. We recently showed (17) that insulin and PDGF can act via ADD-1/SREBP-1c, which might be phosphorylated and activated by MAP-kinase cascade.

Genetic postreceptor defects affecting the gene regulatory MAP-kinase cascade in patients with inherited syndromes of insulin resistance

The genetic basis of insulin resistance or diabetes and coronary heart disease is very heterogeneous. One reason for this "genetic nightmare" of the metabolic syndrome is that its main components, such as hypertension, dyslipidaemia, obesity, and diabetes, are all fairly arbitrarily defined by certain cut off points of physiological variables, i.e., levels of blood pressure, plasma levels of lipids or blood sugar, and body weight, but not by common essential pathogenetic features. Probably, not a single but a diverse sets of genes determine for example whether the degree and specificity of decreased insulin sensitivity or action leads to clinical detectable blood sugar elevation and/or other features of the metabolic syndrome. Brüning et al. (3) have provided direct evidence for a complex pattern of inheritance by generating a novel polygenic model of NIDDM in mice. Transgenic mice being heterozygous for the null-allele of either IRS-1 or the insulin receptor appears to be insulin resistant, but not diabetic. Crossing these animals to develop animals having a heterozygous null- allele for both proteins leads to insulin resistance with consecutive hyperinsulinaemia and 40 % of these heterozygous mice become overtly diabetic at 4 to 6 months of age. White's group et al. (38) have shown recently that the knock-out of the other insulin receptor substrate (IRS-2) leads to clinical overt diabetes characterized not only by insulin resistance but also by decreased insulin secretion. Clinically, different gene loci have been only identified so far in very well-described subtypes of type 2 diabetes, for example, MODY and diabetes associated with mitochondrial mutations. However, decreased insulin sensitivity affects up to 25 % of the western population and will increase with urbanization in the Asian continent. This means that about 20 million people are affected in Germany and that a genetic defect found in 1 % of patients means that up to 200,000 individuals are affected. Therefore, a relatively "rare" genetic component identified in a disease with very high prevalence, like coronary heart disease or insulin resistance, appears to be "frequent" in absolute terms. Therefore, one major aim of genetic approaches is to provide diagnostic markers to identify high-risk individuals to implement effective individual based prevention.

Different genetic approaches have been undertaken to identify gene loci in multifactorial diseases. One basic genetic approach is to investigate whether patients with inherited forms of insulin resistant diabetes have genetic defects in the signaling molecules involved in insulin action. Then, characterization of these defects will help to understand the physiological significance of this signaling molecule in insulin action, its role in insulin resistance, and provides a novel candidate for genetic analysis in different populations or subtypes of diabetes mellitus. One example for this approach is the characterization of genetic defects in the LDL receptor gene in patients with familial hypercholesterolaemia (29). These studies paved the way to understand the physiological significance of the LDL receptor for cellular cholesterol homeostasis, its role in hypercholesterolaemia, and helped to identify genetic components involved in atherogenesis or coronary heart disease. Therefore, we believe that the molecular characterization of signal transduction defects in patients with genetic syndromes of cellular insulin resistance are good examples to identify novel candidate genes, which might play a role in the pathogenesis of the metabolic syndrome.

We have focused on patients with syndromes of insulin resistance on post receptor defects affecting the MAP-kinase cascade, the intracellular signaling cascade coupling the insulin receptor to major gene regulatory events, like cellular cholesterol metabolism as mentioned above. We have found (15, 16) signaling defects in different patients at various levels of the MAP-kinase cascade, which may be related to the degree of clinical insulin resistance in some of these patients. Furthermore, these studies and others indicate that at the postreceptor level several defects may exist in a single patient and that not only the action of insulin, but also of IGF-1 as well as of other growth factors can be affected. This proves that insulin resistance does not only affect glucose metabolism, but can be related to all other pleiotropic effects of insulin including complex gene regulatory events.

References

1. American Diabetes Association (1998) Management of dyslipidaemia in adults with diabetes. Diabetes Care 21: 179–182
2. Brown MS, Goldstein JL (1997) The SREBP-pathway: Regulation of cholesterol metabolism by proteolysis of membrane-bound transcription factor. Cell 89: 331–340
3. Brüning JC, Winnay J, Bonner-Weir S, Taylor SI, Accile D, Kahn CR (1997) Development of a novel polygenic mouse model for NIDDM in mice heterozygous for IR and IRS-10 alleles. Cell 88: 516–527
4. Brun RP, Kim JB, Hu B, Spiegelman BM (1997) Peroxisome proliferator-activated receptor gamma and the control of adipogenesis. Curr Opin Lipidol 8: 212–218
5. Carmeliet P, Collin D (1997) Molecular genetics of the fibrinolytic and coagulation systems in haemostasis, thrombogenesis, restenosis and atherosclerosis. Curr Opin Lipidol 8: 118–125
6. Downs JR, Clearfield M, Wies S, Witney E, Shapiro DR, Beere PA, Langendorfer A, Stein EA, Quyre W, Gotto AM, Jr, for the AFCAPF/TexCAPS Research Group (1998) Primary prevention of acute coronary events with lovastatin in men and women with average cholesterol levels. JAMA 279: 1615–1622
7. Ferra U, Satori C (1997) Insulin as a vascular sympathoexcitatory hormone. Circulation 96: 4104–4113
8. Ferranini E, Buzzigoli G, Bonadonna R (1987) Insulin resistance in essential hypertension. N Engl J Med 317: 350–357
9. Gloom WF, Keass W, Rusher W (1997) Leptin – the voice of adipose tissue. Johann Ambrosius Barth Verlag, Heidelberg, Leipzig
10. Gaudet D, Vohl M-C, Perron P, Tremblay G, Gagne C, Lesiege D, Bergeron J (1998) Relationships of abdominal obesity and hyperinsulaemia to angiographically assessed coronary artery disease in men with known mutations in the LDL receptor gene. Circulation 97: 871–877
11. Haffner SN, Lehto N, Rönnemaa T, Pyörälä K, Laakso M (1998) Mortality from coronary heart disease in subjects with type 2 diabetes and in non-diabetic subjects with and without myocardial infarction. N Engl J Med 339: 229–234
12. Haffner SN, Valdez RA, Hazuda HP, Mitzbell BD, Murales PA, Stern PA (1992) Prospective analysis of the insulin resistance syndrome (syndrome X). Diabetes 41: 7115–7122
13. Kim JB, Spotts GD, Halvorsen YD, Shih HM, Ellenberger T, Tow HC, Spiegelman BM (1995) Dual DNA binding specificity of ADD-1/SREBP-1 controlled by a single aminoacid in the basic helix-loop-helix domaine. Mol Cell Biol 15: 2582–2588

14. Kim JB, Spiegelman BM (1996) ADD1/SREBP-1 promotes adipocyte differentiation in gene expression linked to fatty acid metabolism. Genes Dev 10: 1096–1107
15. Knebel B, Kellner S, Kotzka J, Siemeister G, Dreyer M, Streicher R, Schiller M, Rüdiger HW, Seemanova E, Krone W, Müller-Wieland D (1997) Defects of insulin and IGF-1 action at receptor and postreceptor level in a patient with type A syndrome of insulin resistance. Biochem Biophys Res Com 234: 626–630
16. Knebel B, Kotzka J, Avci H, Schiller M, Zymny S, Krone W, Müller-Wieland D (1998) Postreceptor defects in patients with syndromes of insulin resistance: Gene therapy and culture cells. Diabetes 47 (Suppl 1): a0667
17. Kotzka J, Müller-Wieland D, Kopponen A, Njamen D, Kremer L, Munck M, Knebel B, Roth G, Krone W (1998) ADD1/SREBP-1c: Transcription factor mediating insulin action via MAP-kinase pathway. Biochem Biophys Res Com 249: 375–379
18. Lehmann JM, Moore LB, Smith-Oliver TA, Wilkison WO, Wilsson TM, Kliewer SA (1995) An antidiabetic thiazolidinedione as a high affinity ligand for the nuclear receptor PPAR-g. J Biol Chem 270: 12953–12956
19. Müller-Wieland D, Kotzka J, Krone W (1997) Stabilization of atherosclerotic plaque during lipid lowering. Curr Opin Lipidol 8: 348–353
20. Müller-Wieland D, Krone W (1997) Adipositas und Hypertonie. Internist 38: 237–243
21. Müller-Wieland D, Krone W (1995) Insulinresistenz und Fettstoffwechselstörungen. Herz 20: 33–46
22. Pyörälä K, Pedersen TR, Kjekshus J, Faergeman O, Olsson AG, Thorgeirsson G (1997) Cholesterol lowering with simvastatin improves prognosis of diabetic patients with coronary heart disease: A subgroup analysis of the Scandinavian Simvastatin Survival Study (4S). Diabetes Care 20: 614-620 [Eratum (1997) Diabetes Care 20: 1048]
23. Ristow M, Müller-Wieland D, Pfeiffer A, Krone W, Kahn CR (1998) Obesity associatted with a mutation in peroxisome-proliferator activated receptor gamma 2 (PPAR-γ2), a regulator of adipocited differentiation. N Engl J Med 339: 953–959
24. Roth G, Kotzka J, Meyer HE, Munck M, Müller-Wieland D, Krone W (1998) Role of the transcription factors SREBP-1 and SREBP-2 in the regulation of the LDL receptor (LDLR) gene by insulin and growth factors. Diabetes 47 (Suppl 1): a0283
25. Sachs FM, Pfeffer MA, Moye LA et al. (1996) The effect of pravastatin and coronary events after myocardial infarction in patients with average cholesterol levels. N Engl J Med 335: 1001–1009
26. Satow R, Inoue J, Kawabe Y, Kodama T, Takano T, Maeda M (1996) Sterol-dependent transcriptional regulation of sterol regulatory element-binding protein-2. J Biol Chem 273: 26461–26464
27. Scandinavian Simvastatin Survival Study Group (1994) Randomized trial of cholesterol lowering in 4444 patients with coronary heart disease: The Scandinavian Simvastatin Survival Study (4S). Lancet 344: 1383–1389
28. Shepherd J, Cobbe SM, Ford I et al. (1995) For the West of Scotland Coronary Prevention Study Group. Prevention of coronary heart disease with pravastatin in men with hypercholesterolaemia. N Engl J Med 333: 1301–1307
29. Soutar AK (1998) Update on low density lipoprotein receptor mutations. Curr Opin Lipidol 9: 141–145
30. Spiegelman BM (1997) Peroxisome proliferator-activated receptor gamma: A key regulator of adipogenesis and systemic insulin sensitivity. Eur J Med Res 2: 257–264
31. Spiegelman BM (1998) PPAR-γ: Adipogenic regulator in thiazolidinedione receptor. Diabetes 47: 507–514
32. Spiegelman BM, Flyer JS (1996) Adipogenesis and obesity: Rounding out the big picture. Cell 87: 377–389
33. Stamler J, Vaccaro O, Neaton JD, Wetworth D for the Multiple Risk Factor Intervention Trial Research Group (1993) Diabetes, other risk factors and 12-yr cardiovascular mortality for men screened in the multiple risk factor intervention trial. Diabetes Care 16: 434–444
34. Streicher R, Kotzka J, Müller-Wieland D, Siemeister G, Munck M, Avci H, Krone W (1996) SREBP-1 mediates activation of the low density lipoprotein receptor promoter by insulin and insulin-like growth factor-1. J Biol Chem 271: 7128–7133
35. Tonkin A (1997) LIPID Plenary Session XII: Late-breaking clinical trials. 17th Scientific Sessions of the American Heart Association.
36. Tontonoz P, Kim JB, Graves RH, Spiegelman BM (1993) ADD1: A novel helix-loop-helix transcription factor associated with adipocyte determination and differentiation. Mol Cell Biol 13: 4753–4759
37. Weidmann P, Müller-Wieland D, Curthen M, Krone W (1995) Insulinresistenz und arterielle Hypertonie. Herz 20: 60–32
38. Withers DJ, Gutierrez JS, Towery H, Burks J, Ren JM, Preves S, Zhang Y, Bernard D, Pons S, Schulman GI, Bonner-Wier S, White MF (1998) Dysruption of IRS-2 causes type 2 diabetes in mice. Nature 391: 900–904

Author's address:
Prof. Dr. D. Müller-Wieland
Klinik II und Poliklinik für Innere Medizin
der Universität zu Köln
D-50924 Köln

Genetic control of hemostatic factors in relation to atherosclerosis

J. Schüttrumpf, H. H.Watzke

Department of Medicine I, Division of Hematology and Hemostaseology
University of Vienna, Austria

Abstract

Increased levels of coagulation factors VII and fibrinogen were identified as risk factors for acute coronary syndromes many years ago. Analysis of the genes coding for these proteins suggest a genetic component in the determination of their plasma level. More than ten different genetic polymorphisms have been described in the fibrinogen gene. They influence the fibrinogen level at varying intensities and show a heterogenous association with coronary heart disease. A similar picture evolves from the analysis of the factor VII gene. Associations with a change in factor VII levels have been reported from all polymorphisms. However, they are in a strong linkage disequilibrium. The association with coronary heart disease is still controversial. Similar results have been obtained by analysis of many other coagulation factors like prothrombin, factor V, and factor XIII.

Introduction

Increased levels of coagulation factors are well known risk factors for acute coronary syndromes. Particularly, high levels of coagulation factor VII or fibrinogen were associated with acute myocardial infarction (MI) in a large epidemiologic study. The plasma levels of these and other coagulation factors is mainly determined genetically. Genetic polymorphism within the regulatory sequences necessary for gene transcription and protein expression modulate the protein levels in plasma. Studies have been performed investigating the connection of polymorphisms with the plasma levels of coagulation factors (Fig. 1). Others have focussed on the direct link of polymorphisms and the risk of acute coronary syndromes (Fig. 1).

This short overview is focused on these association studies only. The partly contradictory results among these studies may result from differences of the study populations: age, the survived time after a myocardial infarction, gender, smoking or metabolic risk factors, and many other special conditions may have influence on the outcome of such a study.

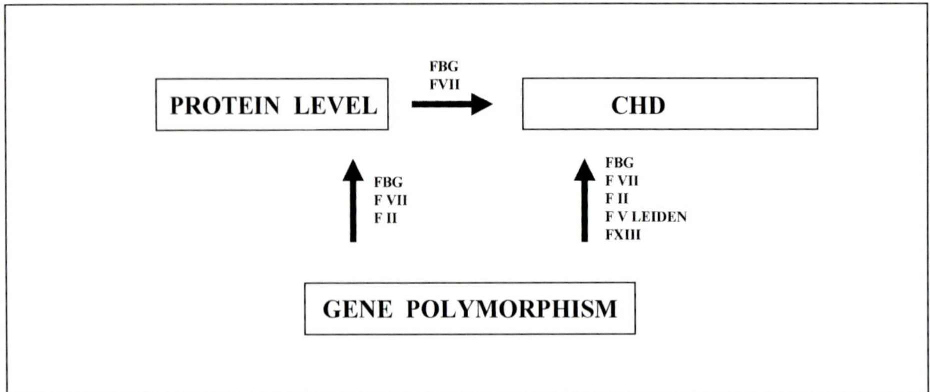

Fig. 1. Associations of genetic polymorphisms of coagulation factors with coronary heart disease (CHD) and protein levels. Arrows indicate possible associations. Coagulation factors for which at least one study has shown a significant association are listed next to arrows.

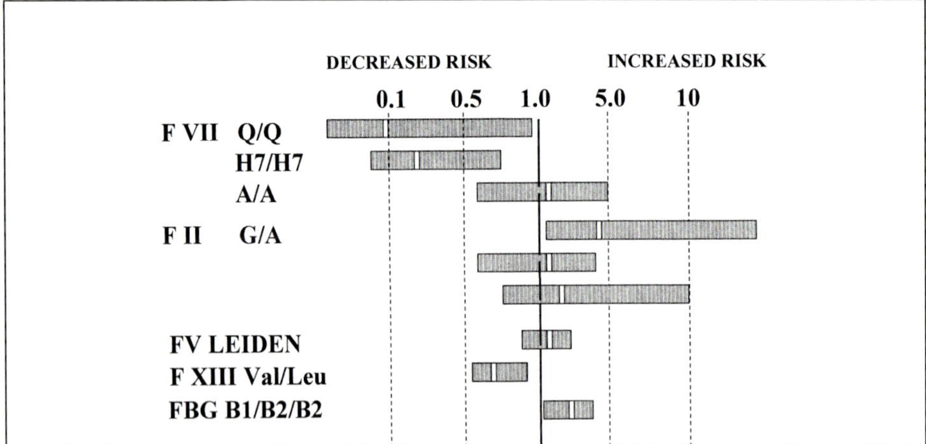

Fig. 2. Odds ratios and 95 % confidence intervals of relative risks of coronary heart disease in carriers of genetic polymorphisms of coagulation factors. Data are taken from the following authors: Factor VII from (16); Factor II from (8, 26, 27, 36); Factor V Leiden from (25); Factor XIII from (18, 19); Fibrinogen from (38).

Data on the association of coronary heart disease (CHD) and genetic polymorphisms are available from the following clotting factors: fibrinogen, prothrombin, factor V, factor VII, and factor XIII (Fig. 2). The review will therefore focus on these proteins and their genes.

Fibrinogen

Different polymorph alleles in the fibrinogen genes were candidates for an association with CAD and MI.

The β-fibrinogen G/A-455 polymorphism (HaeIII RFLP)

Thomas et al. (31) described a *Hae*III restriction fragment length polymorphism (RFLP) caused by a A for G substitution at position –455 or –453 (different denomination in the various studies) in the 5'-untranslated region of the β fibrinogen gene. They showed an association of the H2 allele (the allele which has lost the *Hae*III restriction side) with raised plasma fibrinogen levels.

The first study investigating a direct association between a genetic polymorphism and MI was the ECTIM Study (29), in which the *Hae*III RFLP of the -fibrinogen gene (31) was analyzed. The prevalence of the polymorphismus was determined in 533 male patients with MI aged 25 to 64 years and in 648 healthy male controls from the same geographic region. Plasma fibrinogen levels were significantly higher in individuals (patients and controls) carrying the H2 allele, particularly among smokers. In addition, fibrinogen levels were higher in patients (overall mean of 343 mg/dl) compared to controls (300 mg/dl; P < 0.0001). However, no difference in the distribution of the H2 allele could be found between the two groups (frequency of the H2 allele among patients vs. controls: 0.19 vs. 0.21; relative risk: 0.89 with 95 % CI from 0.69 to 1.13).

Similar results concerning the *Hae*III RFLP were reported by Green et al. (11) from Sweden (31). The frequency of the A allele (H2) was 0.25 in both the group of 123 patients with MI before the age of 45 and the group of 86 age matched controls. Also the measured Distribution of plasma fibrinogen levels between the groups was similar to the ones reported in the ECTIM Study (29).

Yu et al. (37) compared in the prevalence of the *Hae*III RFLP in 192 caucasian patients (aged 63.7 ± 10.3 SD years) with angiographically confirmed CHD and 331 normal controls. The distribution of the A allele (*Hae*III RFLP) in the two groups was significantly different (patients: 0.16, controls: 0.25; p = 0.0013).

In all of the following studies the effect of the *Hae*III RFLP on the fibrinogen plasma levels was confirmed, but they all failed to show an association between the polymorphism and the CHD. In a sample of 9127 individuals from the general population from the Copenhagen City Heart Study, the genetic effect on the plasma fibrinogen levels appeared stronger in individuals with ischemic heart disease. However, the prevalence of the polymorphism was similar in individuals with the disease and without it (32).

Gardemann et al. (10) studied 923 patients, who underwent coronary angiography for diagnostic purposes. When clinical or chemical signs of an acute phase reaction who were present, fibrinogen levels were higher in individuals being homozygous for the A allele compared with those being homozygous for the G allele. These findings were confirmed by the investigation of a subgroup of 207 patients who underwent aortocoronary bypass surgery. However, a direct association between the prevalence of the A or H2 allele and CHD or MI was not found.

Similar results were obtained in the study from van der Bom et al. (34). No difference in the distribution of the *Hae*III RFLP was found between 139 subjects with previous MI and 287 controls aged 55 years and older.

The β-fibrinogen BclI polymorphism and other polymorphisms of the fibrinogen gene

In another publication from the ECTIM Study (3) the single known polymorphism from the fibrinogen gene and ten polymorphisms from the β fibrinogen gene were analyzed. Five of the polymorphisms in the β fibrinogen gene were detected by single-strand conformation polymorphism analysis (SSCP). 565 patients with CHD (aged 25 to 64 years) and 668 controls from four different centers were enrolled in the study. Some polymorphisms showed an association – positive and negative – or even a complete concordance with each other. Two polymorphisms were excluded from the study after the first 100 subjects because of a complete concordance with the β *Hae*III RFLP. A significant association of plasma fibrinogen levels was found with the β *Bcl*I ($P < 0.015$), β C448 ($P < 0.004$), β *Hae*III ($P < 0.002$), and β-1420 ($P < 0.003$) polymorphisms. An independent association was present in the β *Hae*III ($P < 0.0003$) and the β-854 ($P < 0.01$) polymorphisms. The effect on the plasma fibrinogen levels was only significant in smokers. Taking the number of coronary arteries with a stenosis larger than 50 % as a measure of the severity of CAD, associations of the less frequent alleles of the β *Bcl*I ($P < 0.0003$), β C448 ($P < 0.002$), β *Hae*III ($P < 0.006$), and β-1420 ($P < 0.01$) polymorphisms and the severity of the disease remained significant. In a stepwise logistic regression analysis only the β *Bcl*I polymorphism remained significant. Patients with three-vessel lesions carried more frequently the less common allele of this polymorphism ($P < 0.05$).

The β *Bcl*I polymorphism was studied by Zito et al. (38). 102 patients with AMI and a first degree relative with the a history of the disease or of stroke before the age of 65 years and 173 controls were examined. The frequency of the less frequent B2 allele was higher in patients (28 %) than in controls (17 %; $P = 0.002$). Carriers of the B2 allele were present more often in the group of patients than in controls (odds ratio: 2.4, $P < 0.001$). Furthermore, an association was found between the genotype and the fibrinogen plasma levels in smokers and in non-smokers.

The study from Carter et al. (5) included 405 patients with CAD and 216 healthy controls. No association was found between the β 448 polymorphism and the occurence MI.

Prothrombin

An A/G polymorphism at position 20210 in the 3'-untranslated region of the gene, originaly described by Poort et al. (24), has been investigated as possible risk factor for CHD. In has been shown that elevated prothrombin levels in the blood coincide with the appearance of the A allele.

A study from Watzke et al. (36) determined the prevalence of the A allele in the general Austrian population examining 102 healthy newborns. 1.96 % (2 of 102) of them were carrier of the A allele. In contrast, 5.1 % (5 of 98) of a group of 98 patients with CHD (19 female, age: 53 + 12 SD years and 79 male, age 49 + 8.5 SD years) had the A allele. Although this results did not reach statistical significance they may indicate an association between the polymorphism and the occurence of CHD.

Rosendaal et al. (26) compared in a case control study 79 women (18 to 44 years old) with first myocardial infarction and 381 control women all from western Washington. The A allele was with more common in women with MI (5.1 %) than among controls (1.6 %). In an age-adjusted logistic model, the odds ratio for MI was 4.0 (95 % confidence interval 1.1 to 15.1, $P = 0.038$). The relative risk was even higher, when also another cardiovascular risk factor was present, such as smoking (odds ratio 43.3). From this data it was concluded that an increased risk of MI is associated with the A allele and a synergism exists with other atherosclerotic risk factors.

In a similar study from Doggen et al. (8), 560 male patients from the Netherlands with a first MI before the age of 70 years (age: 56.2 + 9.0 SD years) were analyzed together with 646 control subjects (age: 57.3 ± 10.8 SD years). 1.8 % (10 of 560) of the patients and 1.2 % (8 of 646) of the group of controls were carrying the A allele. The calculated odds ratio was 1.5 (95 % confidence interval 0.6 to 3.8). An increased relative risks could be found in this study when other risk factors for MI were present.

A study from Spain (6) compared 101 patients with CHD and gender and age matched controls in a prospective case control setup. The G/A genotype was present in 4 % of the patients and in 2 % of the controls. However the results did not reach a statistical significance.

In the study from Arruda et al. (2) comparing 220 survivors of a MI with 295 neonates was found a prevalence of 3 % in the patient group and of 0.7% in the neonates. The difference was significant ($P = 0.03$).

Factor V

A G to A point mutation at position 1691of the factor V gene has been identified which results in the substitution of arginin at position 506 by glycine (factor V Leiden). The protein expressed from the mutant gene is resistant to the inactivation by activated protein C (APC) (4, 14, 35, 39). This defect was initially described as a risk factor for venous thrombosis.

Samani et al. (28) found the mutation in only 2 of 60 patients with MI (median age of 47.5 years, range 30–54).

März et al. (22) identified 21 (9 %) subjects with the mutation of 224 CAD patients (median age 58 years, range 32–78) with only 8 (4 %) individuals carrying the mutation of 196 controls. The difference was statistically significant (odds ration: 2.4; $P = 0.032$).

The factor V Leiden mutation was present in a heterozygous form in 33 and in a homozygous in 1 of 643 male patients with previous MI (aged 25–64 years) participating in the ECTIM study (9). Similary, 33 homozygous and 1 heterozygous carrier of the mutation were found in 726 age matched control subjects. Thus, there was no difference in the prevalence of the mutation between patients with MI and healthy controls.

Van Boxmeer et al. (33) analyzed the mutation in a group of CAD patients aged below 50 years. Seven of 149 (4.7 %) patients with MI and 5 of 126 (4 %) control individuals had the mutation. The slight difference was not statistically significant.

From a cohort of 14916 apparently healthy men in the Physicians' Health Study (25) 374 experienced a myocardial infarction during follow-up. The prevalence of the mutation in this group was 6.1 %. In the group of 704 healthy men the prevalence was 6 %. No association between the mutation and the MI was found.

The prevalence of the factor V Leiden genotype was studied in 122 patients with MI younger than 60 years and 138 controls from two different centers in Finland (19). A statistical significant difference was found in one center: 6 of 71 patients (8.5 %) vs 1 of 87 controls (1.1 %) were carriers of the mutation ($P < 0.05$). These results were sharply contrasted by the outcome of in the other participating center. Only 1 of 51 patients (2 %) compared with three of 50 controls (6 %) had the mutation. The result was not statistically significant when both centers pooled their patients. The authors speculated that a possible explanation for the discrepant results between the centers was the different age of the two groups of patients. The mean age of patients from the first center was ten years higher compared to the other center.

Holm et al. (15) found in their study a high prevalence of the Factor V Leiden mutation in Sweden. Of 101 patients with MI before the age of 50 years, 18 % were carriers of the FV Q506 allele, while among a control group of the same size the prevalence was 11 %. A statistical significance of the prevalence was found comparing the 79 male patients and controls (23 % vs. 10 %; $P = 0.03$) with an odds ratio of 2.6 (95 % confidence interval from 1.1 to 6.4).

No difference in the prevalence of the factor V Leiden mutation was found in the studies by Jeffery et al. (7, 17).

The prevalence of the Factor V Leiden mutation and control women was investigated. Rosendaal et al. (27) found a prevalence of the mutation in 84 women younger than 45 years with a history of MI of 9.5 % and of 4.1 % among 388 controls (odds ratio: 2.4 with a 95 % CI from 1.0 to 5.9). Furthermore, the authors reported that there was a trend toward a higher prevalence in women with MI who also have another major risk factor, particularly smoking.

Factor VII

Two common polymorphisms with a known association to factor VII levels in the blood were reported.

Green et al. (12) identified a G to A substitution in the codon for amino acid 353 (R353Q), leading to a change from arginine to glutamine. A high association with the factor VII coagulant activity (factor VIIc) can be seen. Individuals heterozygous showed a mean factor VIIc level of 64 %, while homozygous for the Q allele only had levels of 33 %.

The other polymorphism has been described in the hypervariable region of intron 7 (13, 21).

In the multi-center case-control ECTIM study the R353Q polymorphism was analyzed in case patients with MI and normal controls (20). But no association between polymorphism and MI was found.

Iacoviello et al. (16) involved both the R353Q and the hypervariable region of intron 4 in their study. In a case-control setup 165 patients with familial myocardial infarction (age: 55 ± 9 SD years) and 225 controls without a personal or family history of cardiovascular disease (age: 56 ± 8 SD years) were analyzed. Also factor VII clotting activity and antigen levels were measured. In the hypervariable region 4 three different alleles were concerned; H5, H6, and H7. The allele frequencies in patients and controls were as following; patients: R: 84.5 %, Q: 15.5 %, H7: 26.7 %, H6: 70.6 %, H5: 2.7 %; controls: R: 78.6 %, Q: 21.4 %, H7: 35.6 %, H6: 63.8 %, H5: 0.7 %. The presence of the Q or the H7 allele decreased both the risk of myocardial infarction and the levels of factor VII clotting activity and factor VII antigen. In addition, patients with the lowest level of factor VII clotting activity had a lower risk of MI than with the top levels (odds ratio: 0.13, 95 % confidence interval: 0.05 to 0.34). Individuals with RR genotype for the R353Q polymorphism had the highest risk for MI, followed by RQ and QQ ($P < 0.001$). Looking at the polymorphism in the hypervariable region 4, the decreasing order for the risk of MI was H7H5 respectively H6H5, H6H6, H6H7, and H7H7 genotypes ($P < 0.001$). The lowest risk of MI had individuals with the QQ or H7H7 genotype (odds ratio: 0.08 with 95 % CI from 0.01 to 0.9 and odds ratio: 0.22 with 95 % CI from 0.08 to 0.63).

Factor XIII

A common G to T polymorphism has been reported in codon 34 of exon 2 in the A-subunit near to the thrombin activation side of the human coagulation factor XIII gene (1, 17, 38). The polymorphism causes a replacement of the amino acid valine by leucine (Factor XII-IVal34Leu).

To test an association of this polymorphism with MI was aim of the study of Kohler et al. (18). 398 patients admitted for coronary angiography after a history of chest pain were matched with 196 healthy controls for age and race. From the 398 patients 197 had a confirmed history of MI according to WHO criteria. No significant relation between all patients and controls could be found. The allele distribution found in controls and patients without MI were very similar (genotypes controls: G/G 52 %, G/T 45 %, T/T 7 %; patients without MI: G/G 50 %, G/T 45 %, T/T 5 %), while in the group of patients with MI a significantly lower prevalence of the T allele and an increased appearance of the homozygous wild type was found (G/G 68 %, G/T 27 %, T/T 5 %); patients without MI vs. patients with MI ($P = 0.0009$) and controls vs. patients with MI ($P = 0.005$). In a logistic regression model the odds ratio as a measure of the decreased risk was 0.67.

References

1. Anwar R, Stewart AD, Miloszewski KJ, Losowsky MS, Markham AF (1995) Molecular basis of inherited factor XIII deficiency: Identification of multiple mutations provides insights into protein function. Br J Haematol 91: 728–735
2. Arruda VR, Siquiera LH, Chiaparini LC, Coelho OR, Mansur AP, Ramires, Annichino-Bizzacchi JM (1998) Prevalence of the prothrombin gene variant 20210 G –> A among patients with myocardial infarction. Cardiovasc Res 37: 42–45
3. Behague I, Poirier O, Nicaud V, Evans A, Arveiler D, Luc G, Cambou JP, Scarabin PY, Bara L, Green F, Cambien F (1996) Beta fibrinogen gene polymorphisms are associated with plasma fibrinogen and coronary artery disease in patients with myocardial infarction. The ECTIM Study. Etude Cas-Temoins sur l'Infarctus du Myocarde. Circulation 93: 440–449
4. Bertina RM, Koeleman BP, Koster T, Rosendaal FR, Dirven RJ, de R, van der Velden PA, Reitsma PH (1994) Mutation in blood coagulation factor V associated with resistance to activated protein C [see comments]. Nature 369: 64–67
5. Carter AM, Ossei-Gerning N, Wilson IJ, Grant PJ (1997) Association of the platelet Pl(A) polymorphism of glycoprotein IIb/IIIa and the fibrinogen Beta 448 polymorphism with myocardial infarction and extent of coronary artery disease. Circulation 96: 1424–1431
6. Corral J, Gonzalez-Conejero R, Lozano ML, Rivera J, Heras I, Vicente (1997) The venous thrombosis risk factor 20210 A allele of the prothrombin gene is not a major risk factor for arterial thrombotic disease. Br J Haematol 99: 304–307
7. Demarmels BF, Merlo C, Furlan M, Sulzer I, Binder BR, Lammle (1995) No association of APC resistance with myocardial infarction. Blood Coagul Fibrinolysis 6: 456–459
8. Doggen CJ, Cats VM, Bertina RM, Rosendaal FR (1998) Interaction of coagulation defects and cardiovascular risk factors: Increased risk of myocardial infarction associated with factor V Leiden or prothrombin 20210A. Circulation 97: 1037–1041

9. Emmerich J, Poirier O, Evans A, Marques-Vidal P, Arveiler D, Luc G, Aiach M, Cambien F (1995) Myocardial infarction, Arg 506 to Gln factor V mutation, and activated protein C resistance [letter]. Lancet 345: 321

10. Gardemann A, Schwartz O, Haberbosch W, Katz N, Weiss T, Tillmanns H, Hehrlein FW, Waas W, Eberbach A (1997) Positive association of the beta fibrinogen H1/H2 gene variation to basal fibrinogen levels and to the increase in fibrinogen concentration during acute phase reaction but not to coronary artery disease and myocardial infarction. Thromb Haemost 77: 1120–1126

11. Green F, Hamsten A, Blomback M, Humphries S (1993) The role of beta-fibrinogen genotype in determining plasma fibrinogen levels in young survivors of myocardial infarction and healthy controls from Sweden. Thromb Haemost 70: 915–920

12. Green F, Kelleher C, Wilkes H, Temple A, Meade T, Humphries S (1991) A common genetic polymorphism associated with lower coagulation factor VII levels in healthy individuals. Arterioscler Thromb 11: 540–546

13. Green F, Johansen LG, Grootendorst D, Temple A, Cruickshank JK, Humphries SE, Jespersen J, Kluft C (1994) New alleles in F7 VNTR. Hum Mol Gen 3: 384

14. Greengard JS, Sun X, Xu X, Fernandez JA, Griffin JH, Evatt B (1994) Activated protein C resistance caused by Arg506Gln mutation in factor Va [letter]. Lancet 343: 1361–1362

15. Holm J, Zoller B, Berntorp E, Erhardt L, Dahlback B (1996) Prevalence of factor V gene mutation amongst myocardial infarction patients and healthy controls is higher in Sweden than in other countries. J Intern Med 239: 221–226

16. Iacoviello L, Di CA, de KP, D'Orazio A, Amore C, Arboretti R, Kluft C, Benedetta DM (1998) Polymorphisms in the coagulation factor VII gene and the risk of myocardial infarction [see comments]. N Eng J Med 338: 79–85

17. Jeffery S, Leatham E, Zhang Y, Carter J, Pratel P, Kaski JC (1996) Factor V Leiden polymorphism (FV Q506) in patients with ischaemic heart disease, and in different populations groups. J Hum Hypertens 10: 433–434

18. Kohler HP, Stickland MH, Ossei-Gerning N, Carter A, Mikkola H, Grant PJ (1998) Association of a common polymorphism in the factor XIII gene with myocardial infarction. Thromb Haemost 79: 8–13

19. Kohler HP, Stickland MH, Ossei-Gerning N, Carter A, Mikkola H, Grant PJ (1998) Association of a common polymorphism in the factor XIII gene with myocardial infarction. Thromb Haemost 79: 8–13

20. Lane A, Green F, Scarabin PY, Nicaud V, Bara L, Humphries S, Evans, Luc G, Cambou JP, Arveiler D, Cambien F (1996) Factor VII Arg/Gln353 polymorphism determines factor VII coagulant activity in patients with myocardial infarction (MI) and control subjects in Belfast and in France but is not a strong indicator of MI risk in the ECTIM study. Atherosclerosis 119: 119–127

21. Marchetti G, Patracchini P, Gemmati D, DeRosa V, Pinotti M, Rodorigo G, Casonato A, Girolami A, Bernardi F (1992) Detection of two missense mutations and characterization of a repeat polymorphism in the factor VII gene (F7). Hum Genet 89: 497–502

22. März W, Seydewitz H, Winkelmann B, Chen M, Nauck M, Witt I (1995) Mutation in coagulation factor V associated with resistance to activated protein C in patients with coronary artery disease [letter]. Lancet 345: 526

23. Mikkola H, Syrjala M, Rasi V, Vahtera E, Hamalainen E, Peltonen L, Palotie A (1994) Deficiency in the A-subunit of coagulation factor XIII: two novel point mutations demonstrate different effects on transcript levels. Blood 84: 517–525

24. Poort SR, Rosendaal FR, Reitsma PH, Bertina RM (1996) A common genetic variation in the 3'-untranslated region of the prothrombin gene is associated with elevated plasma prothrombin levels and an increase in venous thrombosis. Blood 88: 3698–3703

25. Ridker PM, Hennekens CH, Lindpaintner K, Stampfer MJ, Eisenberg PR, Miletich JP (1995) Mutation in the gene coding for coagulation factor V and the risk of myocardial infarction, stroke, and venous thrombosis in apparently healthy men [see comments]. N Eng J Med 332: 912–917

26. Rosendaal FR, Siscovick DS, Schwartz SM, Psaty BM, Raghunathan TE, Vos HL (1997) A common prothrombin variant (20210 G to A) increases the risk of myocardial infarction in young women. Blood 90: 1747–1750

27. Rosendaal FR, Siscovick DS, Schwartz SM, Beverly RK, Psaty BM, Longstreth WTJ, Raghunathan TE, Koepsell TD, Reitsma PH (1997) Factor V Leiden (resistance to activated protein C) increases the risk of myocardial infarction in young women [see comments]. Blood 89: 2817–2821

28. Samani NJ, Lodwick D, Martin D, Kimber P (1994) Resistance to activated protein C and risk of premature myocardial infarction [letter]. Lancet 344: 1709–1710

29. Scarabin PY, Bara L, Ricard S, Poirier O, Cambou JP, Arveiler D, Luc, Evans AE, Samama MM, Cambien F (1993) Genetic variation at the beta-fibrinogen locus in relation to plasma fibrinogen concentrations and risk of myocardial infarction. The ECTIM Study. Arterioscler Thromb 13: 886–891

30. Suzuki K, Henke J, Iwata M, Henke L, Tsuji H, Fukunaga T, Ishimoto, Szekelyi M, Ito S (1996) Novel polymorphisms and haplotypes in the human coagulation factor XIII A-subunit gene. Hum Gen 98: 393–395

31. Thomas AE, Green FR, Kelleher CH, Wilkes HC, Brennan PJ, Meade TW, Humphries SE (1991) Variation in the promoter region of the beta fibrinogen gene is associated with plasma fibrinogen levels in smokers and non-smokers. Thromb Haemost 65: 487–490

32. Tybjaerg-Hansen A, Agerholm-Larsen B, Humphries SE, Abildgaard S, Schnohr P, Nordestgaard BG (1997) A common mutation (G-455 –> A) in the beta-fibrinogen promoter is an independent predictor of plasma fibrinogen, but not of ischemic heart disease. A study of 9,127 individuals based on the Copenhagen City Heart Study. J Clin Invest 99: 3034–3039

33. van Bockxmeer F, Baker RI, Taylor RR (1995) Premature ischaemic heart disease and the gene for coagulation factor V [letter]. Nat Med 1: 185

34. van der Bom JG, de MM, Bots ML, Haverkate F, de JP, Hofman, Kluft C, Grobbee DE (1998) Elevated plasma fibrinogen: cause or consequence of cardiovascular disease? Arterioscl Thromb Vasc Biol 18: 621–625

35. Voorberg J, Roelse J, He X, Dalbäck B (1994) Identification of the same factor V gene mutation in 47 out of 50 thrombosis-prone families with inherited resistance to activated proteion C. J Clin Invest 94: 2521–5

36. Watzke HH, Schüttrumpf J, Graf S, Huber K, Panzer S (1997) Increased prevalence of a polymorphism in the gene coding for human prothrombin in patients with coronary heart disease. Thromb Res 87: 521–526

37. Yu Q, Safavi F, Roberts R, Marian AJ (1996) A variant of beta fibrinogen is a genetic risk factor for coronary artery disease and myocardial infarction. J Invest Med 44: 154–159

38. Zito F, Di CA, Amore C, D'Orazio A, Donati MB, Iacoviello (1997) Bcl I polymorphism in the fibrinogen beta-chain gene is associated with the risk of familial myocardial infarction by increasing plasma fibrinogen levels. A case-control study in a sample of GISSI-2 patients. Arterioscl Thromb Vasc Biol 17: 3489–3494

39. Zoller B, Svensson PJ, He X, Dahlback B (1994) Identification of the same factor V gene mutation in 47 out of 50 thrombosis-prone families with inherited resistance to activated protein C. J Clin Invest 94: 2521–2524

Author's address:
Univ. Prof. Dr. H. H. Watzke
Klinik für Innere Medizin I
Abteilung für Hämatologie und Hämostaseologie
Währinger Gürtel 18–20
A-1090 Wien, Austria

Increased platelet aggregability associated with platelet GPIIIa PI[A2] polymorphism: the Framingham Offspring Study

D. Feng[1], K. Lindpaintner[2,3], M. G. Larson[4], V. S. Rao[2], C. J. O'Donnell[4],
I. Lipinska[1], C. Schmitz[2], P. A. Sutherland[4], H. Silbershatz[5], R. B. D'Agostino[5],
J. E. Muller[6], R. H. Myers[7], D. Levy[4], G. H. Tofler[1]

[1] The Institute for Prevention of Cardiovascular Disease, Beth Israel Deaconess Medical Center, and [2] Cardiovascular Division, Brigham & Women's Hospital, and the [3] Department of Cardiology, Children's Hospital, Harvard Medical School; [4] National Heart, Lung and Blood Institute's Framingham Heart Study; [5] Statistics and Consulting Unit, Department of Mathematics, Boston University; [6] Cardiology Division, University of Kentucky Medical Center; [7] Department of Neurology, Boston University, USA

Abstract

The platelet glycoprotein *IIb/IIIa (GP IIb/IIIa)* plays a pivotal role in platelet aggregation. Recent data suggest that the *PI[A2]* polymorphism of *GPIIIa* may be associated with an increased risk for cardiovascular disease. However, it is unknown if there is any association between this polymorphism and platelet reactivity. We determined *GPIIIa* genotype and platelet reactivity phenotype data in 1422 subjects from the Framingham Offspring Study. Genotyping was performed using PCR based restriction fragment length polymorphism analysis. Platelet aggregability was evaluated by the Born method. The threshold concentrations of epinephrine and adenosine diphosphate (ADP) were determined. Allele frequencies of *PI[A1]* and *PI[A2]* were 0.84 and 0.16, respectively. The presence of one or two *PI[A2]* alleles was associated with increased platelet aggregability as indicated by incrementally lower threshold concentrations for epinephrine and ADP. For epinephrine, the mean concentrations were 0.9 μmol/L (0.9–1.0) for homozygous *PI[A1]*, 0.7 μmol/L (0.7–0.9) for the heterozygous *PI[A1]/PI[A2]*, and 0.6 μmol/L (0.4–1.0) for homozygous *PI[A2]* individuals, p = 0.009. The increase in aggregability induced by epinephrine remained highly significant (p = 0.007) after adjustment for covariates. For ADP-induced aggregation, the respective mean concentrations were 3.1 μmol/L (3.0–3.2), 3.0 μmol/L (2.9–3.2), and 2.8 μmol/L (2.4–3.3), p = 0.19 after adjustment for covariates. Our findings indicate that molecular variants of the gene encoding *GPIIIa* play a role in platelet reactivity *in vitro*. Our observations are compatible with and provide an explanation for the reported association of the *PI[A2]* allotype with increased risk for cardiovascular disease.

Introduction

Myocardial infarction results from the formation of a platelet-rich thrombus at the site of a ruptured coronary atherosclerotic plaque (10, 11). The platelet surface receptor glycoprotein *IIb/IIIa* (GP *IIb/IIIa*) plays a key role in the formation of such thrombus by binding fibrinogen and von Willebrand factor. The importance of the GP *IIb/IIIa* receptor has been further supported by recent clinical trials in which GP *IIb/IIIa* antagonists have been shown to reduce restenosis rate following angioplasty (35) and also to reduce the morbidity and mortality associated with unstable angina (32), high-risk coronary angioplasty (33), and acute myocardial infarction (19).

Although the Pl^{A1} and Pl^{A2} variants of *GP IIIa* have long been recognized as alloantigens and most frequently implicated in syndromes of immune-mediated platelet destruction, until recently little attention has been paid to their role in coronary heart disease. Weiss and colleagues (38) first reported that patients with acute coronary syndromes were more likely than were controls to carry the Pl^{A2} allele. The risk associated with Pl^{A2} was especially high for those aged ≤ 60 years at the time of infarction. Recently Walter and colleagues reported that patients with the Pl^{A2} allele had an increased risk of coronary stent thrombosis compared with Pl^{A1} homozygous individuals (37). However, the association between the Pl^{A2} allele and cardiovascular disease has not been consistent findings. While Carter et al. supported the early findings of Weiss (7), several other studies failed to detect the association (5, 15, 23, 27, 28, 30), including a large prospective study from the Physicians' Health Study (28).

Importantly, the mechanism for the possibly increased risk has not been determined. We hypothesized that the Pl^{A2} allele might be associated with an increase in platelet aggregability and tested this hypothesis in the Framingham Offspring Study.

Methods

The study population

The study subjects were members of the Framingham Offspring Study, a long-term, prospective evaluation of risk factors for cardiovascular disease. The design and methodology of the Framingham Offspring Study have been described in detail elsewhere (17). The participants are natural or adopted children of the original Framingham Heart Study subjects. For this study, we collected data from consecutive subjects examined between April 3, 1991 and June 29, 1995, during the fifth Offspring Study examination cycle.

Of the 3799 subjects who attended examination cycle 5, blood samples were collected from 3286 subjects for platelet aggregation analysis. For the present analysis, we excluded subjects who were not members of a sibship (n = 1298) since linkage analysis was also performed. We also excluded subjects in whom platelet aggregation data were not available or who were under treatment with anticoagulant or antiplatelet drugs (n = 536). Finally, we excluded subjects in whom genotyping could not be successfully accomplished (n = 30). A total of 1422 subjects fulfilled all inclusion criteria.

Determination of platelet aggregability

Blood samples were always obtained in the morning to avoid the circadian change of platelet aggregability. Blood was drawn in 3.8 % sodium citrate solution (1:9). Platelet rich plasma was separated by centrifugation for 10 minutes at 160 g. Platelet aggregation was measured on a 4-channel aggregometer according to the method of Born (2). The aggregation agents tested were epinephrine and adenosine diphosphate in varying concentrations (0.01–30 μmol/l) and a fixed concentration of arachidonic acid (1.6 mmol/l). The lowest concentrations of adenosine diphosphate and epinephrine required to produce a biphasic response with greater than 50 % aggregation (threshold concentration) were determined. A decreased threshold concentration indicates an increase in platelet aggregability. In addition, the presence or absence of an aggregation in response to arachidonic acid was determined.

Genotyping

To detect the substitution of cytosine for thymidine at position 1565 in exon 2 of the glycoprotein *IIIa* gene that is responsible for the *Pl^{A2}* polymorphism, we used a modified PCR-based restriction fragment length polymorphism (RFLP) analysis (26). Genomic DNA was isolated from whole blood. Genomic DNA (10–20 ng in 5 μl volume) was incubated at 96 °C for 3 minutes, followed by addition of master-mix (10 μl) to yield a final reagent concentration of 333 nmol/l for sense and anti-sense primer, 167 nmol/L of each of dATP, dTTP, dCTP, and dGTP, 2.5 mmol/L magnesium chloride, 50 mmol/L potassium chloride, 10 mmol/L Tris-HCl (pH 8.4 at 25 °C), 0.1 % Triton X-100, 0.02 mmol/L cresol red, and 83 mmol/L sucrose, as well as 0.15 units of Taq polymerase. The sequences of the sense and anti-sense primers were 5'tgggacttctctttgggctcctgacttac3' and 5'ccttcagcagattctc-cttcaggtcac3', respectively. DNA was amplified by 39 cycles of denaturing at 96 °C for 20 seconds, annealing at 56 °C for 40 seconds, and extension at 72 °C for 30 seconds.

Restriction buffer (10 μl) was added to yield a final concentration of 10 mmol/L Tris-HCl, 5.5 mmol/L magnesium chloride, 12.5 mmol/L sodium chloride, 30 mmol/L potassium chloride, 0.4 mmol/L dithiothreitol, and 0.1 % Triton X-100. The samples were incubated at 37 °C with 4 units of restriction endonuclease *MspI* overnight. This step was then repeated for complete digestion. In the presence of the *Pl^{A2}*, but not *Pl^{A1}* allele, the 82 base pair (bp) amplification product was cleaved into fragments of 39 bp and 43 bp.

Msp I digested amplification product (8 μl) was loaded onto 2 % agarose gel slabs containing 40 mmol/L Tris acetate and 2 mmol/L EDTA. Samples were size-fractionated at 6 V/cm for 30 minutes. Bands were visualized after staining with ethidium bromide by 300 nM ultraviolet transillumination. PCR results were scored without knowledge of platelet aggregability results. When there was any ambiguity, genotyping was repeated. Ninety-eight percent of the subjects were successfully genotyped.

Statistical analysis

Demographic and clinical characteristics were compared among genotype groups by one-way analysis of variance (ANOVA) or by chi-square test. Chi-square test was also used to compare the observed allele and genotype frequencies against Hardy-Weinberg equilibrium prediction. Data on epinephrine and ADP threshold concentrations were log-transformed and compared among genotype groups by one-way ANOVA (18) as well as nonparametric

Kruskall-Wallis test. Post-hoc pair-wise comparisons among genotypes were performed using Scheffe's adjustment. Multiple regression was used to adjust for age, sex, body mass index, diabetes, triglyceride, total cholesterol and HDL cholesterol, the presence of cardiovascular disease, menopausal status and estrogen replacement status (18, 31). Using appropriate dummy variables, separate models for recessive, dominant, and additive genetic effects were evaluated. Generalized estimating equation algorithms were used to correct for intra-family correlations (21). Data on platelet aggregation were expressed as geometric mean ± 95 % confidence interval. P < 0.05 was regarded as statistically significant.

Finally, a test of genetic linkage based on excess allele sharing for the quantitative traits (epinephrine and ADP threshold concentrations) with *GP IIIa* genotype was carried out, using SIBPAL version 2.7 of S.A.G.E (1996) (1, 4). This program provides an estimate of the proportion of alleles shared identical by descent at the *GP IIIa* locus using the sib-pairs under study. Under this algorithm, linkage between marker and phenotype results in a negative value for the slope of the regression of the squared trait difference on the estimated proportion of alleles.

Results

Subject characteristics

There were no significant differences among individuals within each genotype group for age, sex, body mass index, diabetes mellitus, smoking, cardiovascular disease, hypertension, triglyceride level, total and HDL cholesterol levels or alcohol consumption (Table 1).

Table 1. The demographic characteristics*

	PL^{A1}/PL^{A1}	PL^{A1}/PL^{A2}	PL^{A2}/PL^{A2}	P
Number	n = 1017	n = 369	n = 36	–
Sex (% male)	46	46	47	0.98
Age	53.4 ± 0.3	54.0 ± 0.5	51.4 ± 1.7	0.30
Hypertension (%)	33	29	33	0.38
Cardiovascular Disease (%)	6.7	7.9	8.3	0.72
Diabetes (%)	6.2	5.2	11.1	0.34
Smoker (%)	21	16	11	0.08
BMI (kg/m²)	27.4 ± 0.2	27.9 ± 0.3	26.8 ± 0.9	0.24
Triglyceride (mmol/l)	1.66 ± 0.03	1.57 ± 0.06	1.54 ± 0.19	0.40
Total cholesterol (mmol/l)	5.28 ± 0.03	5.33 ± 0.05	5.35 ± 0.16	0.70
HDL cholesterol (mmol/l)	1.27 ± 0.01	1.32 ± 0.02	1.27 ± 0.06	0.23
Alcohol (oz/wk)	2.9 ± 0.1	2.6 ± 0.2	1.4 ± 0.7	0.06

* Data are expressed as mean ± SEM or percentages

The allele frequencies of *Pl^{A1}* and *Pl^{A2}* were 0.84 and 0.16, respectively, and are in accord with those predicted by the Hardy-Weinberg equilibrium (p = 0.44).

The genotype frequencies were similar between subjects excluded from the present analysis in whom genotyping was performed and those included in the present analysis. The frequencies of *Pl^{A1}* homozygous, heterozygous and *Pl^{A2}* homozygous were 72.9 %, 24.3 %, and 2.8 % among subjects excluded, and 71.5 %, 26.0 %, and 2.5 %, respectively, among subjects included in the present analysis, p = 0.74.

Pl^A Polymorphism and platelet aggregability: association analysis (Table 2)

Epinephrine-induced platelet aggregation

The presence of one or two *Pl^{A2}* alleles was associated with an incrementally lower threshold concentration for epinephrine-induced aggregation (unadjusted ANOVA p = 0.009 and Kruskall-Wallis p = 0.0008). This increase in platelet aggregability associated with *Pl^{A2}* allele remained significant (ANOVA, p = 0.007) after adjustment for age, sex, body mass index, diabetes, triglyceride, total and HDL cholesterol, presence of cardiovascular disease, menopausal status, and estrogen replacement therapy. There was no difference in results in analyses which included or excluded subjects with cardiovascular disease.

Post-hoc analysis (Scheffe's test) was performed to compare genotype group pair-wisely. The difference of epinephrine threshold concentration between *Pl^{A1}* homozygous and *Pl^{A1}*/*Pl^{A2}* heterozygous was significant, p = 0.02. Due to the small sample size with the *Pl^{A2}* homozygous group (n = 36), the difference between *Pl^{A2}* homozygous and *Pl^{A1}* homozygous or *Pl^{A1}*/*Pl^{A2}* heterozygous were statistically insignificant, p = 0.18 and 0.69, respectively.

Regression models with dummy variables were used to test different modes of genetic transmission, in each case accounting for the above-mentioned possible confounders. The additive model (i.e., a gene-dose model) yielded the best fit with p = 0.002, followed by the dominant model (p = 0.003). But in the recessive model, no statistically significant effect was seen (p = 0.16). The threshold concentration of epinephrine decreased by 19 % per "dose" of *Pl^{A2}* allele (by 35 % for *Pl^{A2}* homozygous) relative to the *Pl^{A1}* homozygote.

ADP-induced platelet aggregation

There was a trend toward the *Pl^{A2}* allele being associated with a decreased threshold concentration for ADP, which was directionally consistent with the results seen with epinephrine-induced aggregation. However, the differences observed were not statistically

Table 2. Platelet aggregability induced by epinephrine and ADP

	Pl^{A1}/Pl^{A1}	Pl^{A1}/Pl^{A2}	Pl^{A2}/Pl^{A2}	P*
Epinephrine (μmol/l)	0.9 (0.9–1.0)	0.7 (0.7–0.9)	0.6 (0.4–1.0)	0.007
ADP (μmol/l)	3.1 (3.0–3.2)	3.0 (2.9–3.2)	2.8 (2.4–3.3)	0.190

* P values were ANOVA, adjusted for age, sex, body mass index, diabetes, triglyceride, total and HDL cholesterol, cardiovascular disease, menopausal status, and estrogen replacement therapy

significant (ANOVA, p = 0.48; Kruskall-Wallis test, p = 0.23); after adjustment for covariates p = 0.19 (ANOVA).

Pl^A polymorphism and platelet aggregability: linkage analyses result

A negative regression coefficient (–0.1926), consistent with genetic linkage but not statistically significant (p = 0.35), was observed for epinephrine-induced platelet aggregation. The regression coefficient for ADP threshold concentration was 0.2777, p = 0.60. The heterozygosity index of this dimorphic marker was 0.27.

Contribution of genetic and traditional risk factors to platelet aggregation
(Table 3)

In the model for epinephrine-induced aggregation, sex accounted for 2.7 % of the variance (p < 0.0001), triglyceride 1.1 % (p < 0.0001), *GP IIIa* genotype 0.7 % (p = 0.007), and age 0.5 % (p = 0.08). The remaining variables contributed less than 0.2 % each.

Table 3. Contribution of genetic and traditional risk factors to platelet aggregation

	Factors	Contribution	P Value	Note
Epinephrine-induced aggregation*	Sex	2.7 %	< 0.0001	Female associated with an increased aggregability
	Triglyceride	1.1 %	< 0.0001	Lower triglyceride associated with an increased aggregability
	GPIIIa genotype	0.7 %	0.007	Pl^{A2} allele associated with an increased aggregability
ADP-induced aggregation@	Sex	3.1 %	< 0.0001	Female associated with an increased aggregability
	Age	0.9 %	0.003	Increased age associated with an increased aggregability
	Triglyceride	0.8 %	0.0006	Lower triglyceride associated with increased aggregability
	HDL-cholesterol	0.5 %	0.006	Lower levels associated with increased aggregability
	HRT#	0.3 %	0.03	Therapy associated with increased aggregability
	GP IIIa genotype	0.2 %	0.21	Pl^{A2} allele associated with increased aggregability

*: In the epinephrine-induced aggregation, the remaining variables, including age, CVD, BMI, diabetes, total and HDL cholesterol, menopausal status, and HRT were not significantly associated with platelet aggregability. @: In the ADP-induced platelet aggregation, CVD, BMI, diabetes, total cholesterol levels, and menopausal status were not significantly associated with platelet aggregability. # HRT = hormone replacement therapy

In the model for ADP-induced aggregation, sex accounted for 3.1 % of the variance (p < 0.0001), age 0.9 % (p = 0.003), triglyceride 0.8 % (p = 0.0006), HDL-cholesterol 0.5 % (p = 0.006), hormone replacement therapy 0.3 % (p = 0.03), and *GP IIIa* genotype 0.2 % (p = 0.21). The remaining variables contributed less than 0.2% each.

Discussion

In the Framingham Offspring Study, the presence of one or two *Pl^{A2}* alleles of the platelet GP IIIa receptor was associated with an incrementally lower platelet threshold concentration in response to epinephrine and a trend toward lower threshold concentration in response to ADP. The increase in aggregability induced by epinephrine remained highly significant after adjustment for covariates. For epinephrine-induced aggregation, *GPIIIa* genotype explained 0.7 % of the variance, while age, sex, and triglyceride accounted for an additional 4.3 % of the variance.

GP IIIa polymorphism and cardiovascular disease

The familial clustering of coronary heart disease and the presence of a higher concordance in mortality among monozygotic twins compared with dizygotic twins suggest an important pathogenic role for genetic factors (22). Although a small proportion of coronary heart disease can be attributed to single gene defects (e.g, familial hypercholesterolemia or homocysteinuria), the nature of additional contributing genetic factors remains largely unknown. Since platelets play a central role in the pathogenesis of acute cardiovascular disease, it is possible that inherited platelet variants may contribute to cardiovascular disease risk. Knowledge of such variants and their phenotypic expression may lead to progress in coronary disease risk assessment and therapeutic intervention.

Weiss and colleagues (38) showed that patients with acute coronary syndromes were more likely than were controls to carry the *Pl^{A2}* allele. In their study, the prevalence of the *Pl^{A2}* allele was 2.1 times higher in the patients than among the controls. These findings, coupled with an anecdotal report about the sudden death of a 28 year old Olympic skater who had severe coronary artery disease and carried the *Pl^{A2}* allele, but no other traditional risk factors, resulted in the *Pl^{A1}/Pl^{A2}* dimorphism receiving widespread attention (13). Further studies of this genetic marker are warranted since, while there has been some support for the findings of Weiss et al. (6, 7), results from several other groups found no association between the *Pl^{A2}* allele and cardiovascular disease, including an analysis by Ridker et al. of the Physicians' Health Study (5, 15, 23, 27, 28, 30).

GP IIIa polymorphism and platelet aggregability

Platelet *GP IIb/IIIa* is the most abundant platelet receptor, with an estimated 50,000 copies per cell (16). It is present in the platelet membrane as a heterodimeric complex whose formation requires the presence of divalent cations. The receptor is highly polymorphic and has long been recognized as having alloantigens (20). *Pl^{A}* alloantigens have been most frequently considered for their role in syndromes of immune-mediated platelet destruction, such as post-transfusion purpura and neonatal alloimmune thrombocytopenic purpura (20). Newman and colleagues (26) identified the molecular basis of this polymorphism. The Pl^{A1}-allotype carries a leucine at position 33 of glycoprotein *IIIa* whereas the Pl^{A2}-allotype has a proline at position 33, due to a thymidine to cytosine substitution at 1565 in exon 2 of the glycoprotein *IIIa* gene.

The functional influence of the polymorphism on platelet reactivity is largely unknown. Using epinephrine as a platelet agonist, we found that the presence of the Pl^{A2} allele was associated with heightened platelet aggregability. Furthermore, the Pl^{A2} associated increase in aggregability remained significant after adjustment for traditional risk factors that could influence platelet aggregability. The effect of the *GP IIIa* polymorphism on epinephrine induced aggregation is in according with additive model, with threshold concentration decreased by 19 % per "dose" of Pl^{A2} allele (35 % for Pl^{A2} homozygous) comparing with the Pl^{A1} homozygote. Using multiple regression analysis, we found that the polymorphism explained a small, but significant percentage of variance of aggregability induced by epinephrine.

The platelet Pl^{A} antigen system is not in the two putative RGD sequence binding regions of *GP IIIa*, which are located within residues 107–179 and 211–222 from the amino terminal, respectively (8, 12). However, according to Calvete (3), the Leu33/Pro33 polymorphism is enclosed within a small 13 amino acid loop formed by the pairing of Cys26 with Cys38. In addition, a long-range disulfide bond linking Cys5 and Cys435 has been identified which could bring the amino terminal region of *IIIa*, including the small loop that contains the Pl^{A} polymorphic residue, into immediate proximity with the binding regions of *IIIa* (8, 12). Due to proline's unique structure, proline substitutions are well recognized for their propensity to induce conformational changes. Such changes can create alloantigenic determinants recognizable by T cell and B cells and induce the production of antibody (24). The conformational changes could also influence activation of the *GP IIb/IIIa* receptor and alter platelet aggregability. Equally possible, the Pl^{A} polymorphism may be in linkage disequilibrium with other as yet undefined molecular variants of the gene that influence platelet reactivity.

Goldschmidt-Clermont and colleagues (14) quantitated fibrinogen binding to platelets of different allotypes. The investigators found that platelets with the Pl^{A2} allele bound significantly less fibrinogen than did platelets that were homozygous for Pl^{A1}. Differences in methodology used to evaluate platelet reactivity in the study make it difficult to compare with our data. Additional larger and more comprehensive investigations will be required to resolve the issue. In a recent study, Cooke et al. found that platelets with the Pl^{A2} allele were more sensitive to aspirin inhibition (9).

Finally, we studied the relation between the Pl^{A} polymorphism and an intermediate phenotype, i.e., platelet aggregability, rather than coronary heart disease. Although it has not been demonstrated that epinephrine-induced platelet aggregation is an independent risk factor for coronary heart disease, there is considerable evidence linking platelet reactivity to cardiovascular disease (29, 34, 36). In the Framingham Heart Study, we will prospectively follow the population to determine whether epinephrine-induced platelet aggregability and the Pl^{A2} allele are risk factors for CVD.

Limitations of the study

First, our analysis was based on a single measurement of platelet aggregation. However, any random variation or misclassification would introduce bias that favors the null hypothesis and an underestimation of the genetic contribution to platelet aggregability.

Additional measures of platelet function should be evaluated in future studies. Second, our analysis was based on the subset of Framingham subjects in whom both genotype and phenotype data were available. However, the genotype distribution was similar between subjects excluded from analysis and those included in the present analysis. Third, a dimorphic marker was used for linkage analysis. While not statistically significant, the results of the linkage analysis are consistent with the findings for the association studies as indicated by the negative slope of the regression line. The failure to reach statistical significance is not too surprising. Due to the limited informativity of the marker used (heterozygosity index = 0.27) and the limited extent to which parental (i.e., identity by descent) information was available, we had limited power to detect a statistically significant linkage. In future studies, a more informative marker should be used for linkage analysis. Finally, we used platelet aggregability to evaluate the relation between the Pl^A polymorphism and platelet function. Although platelet aggregation studies in platelet rich plasma can assess the effect of platelet inhibitors such as aspirin, the *in vivo* correlates and clinical significance of changes in platelet aggregation need to be more fully defined.

Implications of the study

We found that the Pl^{A2} allele was associated with increased platelet aggregability in the Framingham Offspring Study. Our results support the hypothesis that Pl^{A2} might be a genetic risk factor for cardiovascular disease (7, 37, 38), and provide a mechanism for the link. Since epinephrine-induced aggregation was increased with the Pl^{A2} allele and since increased aggregability has been described following assumption of the upright posture (34) and strenuous exercise (39), it would be of interest to determine if subjects with different Pl^A alleles react differently to strenuous exercise. Such a study may not only provide additional insights into the mechanism by which strenuous exercise triggers the onset of cardiovascular events (25), but may also help in selecting individuals for appropriate preventive therapy. In addition, further prospective studies are needed to test if this genetic marker is an independent risk factor for cardiovascular disease. If individuals with the Pl^{A2} allele have a higher incidence of cardiovascular disease, they may benefit from more aggressive measures for preventing and treating cardiovascular disease, including therapy with antiplatelet agents such as *GP IIb/IIIa* receptor antagonists.

Acknowledgments   This study was supported by NIH/NHLBI No1-38038 to Dr. Tofler and by Research Development Award K04-HL-03138-01 from the National Heart, Lung, and Blood Institute to Dr. Lindpaintner. Linkage analysis was performed using S.A.G.E., which is supported by a USPHS Resource Grant (1P41 RR03655) from the National Center for Research Resources.

References

1. Bishop D, Williamson J (1990) The power of identity-by-state methods for linkage analysis. Am J Hum Genet 46: 254–265
2. Born G (1964) Aggregation of platelet by adenosine diphosphate and its reversal. Nature 194: 927–929
3. Calvete JJ, Henschen A, Gonzalez-Rodriguez J (1991) Assignment of disulphide bonds in human platelet GPIIIa. A disulphide pattern for the beta-subunits of the integrin family. Biochem J 274: 63–71
4. The Case Western Reserve University C, OH. S.A.G.E. Statistical Analysis for Genetic Epidemiology. Release 2. 2. 1996.
5. Carlsson LE, Greinacher A, Spitzer C, Walther R, Kessler C (1997) Polymorphisms of the human platelet antigens HPA-1, HPA-2, HPA-3, and HPA-5 on the platelet receptors for fibrinogen (GPIIb/IIIa), von Willebrand factor (GPIb/IX), and collagen (GPIa/IIa) are not correlated with an increased risk for stroke. Stroke 28: 1392–1395

6. Carter AM, Ossei-Gerning N, Grant PJ (1996) Platelet glycoprotein IIIa PlA polymorphism and myocardial infarction. N Engl J Med 335: 1072–3

7. Carter AM, Ossei-Gerning N, Wilson IJ, Grant PJ (1997) Association of the Platelet PlA Polymorphism of Glycoprotein IIb/IIIa and the Fibrinogen Bβ 448 Polymorphism with Myocardial Infarction and Extent of Coronary Artery Disease. Circulation 96: 1424–1431

8. Charo IF, Nannizzi L, Phillips DR, Hsu MA, Scarborough RM (1991) Inhibition of fibrinogen binding to GP IIb-IIIa by a GP IIIa peptide. J Biolog Chem 266: 1415–1421

9. Cooke GE, Bray PF, Hamlington JD, Pham DM, Goldschmidt-Clermont PJ (1998) PLA2 polymorphism and efficacy of aspirin. Lancet 351: 1253

10. Davies MJ, Richardson PD, Woolf N, Katz DR, Mann J (1993) Risk of thrombosis in human atherosclerotic plaques: role of extracellular lipid, macrophage, and smooth muscle cell content. Br Heart J 69: 377–381

11. DeWood MA, Spores J, Notske R, Mouser LT, Burroughs R, Golden MS, Lang HT (1980) Prevalence of total coronary occlusion during the early hours of transmural myocardial infarction. New Eng J Med 303: 897–902

12. D'Souza SE, Ginsberg MH, Burke TA, Lam SC, Plow EF (1988) Localization of an Arg-Gly-Asp recognition site within an integrin adhesion receptor. Science 242: 91–93

13. Goldschmidt-Clermont PJ, Shear WS, Schwartzberg J, Varga CF, Bray PF (1996) Clues to the death of an Olympic champion. Lancet 347: 1833

14. Goldschmidt-Clermont P, Weiss E, Shear W, Kennedy S, Kickler T, Becker L, Bray D (1996) Platelets from PLA2 (–) individuals bind more exogenous fibrinogen than platelet from PLA2 (+) individuals. Blood 88: 26a

15. Herrmann SM, Poirier O, Marques-Vidal P, Evans A, Arveiler D, Luc G, Emmerich J, Cambien F (1997) The Leu33/Pro polymorphism (PlA1/PlA2) of the glycoprotein IIIa (GPIIIa) receptor is not related to myocardial infarction in the ECTIM Study. Etude Cas-Temoins de l'Infarctus du Myocarde. Thromb Haemost 77: 1179–1181

16. Isenberg W, McEver R, Phillips D, Shuman M, Bainton D (1987) The platelet fibrinogen receptor: An immunogold-surface replica study of agonist-induced ligand binding and receptor clustering. J Cell Biol 104: 1655–1663

17. Kannel W, Feinleib M, McNamara J, Garrison R, Castelli W (1979) An investigation of coronary heart disease in families: the Framingham Offspring Study. Am J Epidemiol 110: 281–290

18. Kleinbaum DG, Kupper LL, Muller KE (1988) Applied Regression Analysis and Other Multivariable Methods. Second ed. Boston, MA: PWS-Kent Publishing Company, pp 102–340

19. Kleiman NS, Ohman EM, Califf RM, George BS, Kereiakes D, Aguirre FV, Weisman H, Schaible T, Topol EJ (1993) Profound inhibition of platelet aggregation with monoclonal antibody 7E3 Fab after thrombolytic therapy. Results of the Thrombolysis and Angioplasty in Myocardial Infarction (TAMI) 8 Pilot Study. J Am Coll Cardiol 22: 381–389

20. Kunicki T, Newman P (1992) The molecular immunology of human platelet proteins. Blood 80: 1386–1404

21. Liang KY, Zeger SL (1986) Longitudinal data analysis using generalized estimating linear models. Biometrika 73: 12–22

22. Marenberg ME, Risch N, Berkman LF, Floderus B, de Faire U (1994) Genetic susceptibility to death from coronary heart disease in a study of twins. N Engl J Med 330: 1041–1046

23. Marian AJ, Brugada R, Kleiman NS (1996) Platelet glycoprotein IIIa PlA polymorphism and myocardial infarction. N Engl J Med 335: 1071–2

24. Maslanka K, Yassai M, Gorski J (1996) Molecular identification of T cell that respond in a primary bulk culture to a peptide derived from a platelet glycoprotein implicated in neonatal alloimmune thrombocytopenia. J Clin Investig 98: 1802–1808

25. Mittleman MA, Maclure M, Tofler GH, Sherwood JB, Goldberg RJ, Muller JE (1993) Triggering of acute myocardial infarction by heavy physical exertion. Protection against triggering by regular exertion. Determinants of Myocardial Infarction Onset Study Investigators. N Engl J Med 329: 1677–1683

26. Newman PJ, Derbes RS, Aster RH (1989) The human platelet alloantigens, PlA1 and PlA2, are associated with a leucine33/proline33 amino acid polymorphism in membrane glycoprotein IIIa, and are distinguishable by DNA typing. J Clin Investig 83: 1778–1781

27. Osborn SV, Hampton KK, Smillie D, Channer KS, Daly ME (1996) Platelet glycoprotein IIIa gene polymorphism and myocardial infarction. Lancet 348: 1309–1310

28. Ridker PM, Hennekens CH, Schmitz C, Stampfer MJ, Lindpaintner K (1997) PIA1/A2 polymorphism of platelet glycoprotein IIIa and risks of myocardial infarction, stroke, and venous thrombosis. Lancet 349: 385–388

29. The RISC Group (1990) Risk of myocardial infarction and death during treatment with low dose aspirin and intravenous heparin in men with unstable coronary artery disease. Lancet 336: 827–830

30. Samani NJ, Lodwick D (1997) Glycoprotein IIIa polymorphism and risk of myocardial infarction. Cardiovasc Res 33: 693–697

31. SAS Institute Inc. GLM Procedure, and REG Procedure (1996) In: SAS/STAT Software: Changes and Enhancements through Release 6.11. Cary, NC. SAS Institute, Inc. pp 317–324

32. Simoons ML, de Boer MJ, van den Brand MJ, van Miltenburg AJ, Hoorntje JC, Heyndrickx GR, van der Wieken LR, de Bono D, Rutsch W, Schaible TF, Weisman HF, Klootwijk P, Nijssen KM, Stibbe J, de Feyter PJ (1994) Randomized trial of a GPIIb/IIIa platelet receptor blocker in refractory unstable angina. European Cooperative Study Group. Circulation 89: 596–603
33. Tcheng JE, Harrington RA, Kottke-Marchant K, Kleiman NS, Ellis SG, Kereiakes DJ, Mick MJ, Navetta FI, Smith JE, Worley SJ, Miller JA, Joseph DM, Sigmon KN, Kitt MM, du Mee CP, Califf RM, Topol EJ (1995) Multicenter, randomized, double-blind, placebo-controlled trial of the platelet integrin glycoprotein IIb/IIIa blocker Integrelin in elective coronary intervention. IMPACT Investigators. Circulation 91: 2151–2157
34. Tofler GH, Brezinski D, Schafer AI, Czeisler CA, Rutherford JD, Willich SN, Gleason RE, Williams GH, Muller JE (1987) Concurrent morning increase in platelet aggregability and the risk of myocardial infarction and sudden cardiac death. N Engl J Med 316: 1514–1518
35. Topol EJ, Califf RM, Weisman HF, Ellis SG, Tcheng JE, Worley S, Ivanhoe R, George BS, Fintel D, Weston M, Sigmon K, Anderson KL, Lee KL, Willerson TJ (1994) Randomized trial of coronary intervention with antibody against platelet IIb/IIIa integrin for reduction of clinical restenosis: results at six months. The EPIC Investigators. Lancet 343: 881–886
36. Trip MD, Manger Cats V, van Capelle FJL, Vreeken J (1990) Platelet hyperreactivity and prognosis in survivors of myocardial infarction. N Engl J Med 322: 1549–1554
37. Walter D, Schachinger V, Elsner M, Dimmeler S, Zeiher A (1997) Platelet glycoprotein IIIa polymorphisms and risk of coronary stent thrombosis. Lancet 350: 1217–1219
38. Weiss EJ, Bray PF, Tayback M, Schulman SP, Kickler TS, Becker LC, Weiss JL, Gerstenblith G, Goldschmidt-Clermont PJ (1996) A polymorphism of a platelet glycoprotein receptor as an inherited risk factor for coronary thrombosis. N Engl J Med 334: 1090–1094
39. Winther K, Hillegass W, Tofler GH, Jimenez A, Brezinski DA, Schafer AI, Loscalzo J, Williams GH, Muller JE (1992) Effects on platelet aggregation and fibrinolytic activity during upright posture and exercise in healthy men. Am J Cardiol 70: 1051–1055

Author's address:
Geoffrey H. Tofler, MD
Institute for Prevention of Cardiovascular Disease
Beth Israel Deaconess Medical Center
Harvard Medical School
One Autumn Street, 5th Floor
Boston, MA 02215, USA
E-mail: gtofler@bidmc.harvard.edu

Genetic aspects of chronobiologic rhythms in cardiovascular disease

B. Lemmer

Institute of Pharmacology and Toxicology, Ruprecht-Karls-University Heidelberg, Mannheim, Germany

Abstract

Daily variations in the cardiovascular system are well documented from the carcadian rhythm in blood pressure and heart rate, pathophysiological events such as coronary infarction, angina pectoris down to the receptor-mediated processes of signal transduction. Telemetric data on blood pressure and heart rate profiles in animal models of human primary and secondary hypertension together with biochemical and molecular biological findings can help to get a better understanding of the mechanisms involved in the circadian organization of the cardiovascular system. From animal data of genetically different strains of rats (normotensive, hypertensive, transgenic hypertensive rats), we have good evidence that the master clock located in the nucleus suprachiasmaticus (SCN) is involved in the rhythmic organization. Chronopharmacological studies with different kinds of antihypertensive drugs also point to a genetically bound variation in the circadian pattern of blood pressure and its regulation.

Introduction

The most ubiquious feature of nature is that of rhythmicity. Circadian rhythms have been documented throughout the plant and animal kingdom at every level of eukariotic organization. Circadian rhythms by definition are endogenous in nature, driven by oscillators or clocks (1), and persist under free-running conditions. In various species (Drosophila melongaster, Neurospora, Mouse, Golden hamster) even the genes controlling circadian rhythms have been identified.

In general, the endogenous clock does not run exactly at a frequency of 24 h but somewhat slower. The rhythm in, for example, human body temperature which is timed by the biological clock has an about 25-h period under free-running conditions, i.e., without environmental time-cues or Zeitgebers (e.g. light, temperature). Zeitgebers (2) entrain the biological oscillator or clock, and thereby the "arms" of the the clock, the circadian rhythms, to a precise 24-h period of the solar day (Fig. 1). Endogenous biological rhythms are anticipatory in nature. Thereby, the biological clock allows one to adapt more easily and to

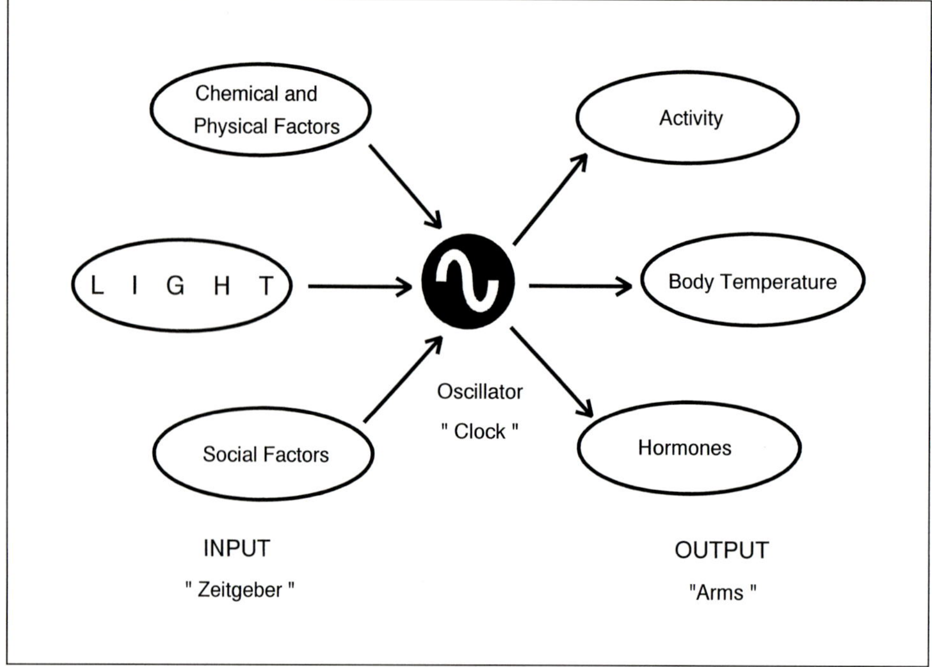

Fig. 1. Inputs and outputs of the clock and entrainment by Zeitgebers.

better survive under changing environmental conditions during the 24 h of a day as well as during varying conditions of the changing seasons.

Chronobiology and chronopharmacology of the cardiovascular system

In man ambulatory blood pressure monitoring [ABPM] is now regarded as the method of choice to assess the 24-h pattern in blood pressure and heart rate and the effectiveness of an antihypertensive therapy (3, 9, 11, 26, 30). ABPM demonstrated that the blood pressures in normotensive and in hypertensive patients are clearly dependent on the time of day (11). Moreover, different forms of hypertension may exhibit different circadian patterns; in normotension as well as in primary hypertension there is in general a nightly drop in blood pressure (dippers), whereas in forms of secondary hypertension due to, e.g., renal disease, gestation, Cushing's disease, diabetes mellitus or the prion disease of fatal familial insomnia (27), the rhythm in blood pressure is in about 70 % of the cases abolished or even reversed with highest values at night (non-dippers) (4, 10, 18, 24). This is of particular interest since the loss in nocturnal blood pressure fall correlates with increased end organ damage in cardiac, cerebral, vascular, and renal tissues (5, 29).

In man pathophysiological events within the cardiovascular system do also not occur at random (8, 18, 31). Thus, the onset of non-fatal or fatal myocardial infarction predominates between 06.00 h – 12.00 h. A similar circadian time pattern has been shown for sudden cardiac death, stroke, ventricular arrhythmias, and arterial embolism. Symptoms in coronary heart diseased patients such as myocardial ischemia, angina attacks or silent ischemia are also significantly more frequent during the daytime hours than at night, whereas the onset of angina attacks in variant angina peaks around 04.00 h during the night. During the early morning hours not only do cardiovascular events predominate but there is also the rapid rise in blood pressure, a rapid increase in sympathetic tone and in the concentrations of pressure hormones, and the highest values in peripheral resistance (18). Thus, it appears that the early morning hours are the hours of highest cardiovascular risk.

Drug treament of human hypertension includes various types of drugs such as diuretics, alpha- and beta-adrenoceptor blocking drugs, calcium channel blockers, converting enzyme inhibitors, diuretics, angiotensin receptor antagonists, and others which differ in their sites of action. Since the main steps in the mechanisms regulating the blood pressure are circadian phase-dependent (10, 18) it is not a surprise that antihypertensive drugs may also exhibit a circadian time-dependency in their effects and/or their pharmacokinetics (for review see 8–11, 13, 18). From these studies it appears that, in primary hypertension antihypertensive drugs should be given at early morning hours, whereas in secondary hypertension it can be necessary to add an evening dose or to apply a single evening dose in order not only to reduce high blood pressure but also to normalize a disturbed blood pressure pattern (10, 11).

However, we still insufficiently understand the mechansism of the circadian regulation of blood pressure and heart rate as well as the circadian phase-dependency of the effects and/or kinetics of antihypertensive drugs. Therefore, we need animal models which allow one to investigate cardiovascular functions "around the clock" in unrestrained freely moving animals as well as drugs effects thereupon. This implies that possible differences in the genetic background of the animals used have to be taken into account.

Animal models of hypertension

The advent of radiotelemetry can be regarded as a breakthrough for studying cardiovascular functions in unrestrained animals of different breedings and different genetic background under well-defined environmental conditions. The use of radiotelemetry can, therefore, help to get a better understanding of the mechanisms of regulation of the rhythms in blood pressure and heart rate and their strain dependency. In addition, the dose- and circadian phase-dependency of drugs can be studied in animals bearing radiotransmitters.

Using radiotelemetry for continuous blood pressure monitoring, we studied the rhythmic patterns in systolic and diastolic blood pressure, heart rate, and motor activity in strains of normotensive rats (outbred: Wistar WISW BOR; inbred: Wistar-Kyoto (WKY), Sprague-Dawley (SPRD)) and of hypertensive rats (spontaneously hypertensive (SHR), transgenic hypertensiv (TGR(m-Ren-2)27)) (17). The latter rats which were derived from SPRD were made hypertensive by transfection of the salivary mouse renin gene.

Entrained to a light-dark cycle of 12 h:12 h (LD 12:12), the different rat strains exhibited clearly strain-dependent differences in the 24 h patterns of cardiovascular functions,

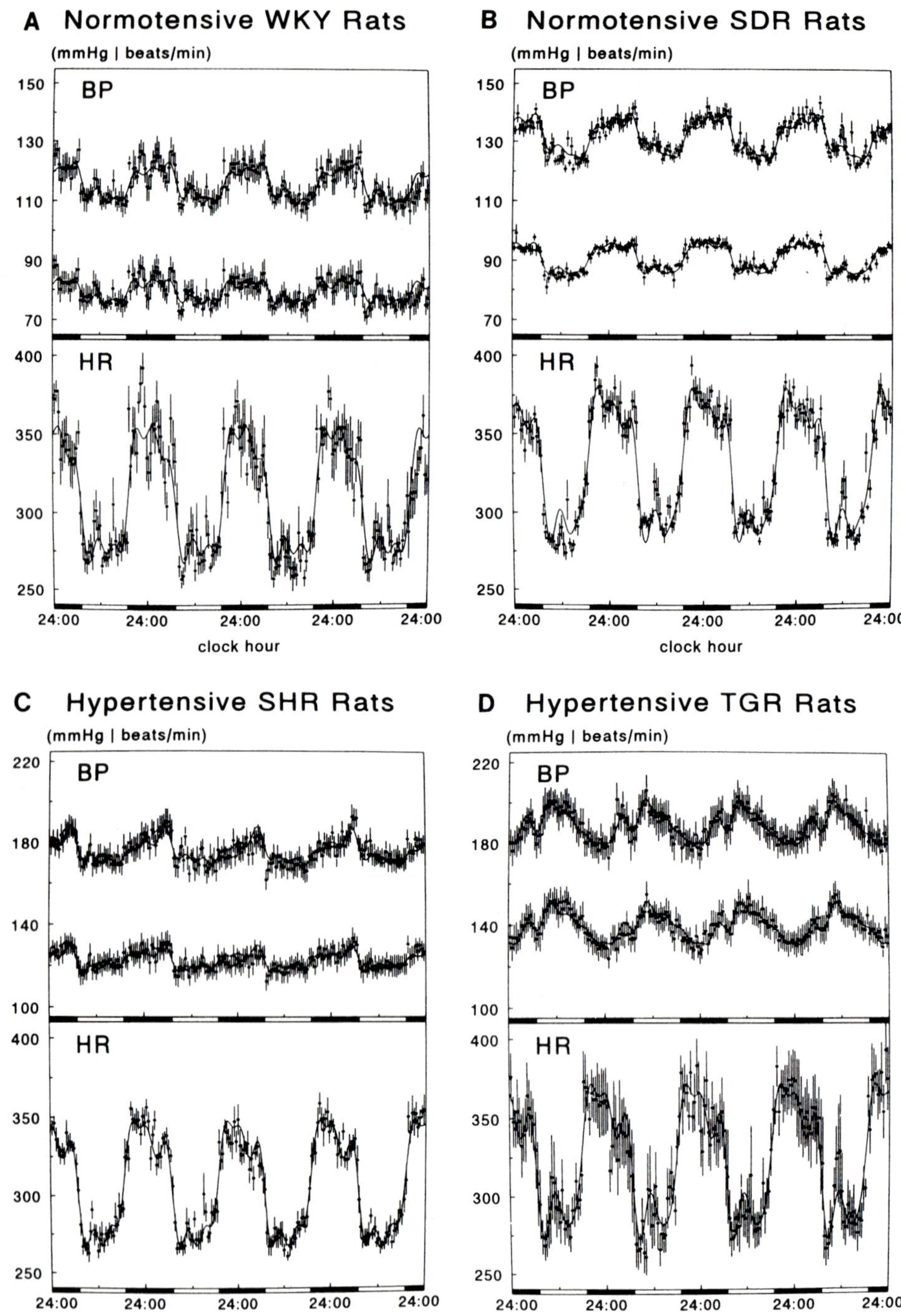

Fig. 2. 24-Hour rhythms in blood pressure and heart rate in male normotensive Wistar-Kyoto (WKY), Sprague-Dawley (SPRD) rats and in spontaneously hypertensive (SHR) and hypertensive transgenic TGR(mRen2)27 rats (TGR) as monitored by telemetry. Telemetric data on systolic and diastolic blood pressure (BP) and heart rate (HR) were registered four days in sequence. Shown are mean values ± SEM of 30-min intervals of 11 SHR and 9 TGR rats, the best nonlinear fit by a partial Fourier analysis (23) is given by the solid line. Data from (17).

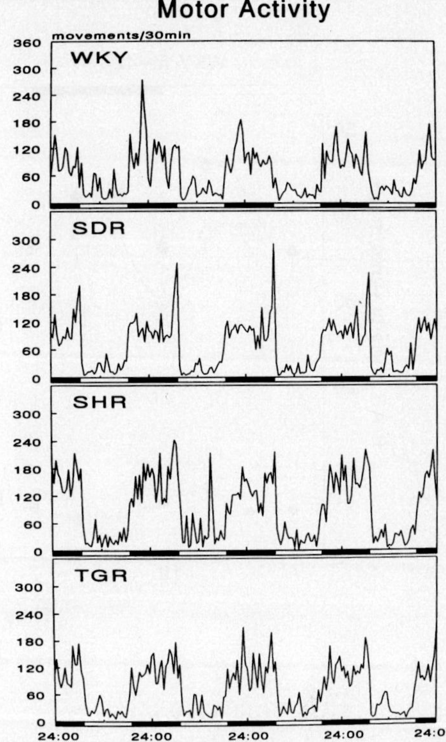

Fig. 3. Circadian rhythm in motor activity in 4 strains of rats, WKY, SPDR, SHR, and TGR (see Fig. 2). Movements were collected for 5 min period intervals and averaged over 30 minutes. Shown are mean values of 8–11 rats monitored for 4 days continuously to demonstrate nocturnal activity in either rat strain. Data from (17).

predominantly in systolic (SBP) and diastolic (DBP) blood pressure as shown in Fig. 2. Normotensive rats, WKY and SPRD, and spontaneously hypertensive rats (SHR), which were derived form WKY and are considered to be an animal model of human primary hypertension, showed normal circadian rhythms in blood pressure, heart rate, and motor activity (Fig. 3) with peaks in the rat's nocturnal activity period (17). In transgenic hypertensive TGR, in contrast, we were able to first describe a significant phase shift in the profile of the circadian rhythms in blood pressure inverse to those in heart rate and motor activity. This demonstrates that expression of an additional single gene brought about a significant modification in the rhythmic pattern of blood pressure and gives further support for a genetic basis of biological rhythms. Due to the peak in blood pressure in the animals' rest phase ("non-dipping"), we proposed TGR to serve as an animal model for the blood pressure pattern observed in human forms of secondary hypertension (17). It is of importance to note that in all strains of rats, including TGR, rhythms in motor activity exhibited the normal circadian pattern with peak values in the animals' activity phase (Fig. 3) giving evidence that activity, which is out of phase with blood pressure in TGR, does not mainly determine the rhythm in blood pressure (17, 21, 25).

The TGR turns out to be a fascinating model in which a single additional mouse renin gene not only resulted in a fulminant hypertension but also significantly changed physiological circadian rhythms. This finding is of great interest because the genetic component of hypertension and, moreover, the mechanisms responsible for a disturbed blood pressure profile in human secondary hypertension are still an open question. Biochemical and pharmacological studies in this animal model can help to increase our understanding and can possibly improve drug treatment.

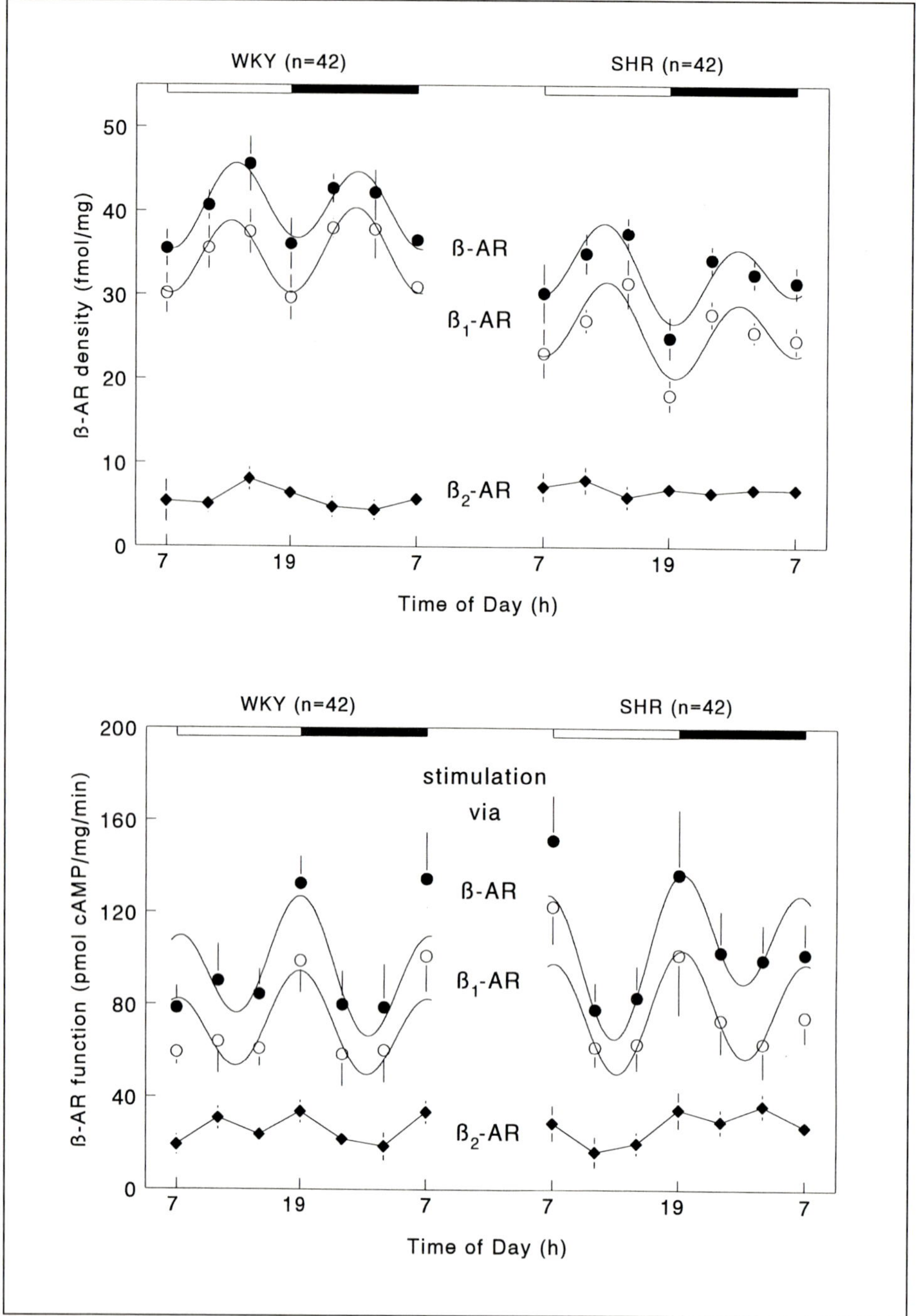

Fig. 4. Rhythms in the density (top) and function (bottom) of β-adrenoceptors and their β_1- and β_2-subtypes in ventricles from normotensive WKY and spontaneously hypertensive SHR animals. Density of β-adrenoceptor subtypes was determined using the non-selective radioligand [^{3}H]CGP 12177 in the absence or presence of the β_1-selective antagonist CGP 20712A. Shown are the densities in total β-adrenoceptors (β-AR) and their subtypes (β_1-AR) and (β_2-AR). Accordingly, function of β-adrenoceptors was determined by the isoprenaline-induced increase in cAMP formation. Data points are means ± SEM, modified from (36).

Genetic differences in signal transduction?

Postsynaptic events of signal transmission such as formation, content, and degradation of the second messenger cAMP were found to exhibit significant daily variation in heart ventricles from Wistar rats (14). Recently, we studied in more detail the postsynaptic signal transduction cascade in the inbred strains of rats (normotensive: WKY, SRPD; hypertensive: SHR, TGR) in order to better understand the mechanisms of regulation of the blood pressure and heart rate rhythms in normo- and hypertension and their strain-dependency (36, for review see 19, 34). In ventricles from WKY and SHR the density of total β-adrenoceptors as well as of the β_1-subtype exhibited significant 12 h-rhythms with peaks occurring around 1:00 h and 13:00 h, i.e., in the middle of the light and dark periods. For the β_2-subtype no significant rhythmicity could be detected (Fig. 4). In SHR cardiac β-adrenoceptor density, calculated as the 24 h mean, was approx. 20 % lower than in WKY due to a loss in the β_1-subtype by 25 %, whereas the density of β_2-adrenoceptors was similar in both strains (Fig. 4, top). In contrast, formation of cAMP was 20–30 % higher in SHR than in WKY under all experimental conditions except after uncoupling of G-proteins by Mn^{2+} (Fig. 5); in cardiac tissue from both strains significant 12 h rhythms were observed in basal adenylyl cyclase activity and after stimulation by GTP, isoprenaline (IPN), and GTP, and a water-soluble forskolin derivative (FOR), respectively. Peaks in basal and stimulated cAMP formation occurred around 7:00 h and 19:00 h, being 6 h apart from those in β-adrenoceptor density (Fig. 4, bottom). The addition of Mn^{2+} instead of Mg^{2+} abolished

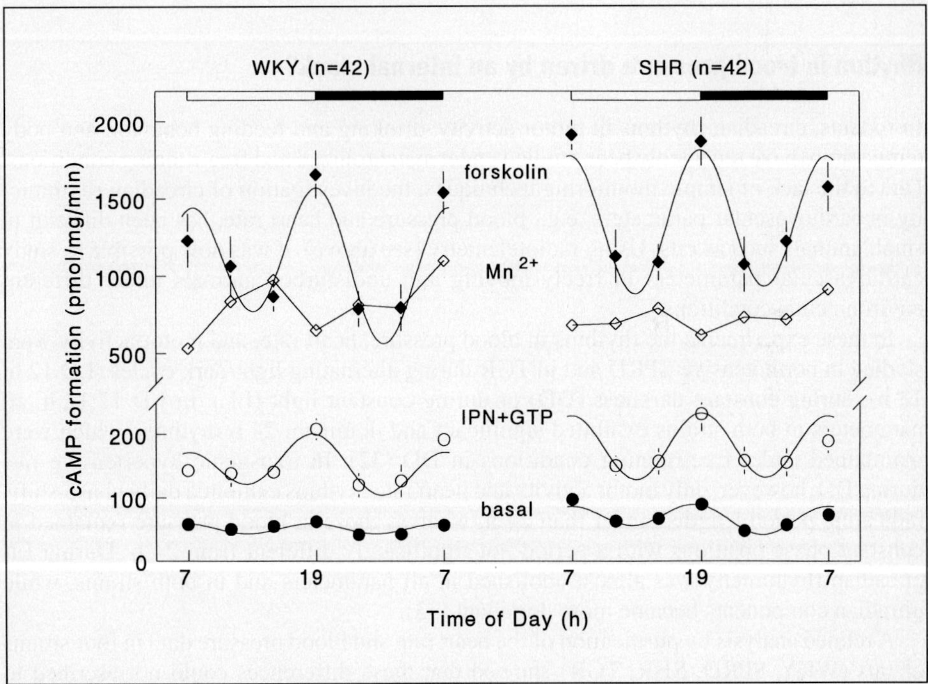

Fig. 5. Circadian variation in basal and stimulated adenylyl cyclase activity in ventricles from WKY rats (left) and SHR (right). Formation of cAMP was measured under basal conditions and after stimulation by isoprenaline 1 μM, Mn^{2+} ions 10 mM, and a forskolin derivative 100 μM. Addition of Mn^{2+} ions abolished the rhythmicity in cAMP formation in both strains, whereas addition of the other activators preserved circadian variation though at a higher level of adenylyl cyclase activity. Data points are means ± SEM, modified from (36).

the circadian rhythmicity in adenylyl cyclase activity (Fig. 5), indicating that G-proteins must be involved in the circadian regulation of cardiac cAMP formation. The discrepancy between the effects of FOR and Mn^{2+}, both of which directly activate the catalytic subunit of the adenylyl cyclase, can be explained by the fact that coupling of $G_{s\alpha}$ to the catalytic subunit is known to potentiate the stimulatory effect of forskolin, probably by increasing the number of high affinity forskolin binding sites. Since coupling of G-proteins is disrupted by addition of Mn^{2+} ions, the resulting stimulation of cAMP formation solely reflects the direct activation of the catalytic subunit. The observation that peaks in cAMP coincided with troughs in β-adrenoceptor density (Fig. 4) could indicate that cAMP dependent desensitization and down-regulation of β-adrenoceptors is involved in the circadian regulation of receptor density. That rhythmicity was lost after uncoupling G-protein by Mn^{2+} from the adenylyl cyclase indicates that G-proteins must be involved in generation of this rhythmic behavior in these rat strains.

It is of interest to note that no circadian phase-dependency was observed in similar experiments in both normotensive SPRD and hypertensive TGR derived from SPRD. Neither total β-adrenoceptor density, nor the subtype distribution, nor basal as well as stimulated adenylyl cyclase activity were found to be rhythmic in cardiac tissues of these two rat strains (33, 37).

Taken together, the data on signal transduction in cardiac tissue of four inbred strains of rats clearly demonstrate a genetic control of these processes. This is of importance to bear in mind when data from different strains are compared without taking into account the presence/absence of rhythmicity.

Rhythm in blood pressure driven by an internal clock?

In rodents, circadian rhythms in motor activity, drinking and feeding behavior, and body temperature have repeatedly been studied under synchronized and free-running conditions. Due to the lack of simple monitoring techniques, the investigation of circadian rhythmicity in cardiovascular parameters, e.g., blood pressure and heart rate, has been difficult in small animals such as rats. Using radiotelemetry (see above), it was now possible to study cardiovascular parameters in freely-moving and undisturbed animals under different environmental conditions.

In these experiments the rhythms in blood pressure, heart rate, and motor activity were studied in normotensive SPRD and in TGR during alternating light-dark cycles (LD 12 h: 12 h), during constant darkness (DD) or during constant light (LL). In LD 12:12 h, all parameters in both strains exhibited significant and dominant 24 h rhythms, which were maintained under free-running conditions in DD (32). In transgenic hypertensive rats during DD, however, only motor activity and heart rate rhythms exhibited daily phase-shifts indicating period lengths longer than 24 h, whereas those in blood pressure remained in constant phase positions with a period not significantly different from 24 h. During LL circadian rhythmicity was almost abolished in all parameters and in both strains, while ultradian components became more dominant (32).

A refined analysis by purification of the heart rate and blood pressure data in four strains of rats (WKY, SPRD, SHR, TGR) showed that these differences could not ascribed to masking effects caused by locomotor activity (21) as already concluded from the original raw data (17). This analysis further adds to the notion that – at least in the rat – the rhythms in blood pressure and heart rate are largely endogenous in origin. Moreover, since the rhythm in blood pressure and motor activity were out of phase in TGR, motility clearly does not determine blood pressure rhythmicity in the rat.

In order to unveil the importance of the central clock, located in the Nucleus supra-chiasmaticus (SCN), for the rhythm generation in blood pressure, electrocoagulation of the SCN was performed followed by telemetric studies (36). Both in normotensive SPRD and in hypertensive TGR circadian rhythms in blood pressure, heart rate, and motor activity were abolished by this treatment. Most interestingly, hypertensive blood pressure values were still present in TGR after SCN lesion, clearly indicating that the SCN is involved in rhythm generation but not in hypertension in this animal model.

These findings clearly indicate that the rhythms in blood pressure and heart rate – as already convincingly described for motor activity - must be under the central control of the SCN. Furthermore, in TGR there is evidence for a disturbance in the circadian regulation of blood pressure (17) which, however, remains responsive to photic input.

It is known that the information of light perception via the retina to the SCN and subsequently the generation of circadian rhythms, e.g., in motor activity, is transmitted by transcription factors such as c-fos and c-jun present in the SCN. Until now neither SCN-mediated regulations of the blood pressure rhythm nor the role of the transcription factors have so far been studied. Therefore, we investigated the mRNA of c-fos and c-jun in the SCN of SPDR and TGR in relation to circadian time (6,7). For the first time these studies gave evidence that c-fos mRNA displays a circadian rhythm in the SCN of normotensive SPDR with peak values at the early light phase (circadian time: CT 2) whereas in TGR no significant rhythm could be detected. No rhythmicity was found for c-jun mRNA in both rat strains. Moreover a one-hour light pulse (at CT 2 or CT 14) increased the expression of c-fos mRNA in SPDR but not in TGR. If c-fos in the SCN is involved in the rhythm generation of also the blood pressure, this observation would go well together with the regulatory role of the SCN under LD and under free-run in SPDR, whereas in TGR blood pressure rhythm has obviously lost its ability to lengthen period under free-running conditions (32).

These studies on the molecular biology of the clock further support the notion of a genetic basis responsible for rhythm generation and its strain-dependency.

Chronopharmacological Implications

The telemetric monitoring of cardiovascular functions also nicely allows one to study in more detail the dose of antihypertensive drugs and their strain-dependent differences in various strains of normotensive and hypertensive rats. Thus, we could demonstrate that the calcium channel blocker amlodipine dose-dependently (1, 3, 10 mg/kg i.p.) decreased SBP, DBP, and HR in 3 strains of rats: In the normotensive strain WISW ED_{50}-values for decreasing SBP/DBP were lower in D (3.7/3.4 mg/kg) than in L (21.9/17.5 mg/kg) (22). In contrast, no circadian phase-dependency was found in SHR and their normotensive WKY controls with ED_{50} values in the range of 4–7 mg/kg in either L or D (15). Most interestingly, the pharmacokinetics of amlodipine in plasma, brain, muscle, heart, liver, and lung of male WISW rats was not circadian phase-dependent (Table 1) (16) clearly indicating that the circadian phase dependency in amlodipine's BP lowering effect cannot be attributed to chronokinetics (t $^1/_2$ ≈ 200 min both in D and L, see Table 1) of the drug. On the other hand, these results demonstrate a circadian phase-dependency in the concentration-effect relationship of this drug.

Concerning strain-dependent differences in blood pressure lowering effects, very similar data were obtained with the alpha1-adrenoceptor blocking drug doxazosin (12, 19). Doxazosin (0.03–1.0 mg/kg i.p.; injected either at 07.00 h or at 19.00 h) decreased BP in WKY during the night without a dose-dependency; only a slight effect was found during daytime

Table 1. Circadian time dependency in the pharmacokinetics of (+)- and (-)-amlodipine in WISW rats. Amlodipine-besylate (2 mg/kg i.v.) was injected i.v. to groups of 4 rats either at 07:00 h or at 19:00 h; groups of four rats were sacrificed 0.25, 0.5, 1, 2, 3, 4, 6, 8, 16, and 24 h later, 10 rats served as untreated controls. Data from (16, and personal comm. Dr. Laufen).

$\mathbf{AUC_{0.25\,h-24\,h}} \pm \mathbf{SEM}$				
i.v. Injection at	07:00 h		19:00 h	
	S(-)-AMLO	R(+)-AMLO	S(-)-AMLO	R(+)-AMLO
Plasma	168 ± 5	143 ± 4	187 ± 7	145 ± 5
Brain	416 ± 13	390 ± 10	395 ± 15	369 ± 13
Muscle	1585 ± 86	1970 ± 110	1631 ± 70	1867 ± 90
Heart	3540 ± 110	4280 ± 170	3940 ± 270	4480 ± 250
Liver	5510 ± 140	7620 ± 210	6700 ± 280	8480 ± 350
Lung	77300 ± 4600	82700 ± 4500	56700 ± 3100	59700 ± 2900
half-life (t ½ min)				
i.v. Injection at	07:00 h		19:00 h	
	S(-)-AMLO	R(+)-AMLO	S(-)-AMLO	R(+)-AMLO
Plasma	225	230	150	109
Heart	255	272	197	229
Brain	231	273	210	266

hours. In SHR the same drug dose-dependently decreased BP to about the same degree during day and night. In TGR, finally, doxazosin reduced BP in a dose-dependent way both during L and D, being, however, more potent in D (Fig. 6).

This data with different antihypertensive drugs clearly demonstrates that drug effects on BP may not only depend on the circadian phase but also on the rat strain studied. Moreover, the telemetric data give further evidence that α-adrenergic mediated regulation of the circadian blood pressure profile plays a different role in different strains of rats.
The AT_1 receptor antagonist losartan reduced BP in SHR and TGR dose-dependently after injection in the morning or in the evening (28). While in SHR losartan was equally effective during D and L, TGR showed a greater reduction in BP after morning dosing of losartan. Moreover, the reductions in TGR were significantly greater and obtained at a 30 fold lower dose than in SHR (28). Similarly, TGR were more sensitive than SHR to the effects of the ACE inhibitor enalaprilat (20). These results demonstrate that the renin-angiotensin system (RAAS) is involved both in the pathomechanisms of hypertension as well as in the inverse circadian BP profile in TGR and that RAS plays a different dominant role in different strains of rats.

Conclusion

Various functions of the cardiovascular system, including blood pressure and heart rate, are highly organized in time. At least in the rat, the rhythms in systolic and diastolic blood pressures are mainly endogenous in nature, i.e., driven by an internal pacemaker, as

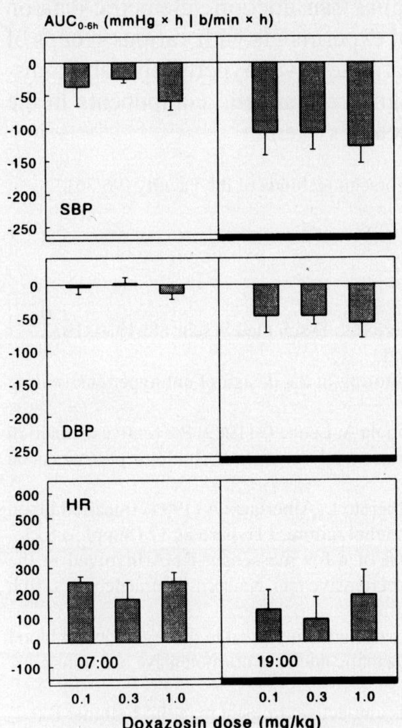

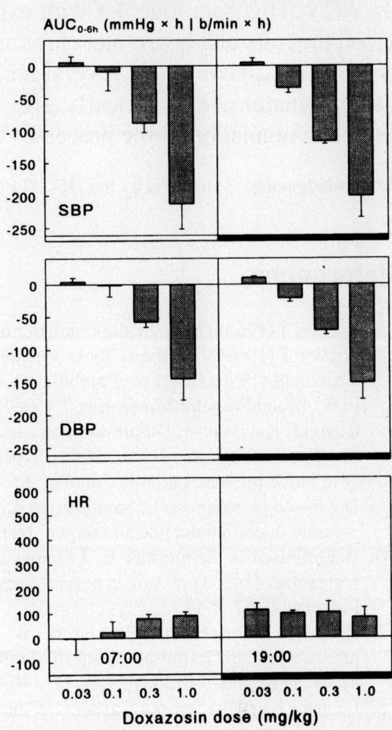

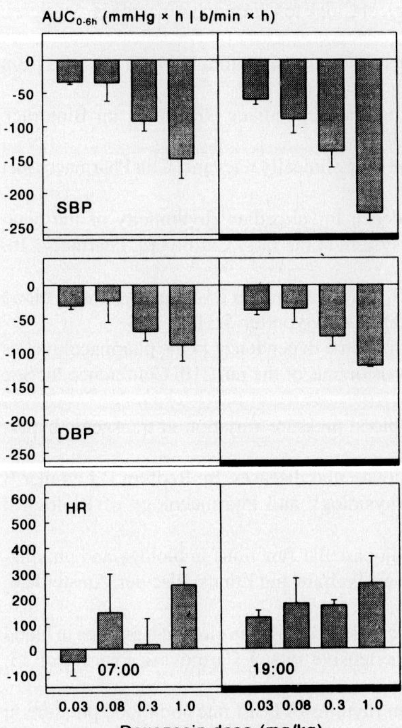

Fig. 6. Dose-dependent decreases in telemetric registered systolic (SBP) and diastolic (DBP) blood pressure and heart rate (HR) by doxazosin (0.03 – 1.0 mg/kg) injected i.p. either at 7.00h or at 19.00h to WKY (A), SHR (B) or TGR (C) rats. Decrease in SBP and DBP and increase in HR is expressed as cumulative differences to individual control values 0–6h after drug injection (delta AUC$_{0-6h}$, mmHg·h) at either injection time. Mean values ± SEM. (12, 19).

evidenced by data under free-running conditions and after lesioning of the central clock in the SCN. This data together with experiments on signal transduction, telemetric data on blood pressure and heart rate, chronopharmacological experiments with various groups of antihypertensive drugs in several inbred strains of normotensive, hypertensive and transgenic hypertensive rats clearly give evidence for significant genetic components in the rhythmic regulation of the processes of the cardiovascular system.

Acknowledgement Supported by the DFG (Le 318/10-1) and the Forschungsfonds of the Faculty (96/36).

References

1. Aschoff J (1963) Gesetzmäßigkeiten der biologischen Tagesperiodik. Dtsch med Wschr 88: 1930–1937
2. Aschoff J (1965) Circadian Clocks. Amsterdam: North-Holland
3. Coats AJS (1996) Benefits of ambulatory blood pressure monitoring in the design of antihypertensive drug trials. Blood Pressure Monitoring 2:157–160
4. Cugini P, Kawasaki T, DiPalma L, Antonicoli S, Battisti P, Coppola A, Leone G (1989) Preventive distinction of patients with primary or secondary hypertension by discriminant analysis of chronobiologic parameters on 24-h blood pressure patterns. Jpn Circ J 53:1363–1370
5. Del Rosso G, Amoroso L, Santoferrara A, Fiederling B, Di LIberato L, Albertazzi A (1994) Impaired blood pressure nocturnal decline and target organ damage in chronic renal failure. J Hypertens 12 (Suppl 3):S15
6. Hauptfleisch S, Schummer B, Lemmer B (1998) Expression of c-fos messenger-RNA involved in the regulation of blood pressure in normotensive and transgenic hypertensive rats. Naunyn-Schmiedeberg's Arch Pharmacol 357, R 17
7. Hauptfleisch S, Schummer B, Lemmer B (1998) Is a neuronal pacemaker involved in the regulation of blood pressure rhythm? Expression pattern of mRNA in the suprachiasmatic nuclei in normotensive and transgenic hypertensive rats. Am J Hyperten 11: 140A
8. Lemmer B (1989) Temporal aspects in the effects of cardiovascular active drugs in man. In: Lemmer B (ed) Chronopharmacology – Cellular and Biochemical Interactions. Marcel Dekker, New York, pp 525–542
9. Lemmer B (1995) of cardiovascular medications - pitfalls and challenges. Brit J Cardiol 2:303–309
10. Lemmer B (1996) Circadian rhythm in blood pressure: Signal transduction, regulatory mechanisms and cardiovascular medication. In: Lemmer B (ed) From the Biological Clock to Chronopharmacology. Stuttgart: Medpharm Publ, pp 91–117
11. Lemmer B (1996) Differential effects of antihypertensive drugs on circadian rhythm in blood pressure from the chronobiological point of view. Blood Pressure Monitoring 1:161–169
12. Lemmer B, Boese S, Mattes A (1993) Wirkung von Doxazosin auf circadiane Rhythmen im Blutdruck normotensiver und hypertensiver Ratten. Z Kardiol Suppl 1:139
13. Lemmer B, Bruguerolle B (1994) Chronopharmacokinetics - are they clinically relevant? Clin Pharmacokinet 26: 419–427
14. Lemmer B, Lang P-H, Schmidt S, Bärmeier H (1987) Evidence for circadian rhythmicity of the beta-adrenoceptor - adenylate cyclase - cAMP -phosphodiesterase system in the rat. J Cardiovasc Pharmacol 10: 138–140
15. Lemmer B, Mattes A, Boese S (1992) Dose-dependent effects of amlodipine on 24-hour rhythms in blood pressure and heart rate in the normotensive and hypertensive rat. Am J Hyperten 5:110A
16. Lemmer B, Mattes A, Boese S, Laufen H (1993) On the circadian time dependency in the pharmacokinetics of the calcium channel blocker amlodipine in plasma and various organs of the rat. 21th Conference Int Soc Chronobiol, Quebec, Canada, Abstr XI-3
17. Lemmer B, Mattes A, Böhm M, Ganten D (1993) Circadian blood pressure variation in transgenic hypertensive rats. Hypertension 22:97–101
18. Lemmer B, Portaluppi F (1997) Chronopharmacology of cardiovascular diseases. In: Redfern P, Lemmer B (eds) Handbook of Experimental Pharmacology, Vol 125 Physiology and Pharmacology of Biological Rhythms. Springer, Heidelberg, New York, pp 251–297
19. Lemmer B, Witte K (1997) Telemetric data acquisition of cardiovascular functions in biology and pharmacology. In: van Zutphen LFM, Balls M (eds) Animal Alternatives, Welfare and Ethics, Elsevier, Amsterdam, New York, pp 311–320
20. Lemmer B, Witte K, Makabe T, Ganten D, Mattes A (1994) Effects of enalaprilat on circadian profiles in blood pressure and heart rate of spontaneously and transgenic hypertensive rats. J Cardiovasc Pharmacol 23: 311–314
21. Lemmer B, Witte K, Minors D, Waterhouse J (1995) Circadian rhythms of heart rate and blood pressure in four strains of rat: Differences due to, and separate from, locomotor activity. Biol Rhythm Res 26: 493–504

22. Mattes A, Lemmer B (1991) Effects of amlodipine on circadian rhythms in blood pressure, heart rate, and motility: A telemetric study in rats. Chronobiol Int 8: 526–538
23. Mattes A, Witte K, Hohmann W, Lemmer B (1991) PHARMFIT – a nonlinear fitting program for pharmacology. Chronobiol Int 8: 460–476
24. Middeke M, Schrader J (1994) Nocturnal blood pressure in normotensive subjects and those with white coat, primary, and secondary hypertension. Brit Med J 308: 630–632
25. Minors D, Witte K, Lemmer B, Atkinson G, Waterhouse J (1998) The correlation between activity, blood pressure and heart rate in freely mobile Sprague-Dawley and transgenic rats. Biol Rhythm Res 29: 213–227
26. Pickering TG (1996) A review of national guidelines on the clinical use of ambulatory blood pressure monitoring. Blood Pressure Monitoring 2: 151–156
27. Portaluppi F, Cortelli P, Avoni P, Vergnani L, Contin E, Maltoni P, Pavani A, Sforza E, degli Uberti EC, Gambetti P, Lugaresi E (1994) Diurnal blood pressure variation and hormonal correlates in fatal familial insomnia. Hypertension 23: 569–576
28. Schnecko A, Witte K, Lemmer B (1995) Effects of the angiotensin II receptor antagonist losartan on 24-hour blood pressure profiles of primary and secondary hypertensive rats. J Cardiovasc Pharmacol 26: 214–221
29. Verdecchia P, Schillaci G, Guerrieri M, Gatteschi C, Benemio G, Boldrini F, Porcellati C (1990) Circadian blood pressure changes and left ventricular hypertrophy in essential hypertension [see comments]. Circulation 81: 528–536
30. White WB (1996) Clinical relevance of ambulatory versus clinic blood pressure when evaluating antihypertensive therapy. Blood Pressure Monitoring 2: 170–173
31. Willich SN, Muller JE (eds) (1996) Triggering of Acute Coronary Syndromes. Kluwer, Dordrecht, The Netherlands
32. Witte K, Lemmer B (1995) Free-running rhythms in blood pressure and heart rate in normotensive and transgenic hypertensive rats. Chronobiol Int 12: 237–247
33. Witte K, Lemmer B (1996) Signal transduction in animal models of normotension and hypertension. Time-dependent structure and control of arterial blood pressure. Ann NY Acad Sci 783: 71–83
34. Witte K, Lemmer B (1997) Rhythms in second messenger mechanisms. In: Redfern P, Lemmer B (eds) Handbook of Experimental Pharmacology, Vol 125 Physiology and Pharmacology of Biological Rhythms. Springer, Heidelberg, New York, pp 135–156
35. Witte K, Parsa-Parsi R, Vobig M, Lemmer B (1995) Mechanisms of the circadian regulation of ß-adrenoceptor density and adenylyl cyclase activity in cardiac tissue from normotensive and spontaneously hypertensive rats. J Mol Cell Cardiol 27: 1195–1202
36. Witte K, Schnecko A, Buijs RM, Vliet J van der, Scalbert E, Delagrange Ph, Guardiola-Lemaître, Lemmer B (1998) Effects of SCN-lesions on circadian blood pressure rhythm in normotensive and transgenic hypertensive rats. Chronobiol Int 15: 135–145
37. Witte K, Schnecko A, Perbandt K, Höfer S, Lemmer B (1998) Signal transduction in cardiac and vascular tissue from normotensive and transgenic hypertensive TGR(mREN2)27 rats. Eur J Pharmacol 341: 337–341

Author's address:
Prof. Dr. med. Dr. h.c. Björn Lemmer
Institut für Pharmakologie und Toxikologie
Ruprecht-Karls-Universität Heidelberg
Fakultät für Klinische Medizin
Maybachstr. 14–16
D-68169 Mannheim, Germany
e-mail: blemmer@rumms.uni-mannheim.de

Is capillary sprouting enough?

I. Buschmann, W. Schaper

Abstract

After birth, the formation of new blood vessels takes place via angiogenesis of arteriogenesis. Angiogenesis is defined as capillary sprouting and results in higher capillary density. It is an important component of various normal and pathological conditions such as wound healing, fracture repair, folliculogenesis, ovulation, and pregnancy. These periods of angiogenesis are tightly regulated. However, if not properly controlled, angiogenesis can also represent a significant pathogenic component of tumor growth and metastasis, rheumatic arthritis, and retinopathies. It is important to recognize that these newly formed capillary tubes lack vascular smooth muscle cells. Any developing new network of endothelial tubes (sprouting capillaries) that is not surrounded by mural cells is fragile and prone to rupture, remains susceptible to hypoxic regulation, fails to become remodeled, and is unable to sustain proper circulation: it cannot adapt to changes in physiological demands of blood supply.

Arteriogenesis defines the growth of arteries from preexisting arterioles and is potentially able to alter significantly the outcome of coronary and peripheral artery disease. Arteriogenesis is by far the most efficient adaptive mechanism for the survival of ischemic limbs or internal organs, like heart and brain, because of its ability to conduct, after adaptive growth, relatively large blood volumes per unit of time. An increased number of capillaries, the result of stimulated angiogenesis, is unable to do that. Arteriogenesis differs from angiogenesis in several aspects, the most important being the dependence of angiogenesis on hypoxia and the dependance of arteriogenesis on inflammation. However, angiogenesis and arteriogenesis share several mechanisms of action, like their dependence on growth factors. Whereas angiogenesis can be largely explained by the actions of VEGF, arteriogenesis is probably a multifactorial process where several growth factors are orchestrated. The role of VEGF in arteriogenesis is not clear, but a chemoattractive role for monocytes and hence an indirect contribution is imaginable.

Three different types of vessel growth

The adult vasculature has a surface area of approximately 1000 square meters, consisting of large arteries, internally lined by endothelial cells and well-ensheathed by smooth muscle cells. These arteries progressively branch into smaller and smaller vessels, terminating in precapillary arterioles that then give rise to capillaries. These vascular tubes are comprised almost entirely of endothelial cells that are only in a few cases coated by smooth muscle cells like pericyte. The capillaries then feed into postcapillary venules that progressively associate into larger and larger venous structures (10).

The development of this vascular tree takes place exclusively during early embryonic stages and is termed *Vasculogenesis* (14). It consists of the differentiation of angioblasts (the precursors of endothelial cells) into blood islands, which then fuse to form primitive capillary plexuses (2). The plexuses subsequently grow by angiogenesis (sprouting and tube formation by single endothelial cells with a preexisting capillary plexus), invade target tissues and give rise to the primitive vascular system of embryonic organs. Some vessels of these primary plexus remain as capillaries while others differentiate into arteries or veins (10).

After birth, the development of new blood vessels (neovascularization) is limited to two distinct processes: *arteriogenesis*, the recuitment and the active proliferation of preexisting collateral arteries and *angiogenesis*, the sprouting of endothelial cells, forming a capillary network. Both processes share common features but differ in many aspects:

Angiogenesis is a process where new capillary blood vessels sprout from a preexisting blood vessel (10). It is an important component of various normal and pathological conditions such as wound healing, fracture repair, folliculogenesis, ovulation, and pregnancy. These periods of angiogenesis are tightly regulated. However, if not properly controlled, angiogenesis can also represent a significant pathogenic component of tumor growth and metastasis, rheumatic arthritis, and retinopathies. Angiogenesis itself is a complex phenomenon consisting of several distinct processes which include endothelial migration and proliferation, extracellular proteolysis, endothelial differentiation (capillary tube formation) and vascular wall remodeling. It is important to recognize that these newly formed capillary tubes lack vascular smooth muscle cells. Any developing new network of endothelial tubes (sprouting capillaries), which is not surrounded by mural cells is fragile and prone to rupture, remains susceptible to hypoxic regulation, fails to become remodeled and is unable to sustain proper circulation: it cannot adapt to changes in physiological demands of blood supply (3, 13).

Arteriogenesis, in contrast, is the rapid profileration of preexisting collateral arteries. During chronic or acute occlusion of a major artery (coronary artery, femoral artery, etc.) preexisting microvascular, thin walled conduits, which are composed of an endothelial lining, an internal elastic lamina, and one or two layers of smooth muscle cells, are recruited in order to bypass the site of occlusion. These vessels, which are not utilized to provide perfusion under normal conditions, have the ability to dramatically increase their lumen by growth so as to provide enhanced perfusion to the jeopardized ischemic regions. Arteriogenesis finally results in fully functional and structurally normal arteries which can ameliorate the ensuing detrimental effects of vessel obstruction in many regions of the body (hind limb, heart, brain, kidney) (5, 8, 11).

What are the first physiological changes during arteriogenesis?

Directly after occlusion of a major artery, a steep pressure gradient along the shortest path within the interconnecting network develops which increases the blood flow velocity, the hydrostatic pressure, cyclic strains, and both laminar and turbulent wall shear forces in these vessels that now assume the new function as "collaterals". Shear stress is defined as force per unit area and may be considered as pressure, frictional wall shear at the cell surface, and tensile or compensatory forces acting to counter an externally applied force. The normal blood flow for instance in a femoral artery shows a shear stress value of 4.8×10^{-3} dyn/cm^2. After occlusion of this artery the blood flow via anastomoses increases more than 200-fold to a value of 889×10^{-3} dyn/cm^2.

What is the first morphologic visible change during arteriogenesis?

The massive increase in shear stress leads to several changes within the newly recruited artery. The most important one is the activation of the endothelium. Some responses occur within seconds, whereas others require several hours before a measurable adaptive change to this stimulus becomes apparent. The transcriptional activity of a number of endothelial genes (12) is upregulated, partially via a protein that binds to the shear stress responsive element [SSRE] that is present in the promoter of several genes (NOS, PDGF, MCP-1). The first step in the activation of the endothelium is the opening of chloride channels that are also responsible for the volume control of endothelial cells. Characteristically stress-activated endothelium appears swollen in scanning electron microscopic images (15). Adhesion molecules are upregulated (4), and the conditions are perfect for the adhesion and invasion of circulating cells. The upregulated expression of the monocyte-chemoattractant-protein-1 [MCP-1] by the endothelium attracts monocytes that adhere to and invade arteriolar collaterals, the first visible morphological change during arteriogenesis (Fig. 1c). They in turn become activated (9), produce tumor necrosis factor alpha and attract more monocytes. Platelets also adhere and produce IL-4 which increases the expression of more adhesion molecules. Upregulation of survival factors for monocytes (granulocyte-macrophage colony-stimulating-factor [GM-CSF]) provide the environment for a stable function of monocytes. These in turn produce fairly large amounts of growth factors, in particular fibroblast growth factor-2 (FGF-2). The adhesion and invasion of monocytes and platelets (also potent producers of growth factors) is soon followed by the first wave of mitosis of the endothelial and smooth muscle cells.

Finally, after a pronounced proliferating and remodeling phase, the collateral artery is no longer distinguishable from a normal artery, except for a slightly higher collagen content between the SM layers.

Role of hypoxia during arteriogenesis

In previous studies, we have shown that chronic intraarterial infusion of the monocyte chemoattractant factor [MCP-1] greatly increased the development of arterial collateral blood vessels (arteriogenesis) following femoral artery occlusion (6, 7). These collaterals were more numerous on angiograms and their ability to conduct blood had increased by a factor of sixfold (Fig. 1a and b). The histological appearance of these typical corkscrew

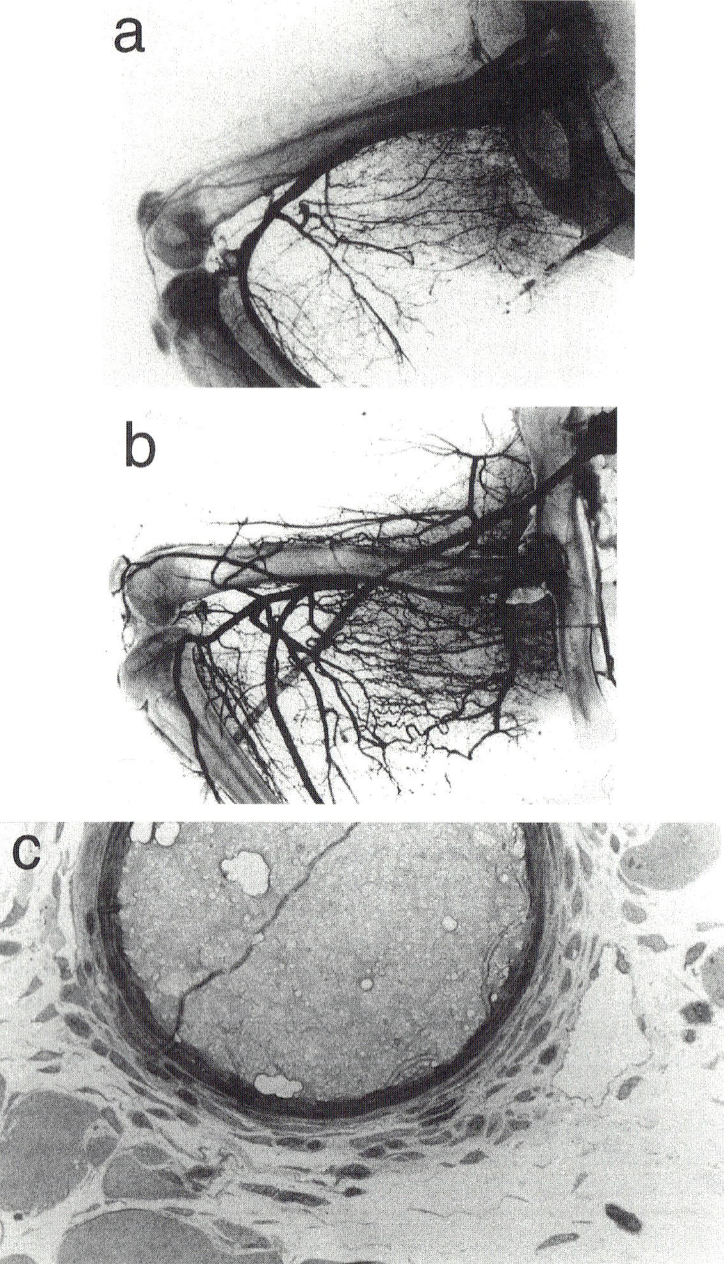

Fig. 1. (a) Angiography of the rabbit hindlimb (7 days PBS-infusion) after femoral artery occlusion; (b) Angiography of the rabbit hindlimb (7 days MCP-1 infusion) after femoral artery occlusion. The number as well as the density of the collateral vessels increased significantly. Collateral arteries show a typical corkscrew pattern; (c) Histological section (midzone of the proliferating collateral artery) after 7 days of MCP-1 infusion. Several macrophages can be observed around the vessel [provided by Dr. Dimitri Scholz and Prof. Dr. Dr. Jutta Schaper].

vessels was that of muscular arteries. In another study, we injected a single dose of lipo-polysaccharide [LPS] intravenously into New Zealand white rabbits 3 days after ligation of the femoral artery (1). This potent stimulator of tumor-necrosis-factor-alpha [TNFalpha] also markedly enhanced the number of monocyte-derived macrophages accumulated around growing collateral arteries. Peripheral and collateral conductances were markedly increased. Nevertheless on a molar basis, MCP-1 is the most potent arteriogenic peptide. The inhibition of monocyte adhesion with monoclonal antibodies against ICAM-1 significantly inhibits collateral artery formation, indicating that monocyte invasion is an obligatory step during arteriogenesis (16).

Other molecules such as vascular endothelial growth factor [VEGF] are endothelial specific mitogens. VEGF is produced by cells in close vicinity of endothelial cells, suggesting paracrine regulation of capillary formation. It is secreted and exerts a direct effect via interaction with endothelial receptors Flk-1 and Flt-1, its chemoattractive action on monocytes is dose-dependent, its expression is highly regulated by hypoxia, and thereby a physiological feedback-mechanism to tissue hypoxia exists. In contrast to angiogenesis which relies on hypoxia, arteriogenesis does not. Hypoxia is known to transcriptionally upregulate the expression of VEGF but post-transcriptional mRNA stabilization may even be more important. VEGF is able to circumvent the hypoxia induced translation inhibition, and we have observed in our rabbit model of hindlimb ischemia that VEGF expression and capillary growth is indeed restricted to ischemic regions. However, collateral artery growth (arteriogenesis) occurs in non-hypoxic tissue. Resting blood flow in the thigh muscles where collaterals develop following femoral artery occlusion is not decreased, its ATP and PCr content is normal and hypoxia-induced gene transcription (LDH-A, VEGF) is not activated. The distance between ischemic regions and the predilection sites for collateral growth can indeed be absurdely large: up to 70 cm between a patient's gangrenous big toe and collaterals spanning a femoral or popliteal occlusion.

Capillaries versus arteries

Arteriogenesis is by far the most efficient adaptive mechanism for the survival of ischemic limbs or internal organs, like the heart and brain, because of its ability to conduct, after adaptive growth, relatively large blood volumes per unit of time. An increased number of capillaries, the result of stimulated angiogenesis, is unable to do that. A capillary network can not efficienty respond to physiological stimuli. A sufficient perfusion of organs and hind limbs depends on large arteries, which are able to transport necessary blood volumes per unit of time. In addition, arteriogenesis differs from angiogenesis in several aspects, the most important being the dependence of angiogenesis on hypoxia and the dependance of arteriogenesis on inflammation. However, angiogenesis and arteriogenesis share several mechanisms of action, like their dependence on growth factors. Whereas angiogenesis can be largely explained by the actions of VEGF, arteriogenesis is probably a multifactorial process where several growth factors are orchestrated. The role of VEGF in arteriogenesis is not clear, but a chemoattractive role for monocytes and hence an indirect contribution is imaginable. Finally, the role of VEGF in clinical studies remains to be clarified, since recent reports described angioma formation after intramyocardial injection of DNA expressing VEGF in a rat model.

References

Owing to space contraints, many relevant primary references have been regrettably omitted.

1. Arras M, Ito WD, Scholz D, Winkler B, Schaper J, Schaper W (1997) Monocyte activation in angiogenesis and collateral growth in the rabbit hindlimb. J Clin Invest 101: 40–50
2. Bussolino F, Mantovani A, Persico G (1997) Molecular mechanisms of blood vessel formation. TIBS 22: 251–256
3. Carmeliet P, Collen D (1998) Vascular development and disorders – molecular analysis and pathogenic insights. Kidney International 53: 1519–1549
4. Chappel DC, Varner SE, Nerem RM, Medford RM, Alexander RW (1998) Oscillatory shear stress stimulates adhesion molecule expression in cultured human endothelium. Circ Res 82: 532–539
5. Fulton WFM (1965) The coronary arteries. Springfield, I.L. Charles C. Thomas Publishers
6. Ito W, Arras M, Scholz D, Winkler B, Htun P, Schaper W (1997) Angiogenesis but not collateral growth is associated with ischemia after femoral artery occlusion. American Journal of Physiology 273 (Heart Circ Physiol 42): H1255–H1265
7. Ito W, Arras M, Winkler B, Scholz D, Schaper J, Schaper W (1997) Monocyte chemotactic protein-1 increases collateral and peripheral conductance after femoral artery occlusion. Circ Res 80: 829–837
8. Longland CJ (1953) The collateral circulation of the limb
9. Polverini PJ, Cotran RS, Gimbrone MA Jr, Unanue ER (1977) Activated macrophages induce vascular proliferation. Nature 269: 804–806
10. Risau W (1997) Mechanisms of angiogenesis. Nature: 671–674
11. Schaper W, Schaper J (1993) Collateral circulation. Kluwer Academic Publishers
12. Shyy Y-J, Hsieh H-J, Usami S, Chien S (1994) Fluid shear stress induces a biphasic response of human monocyte chemotactic protein 1 expression in vascular endothelium. Proc Natl Acad Sci USA 91: 4678–4682
13. Thoma R (1893) Untersuchungen ueber die Histogenese und Histomechanik des Gefaesssystems. F. Enke Stuttgart, Germany
14. Yancopoulos GD, Klagsbrun M, Folkman J (1998) Vasculogenesis, angiogenesis and growth factors: ephrins enter the fray at the border. Cell 93: 661–664
15. Ziegelstein RC, Blank PS, Cheng L, Capogrossi MC (1998) Cytosolic alkalinization of vascular endothelial cells produced by an abrupt reduction in fluid shear stress. Circ Res 82 (7): 803–809
16. Buschmann IR, Hoefer I, Heil M, Schaper W (1999) Monoclonal antibodies against ICAM-1 inhibit arteriogenesis. JACC (Suppl): in press

Author's adress:
Prof. Dr. Dr. h.c. Wolfgang Schaper, MD, PhD · Dr. Ivo Buschmann, MD
Max-Planck-Institute for Physiological and Clinical Research
Department for Experimental Cardiology
Benekestrasse 2
D-61231 Bad Nauheim, Germany

Angiogenesis and gene therapy

P. Schratzberger, J. M. Isner

Departments of Medicine (Cardiology), and Biomedical Research, St Elizabeth's Medical Center, Tufts University School of Medicine, Boston, MA, USA

Abstract

Therapeutic angiogenesis constitutes a fundamental survival mechanism that acts to preserve the integrity of tissues subjected to ischemia. Supplemental administration of angiogenic cytokines – as recombinant protein or plasmid DNA – have been shown to augment collateral development when endogenous angiogenesis is suboptimal for organ function and, thus, constitute a novel therapeutic option for the treatment of cardiovascular disease. These angiogenic cytokines, all of which share in common the ability to act as mitogens for endothelial cells, do not promote angiogenesis in an indiscriminate fashion: thus, angiogenic cytokines selectively produce neovascularization in the ischemic tissues. The purpose of this review is to consider the strategies which have been devised to augment this response as well as to give an overview of the first clinical applications of gene therapy for therapeutic angiogenesis.

Despite major advances in both surgical and percutaneous revascularization techniques, therapeutic options for patients with lower extremity vascular obstructive disease are limited (23). Conventional drug therapy is of no proven benefit for these patients. When vascular obstruction is lengthy and widespread, percutaneous revascularization may not be feasible. Surgical therapy is complicated by a variable morbidity and mortality, and is dependent on long-term graft patency.

Recent investigations have established the feasibility of using recombinant formulations of angiogenic growth factors to expedite and/or augment collateral artery development in animal models of myocardial and hindlimb ischemia (3, 5–7, 49, 55, 63, 79). This strategy has been termed "therapeutic angiogenesis", and constitutes a potential alternative approach for patients with vascular insufficiency of the heart, lower extremities, and other vascular districts as well.

Among the various growth factors which have been shown to promote angiogenesis, vascular endothelial growth factor (VEGF) (25), also known as vascular permeability factor (35) and vasculotropin (VAS) (53), is an endothelial-cell specific mitogen. Because endothelial cells represent the critical cell type responsible for new vessel formation (27), and because smooth muscle cells – one of the critical cell types responsible for the development of certain vascular lesions (14, 51, 57) – would not be directly activated, endothelial-cell specificity has been regarded as an important advantage of VEGF for therapeutic angiogenesis.

Four homodimeric species of VEGF have been identified, each monomer having 121, 165, 189, or 206 amino acids, respectively (66). The secretion pattern of the four isoforms differs markedly. $VEGF_{121}$ is a weakly acidic polypeptide that does not bind to heparin and is freely soluble in the conditioned medium of transfected cells. The heparin-binding capabilities of the remaining three isoforms are progressively augmented as the result of a step-wise enrichment in basic residues. Thus $VEGF_{165}$, the predominant form secreted by a variety of normal and transformed cells (22), is a basic heparin-binding glycoprotein with an isoelectric point of 8.5; while secreted, a significant portion remains bound to the cell surface or extracellular matrix. The $VEGF_{189}$ isoform includes 24 additional amino acids and has been shown not to be freely secreted, but instead remains nearly completely bound to the cell surface and/or extracellular matrix (30). $VEGF_{206}$ is a rare isoform so far identified only in a human fetal liver cDNA library.

No recombinant VEGF protein formulation of any of the three principal isoforms is currently approved or available for human clinical application. Arterial gene transfer constitutes an alternative strategy for accomplishing therapeutic angiogenesis in patients with limb ischemia. In the case of VEGF this is a particularly appealing strategy because the VEGF gene encodes a signal sequence which permits the protein to be naturally secreted from intact cells (66). Previous studies from our laboratory (39, 60) indicated that arterial gene transfer of cDNA encoding for a secreted protein potentially yield meaningful biological outcomes in spite of a low transfection efficiency. Site-specific transfection of rabbit ear arteries with the plasmid pXGH5 encoding the gene for human growth hormone, for example, was found to generate physiologic levels of human growth hormone, despite immunohistochemical evidence of gene expression among < 1 % of cells in the transfected arterial segment (39). While the three principal VEGF isoforms differ markedly with regard to heparin avidity, all include the secretory signal sequence. We therefore performed pre-clinical animal studies to establish the feasibility of site-specific gene transfer of $phVEGF_{121}$, $phVEGF_{165}$, and $phVEGF_{189}$ applied to the hydrogel polymer coating of an angioplasty balloon (56), and delivered percutaneously to the iliac artery of rabbits in which the femoral artery had been excised to cause unilateral hindlimb ischemia (59).

Arterial gene transfer was achieved using "naked DNA", i.e., DNA unassociated with viral or other adjunctive vectors such as liposomes (61). The feasibility of using naked DNA for arterial gene transfer was initially documented in studies employing reporter genes (13, 56); using the hydrogel-polymer-coated balloon catheter, all rabbit arteries transfected with the luciferase gene (33/33, 100 %) expressed luciferase activity. Moreover, luciferase activity was detectable for a minimum of two weeks post-transfection (56). The use of DNA alone clearly simplifies the transfection protocol, obviating, for example, concerns regarding the potential toxicity of viral vectors (78).

Among control animals in which hydrogel-coated balloons were used to deliver pGSVLacZ, gene expression was limited < 0.5 % of total arterial cells (56). Presuming a similarly low transfection efficiency in animals transfected with $phVEGF_{165}$, the demonstration that naked DNA encoding for VEGF could achieve phenotypic modulation of the host circulation confirms previous work suggesting that gene products which are secreted may have profound biologic effects, even when the number of successfully transfected cells remains low. Whether adjunctive use of liposomes or adenoviral vectors might further optimize the functional and/or anatomic results reported to date requires additional study.

Evidence of transgene expression in our animal model of arterial gene transfer has been documented for both VEGF mRNA and protein. Analysis by RT-PCR established that the time course of gene expression in this animal model is < 30 d. This duration of gene expression was nevertheless sufficient to permit augmented collateral vessel development, and is consistent with the time course of collateral development reported previously in this animal model following administration of the recombinant protein (63). Cessation of gene expression by 30 d may be considered to represent a safety feature of the strategy proposed in this report in that the recipient is not exposed indefinitely to increased levels of the gene product. The basis for extinction of gene expression in the present case, along with similar observations made by others using non-viral vectors (38), remains enigmatic. To date, no evidence of an immunological basis has been recognized in animal experiments performed using naked DNA (45, 46).

Analysis of gene expression at the protein level, using an ELISA assay to evaluate blood samples obtained from the rabbit ear artery, documented systemic circulation of the gene product. Thus, while gene transfer was site-specific (no evidence of VEGF mRNA was detected at remote sites), expression of the protein was not. Light microscopic evidence of angiogenesis nevertheless appeared limited to the ischemic hindlimb. The basis for such a site-specific effect may be related to VEGF receptor expression: high-affinity VEGF receptors, particularly KDR (13, 65, 73), are expressed at relatively low levels in quiescent endothelial cells of most adult tissues (10, 11, 19, 52), but are upregulated as much as 13-fold when endothelial cells are exposed to media conditioned by hypoxic myocytes (10).

Augmented vascularity in our animal investigations was documented in vivo by serial angiographic analyses, and ex vivo by analysis of the capillary/myocyte ratio in sections of skeletal muscle obtained from the ischemic limb at the time of necropsy examination. Previous studies from our laboratory (59) documented extensive proliferative activity among endothelial cells comprising the neovasculature of the ischemic hindlimb following administration of recombinant VEGF protein, consistent with the interpretation that angiogenesis contributes to augmented collateral development in the rabbit ischemic hindlimb model following phVEGF$_{165}$ gene transfer.

In vivo studies of blood pressure and blood flow performed pre- and post-gene transfer documented that angiogenesis led to improvement in these physiologic indices (61). The ratio of blood pressure measured in the ischemic versus the normal limb improved to a statistically significant degree among animals transfected with plasmid DNA encoding for all three isoforms compared to LacZ. Likewise, blood flow measured in the ischemic limb with an intra-arterial Doppler guidewire at rest as well as following vasodilator provocation improved in all three VEGF-transfected groups versus the LacZ group. The magnitude of improvement observed in both these hemodynamic and flow indices following arterial gene transfer compares favorably with results obtained previously in this animal model following administration of recombinant VEGF$_{165}$ protein (8, 63).

The teleologic basis for the 121, 165, and 189 isoforms which result from alternative splicing of the VEGF transcript has remained enigmatic. Although VEGF$_{121}$ lacks heparin-binding ability, all three isoforms bind to the flk-1 receptor which transduces the mitogenic signal (36) including VEGF$_{121}$, which binds exclusively to flk-1 (28). Plate et al. speculated that the three principal isoforms might mediate distinct endothelial cell functions (52). We considered that angiogenesis induced by VEGF may be differentially dependent upon the extent to which each particular isoform employed is freely secreted and soluble. The magnitude of freely secreted VEGF$_{121}$ isoform which reaches the ischemic focus from the site of synthesis, for example, might be superior to that achieved with the VEGF$_{165}$ isoform; alternatively, avid binding of the VEGF$_{189}$ isoform to the basement membrane and/or extracellular matrix (48) might result in more protracted bioavailability, and thereby yield an outcome superior to VEGF$_{165}$.

Because it has proved difficult to express affinity-purified recombinant VEGF$_{189}$ protein from mammalian and bacterial systems, we investigated the possibility of hierarchial efficacy among these three isoforms by performing arterial gene transfer of phVEGF$_{121}$, phVEGF$_{165}$, and phVEGF$_{189}$ in the rabbit ischemic hindlimb model. Remarkably, no differences with regard to anatomic or physiologic evidence of angiogenesis could be demonstrated – although all three isoforms yielded statistically significant improvement in every parameter measured compared to the LacZ controls. Moreover, separate experiments performed using 100, 200, and 400 μg of each plasmid failed to disclose a differential dose-response curve among the three isoforms with respect to angiographic score, calf blood pressure ratio, resting/maximum flow or capillary/myocyte ratio (Y. Tsurumi, unpublished data).

These findings represent what is to our knowledge the first demonstration of biological equivalency among the three principal VEGF isoforms for in vivo angiogenesis and may be interpreted to support the observation made previously by Houck et al. (30) regarding the proteolytically clipped VEGF species which result from the action of plasmin on the 165 and 189 isoforms. The size of the resulting monomers, which in each case are mitogenic for endothelial cells and enhance vascular permeability in a Miles assay (42), is similar to the size of the intact 121 isoform. It is therefore possible that the proteolytic cascade of plasminogen activation, a key step during angiogenesis (50), cleaves the longer forms of VEGF, releasing a soluble $VEGF_{121}$-like species that is the final common mediator of angiogenesis in vivo.

Clinical application of arterial gene transfer of phVEGF$_{165}$

We have used our animal studies to develop clinically applicable strategies for therapeutic angiogenesis employing phVEGF$_{165}$. Because recombinant VEGF protein is not yet available for human application, clinical trials of human gene therapy involving percutaneous arterial gene transfer of phVEGF$_{165}$ (34) for patients with critical limb ischemia were undertaken in December, 1994.

Using a dose-escalating design, treatment was initiated with 100 μg of phVEGF$_{165}$. Three patients presenting with rest pain (but no gangrene) and treated with 1000 μg were subsequently shown at 1-year follow-up to have improved blood flow to the ischemic limb and remain free of rest pain. We considered the possibility that VEGF could produce flow augmentation simply as a result of its ability to act as a potent stimulus for the release of nitric oxide (69); this explanation, however, seemed unlikely in view of the demonstration that augmented flow was documented on serial studies performed well beyond the time (21–30 d) that the transferred gene is actively expressed (61). With the increase in dose of phVEGF$_{165}$ to 2000 μg, angiographic evidence of new blood vessel formation became apparent (33). Moreover, patient 8 developed three spider angiomata in the foot and ankle distal to the site of gene transfer; immunohistochemical staining of the lesion which was resected documented extensive proliferative activity among the endothelial cells comprising the lesion. These lesions were first observed 1 week post-gene transfer and regressed completely by 8 weeks later. The lesions were limited to the distal portion of the ischemic extremity. The time-course and distribution of these lesions strongly suggests that these vascular malformations developed as a consequence of phVEGF$_{165}$ expression. These lesions are in fact reminiscent of supernumerary vessels described previously following injection of VEGF recombinant protein into quail embryos (21, 32). The development of these lesions constitutes strong, albeit indirect, evidence of gene expression in this patient. These lesions, although benign and in this case self-limited, may be considered evidence of unwanted angiogenesis and, thus, warrant careful monitoring in future patients receiving angiogenic therapy.

These findings, thus, established proof of principle for two concepts. The first is the potential for the administration of angiogenic growth factors to promote development of new collateral blood vessels in human patients. The second concept is the feasibility of arterial gene transfer of naked DNA.

In the patient with angiographic and histologic evidence of neovascularization, as in several of the patients treated with the 1000 μg dose of plasmid DNA, lower extremity edema developed for the first time post-gene therapy and resolved by week 5 post-gene transfer – 1 week beyond the 21–30 d during which the transgene has been shown to be actively expressed (44) – suggesting that this finding was a consequence of phVEGF$_{165}$ gene transfer. VEGF increases vascular permeability when assessed by the Miles assay (42), accounting for its alternative designation, vascular permeability factor or VPF (16, 22, 35). The association between neovascularity and edema in this patient is consistent with previously reported evidence (22, 32) linking functions of VEGF as a vascular growth factor and permeability factor.

Because the technique employed for local gene delivery in this case involves balloon inflation and thus the potential for endothelial disruption of the arterial wall, the gene transfer site was serially examined by intravascular ultrasound (IVUS). In neither of the examinations performed post-gene therapy was there evidence that hydrogel balloon arterial gene transfer provoked intimal thickening. It is indeed likely that phVEGF$_{165}$ gene transfer accelerates re-endothelialization, and thereby obviates luminal compromise of the transfected segment (2, 4).

Intra-muscular gene transfer of phVEGF$_{165}$

Despite these encouraging preliminary findings, evaluation of candidates for phVEGF$_{165}$ arterial gene therapy exposed certain potential limitations of arterial gene transfer, particularly for lower extremity ischemia. By definition, arterial gene transfer requires access to a satisfactory arterial donor site in the lower extremity circulation. In patients with critical limb ischemia, several factors may conspire to compromise such access. Lower extremity vascular disease is often so extensive that conventional sites for arterial puncture cannot be accessed percutaneously. Arterial sites which are patent may be nevertheless diffusely diseased by atherosclerosis (24). Even in the absence of a thickened neointima, extensive calcific deposits at the intimal/medial interface (so-called "Monckeberg's disease" (37) may limit gene transfer to the smooth muscle cells of the arterial media and/or make the vessel so brittle that balloon inflation fractures the calcified vessel (26), leading to unpredictable abrupt vessel closure; this complication may be devastating if the involved artery is the major donor of pre-existing collaterals or the only patent vessel supplying the ischemic limb. Even if arterial access is possible in such patients, it is often limited to the upper-most portion of the limb, 60 cm or more from sites in the distal limb where ischemia and/or necrosis is most profound. Because recent studies have demonstrated evidence of paracrine mediated endothelial cell upregulation of VEGF receptors by conditioned media of hypoxic muscle (10), there may be a tactical advantage to positioning the putative sites of constitutive VEGF synthesis in closer proximity to the ischemic focus.

Intramuscular (IM) gene transfer, pioneered by Wolff and colleagues (75–77), represents a less invasive alternative to arterial transfection. Striated muscle has been shown to take up and express foreign genes transferred in the form of "naked" plasmid DNA, i.e., DNA unassociated with viral or other adjunctive vectors. As indicated above, IM gene transfer of naked plasmid DNA would be potentially advantageous since it obviates immunologic concerns associated with adenoviral vectors (78). Because naked plasmid DNA injected IM remains in a non-replicative, unintegraded, circular form (76), this strategy also is unlikely to be complicated by insertional mutagenesis.

While IM gene transfer of naked DNA would, thus, appear to address the technical limitations of arterial gene transfer in particular and certain safety issues relevant to cardiovascular gene therapy in general, the magnitude of gene expression resulting from IM transfection has been a subject of further concern. Wolff et al. documented reporter gene expression up to 19 months following IM transfection with naked DNA (75), but concluded that the use of this approach for Duchenne's myopathy did not achieve satisfactory levels of dystrophin (1). Subsequent investigators have been more optimistic when naked DNA was administered IM for use as a vaccine (31, 41, 64, 68). In the case of phVEGF$_{165}$, we considered that the secreted features of the gene product might permit a level of gene expression sufficient to achieve therapeutic angiogenesis. Accordingly, we again used the rabbit model of hindlimb ischemia to test the hypothesis that IM injection of naked plasmid DNA encoding the 165-amino acid isoform of VEGF could augment collateral development and tissue perfusion in the setting of experimentally induced hindlimb ischemia. In fact, we documented successful transfer and expression of phVEGF$_{165}$ in skeletal muscles of the ischemic limb, with evidence of increased collateral vessel development, and consequent amelioration in hemodynamic and physiologic deficits induced by ischemia (67). Previous studies have shown that such improvements in perfusion are associated with improved performance of skeletal muscle groups in the treated limb (72). These findings, thus, demonstrated for the first time the feasibility of the intramuscular (IM) gene transfer with naked DNA encoding VEGF for therapeutic angiogenesis, in particular, and for the first time indicated bioactivity of naked DNA following IM transfection for cardiovascular gene therapy in general. From a clinical standpoint, these findings suggest that IM transfection represents a suitable alternative to arterial gene transfer of phVEGF$_{165}$ in patients with proximal obstruction of the lower extremity vasculature which precludes catheter access.

Many of the previous successful applications of IM gene transfer were achieved in young (4–6 weeks) mice, in which transgene uptake appears to be highest (74). Our findings suggest that IM transfer of naked DNA is neither age nor species specific. VEGF expression was sufficient to yield augmented collateral vessel development associated with improved pressure, flow and perfusion in adult rabbits with hindlimb ischemia. The increase in angiographically apparent vessels and capillary density has been previously shown to result from VEGF-induced increase in endothelial cell proliferation (59). Consequently, the magnitude of improvement in calf blood pressure, blood flow (measured by intravascular Doppler analysis), and tissue perfusion (measured by an increase in microsphere distribution to the ischemic thigh and calf muscles) were all statistically significant in comparison to controls.

Several factors likely contributed to the success of phVEGF$_{165}$ IM gene transfer. As was the case with intra-arterial gene transfer, the secreted nature of the gene product constitutes the most important factor. This is further facilitated in the case of skeletal muscle by the inherently well vascularized nature of this tissue.

Second, plasmid DNA was delivered in a relatively large volume of fluid, directly into the target muscle; the injection was performed slowly to prevent fluid loss from the epimysium. This approach may have allowed for more uniform distribution of the transgene. Wolff et al. previously demonstrated that higher and less variable levels of gene expression could be achieved by injecting a larger rather than a smaller volume of plasmid (77). Similarly, Davis et al. showed that pre-injection of muscles with a relatively large volume of hypertonic sucrose facilitated more uniform distribution and less variable expression of reporter genes (18).

Third, the skeletal muscle which was the site of gene transfer was ischemic. Recent work by Takeshita et al. (58) has shown that the transfection efficiency of IM gene transfer is augmented more than five-fold when the injected muscle is ischemic. This finding may be the result of the skeletal muscle regeneration, including stem cell (myoblast) proliferation. Vitadello et al. (71) have reported an 80-fold increase in chloramphenicol acetyltransferase (CAT) activity following transfection of regenerating versus control muscle. Consistent with this concept, Danko et al. (17) found that bupivacaine, which produce myonecrosis followed by satellite cell (muscle stem cell) proliferation and myotube formation 1–3 d later, may be used to enhance the expression of naked DNA injected IM into striated muscles.

Interestingly, the histologic features of muscle retrieved from the ischemic limbs of animals used for the current series of experiments were similar in many respects to findings reported previously for bupivacaine-treated muscle, featuring myonecrosis, mononuclear cell infiltration, muscle stem cell proliferation, and myotube formation (29). Evidence of myocyte regeneration was in fact demonstrable in the current experiments at the time of IM plasmid administration; this finding may be related to the nearly 7-fold higher transfection efficiency suggested by morphometric analysis β-galactosidase gene expression. Taken together, it is likely that ischemic myonecrosis – a predictable feature of hindlimb ischemia in this animal model (5) – led to spontaneous muscle regeneration, and coincidently augmented uptake of the transgene.

The ischemic milieu of the transfected hindlimb muscle further contributes to the success of therapeutic angiogenesis, independent of transgene uptake, by modulating VEGF receptor expression. Recent work from our laboratory has demonstrated paracrine induction of the KDR receptor (13-fold increase in KDR receptor/cell) in endothelial cells exposed to media conditioned by hypoxic myoblasts (10). This finding presumably acts not only to amplify the impact of any given concentration of VEGF, but potentially accounts as well for the site-specific nature of the angiogenic response in this animal model (9).

Expression of the human VEGF transgene was detected by RT-PCR for up to 14 days after gene transfer in the present study. It is assumed, although not yet documented, that expression at the protein level is limited to a similar time frame. This relatively brief duration of transgene expression is likely related to the CMV promoter employed in the phVEGF165 plasmid construct. Previous work by Wolff (75, 76) and others (17, 74) demonstrated that naked DNA constructs which include the Rous sarcoma virus (RSV) promoter appear to express for considerably longer periods of time, although the level of expression obtained may be lower than that obtained with CMV. Addition of selected introns and/or regulatory sequences in the 3' non-coding region of CMV constructs, however, may augment both the magnitude and temporal stability of transgene expression (15, 40).

Use of a skeletal muscle-specific promoter represents another potential consideration for enhancing the efficiency of IM gene transfer. It is not clear, however, that this strategy would necessarily augment gene expression for the application described in the current series of experiments. Buttrick et al. (12), for example, have previously shown that cardiac-specific expression from the rat myosin heavy chain gene was 20-fold less active than expression from RSV regulatory sequences. Likewise, Vincent et al. (70) have documented similar levels of expression for a pRSV-CAT construct and an MCK-CAT construct (containing the promoter and enhancer of the rabbit creatinin kinase-M gene) in transfection of rat cardiac and skeletal muscles More recently, Vincent and Walsh (unpublished data) have found that 198.3 chicken skeletal actin promoter (–198 to –1 and +1 to 313 fragment) was 1 % as active as RSV-LTR or CMV promoters in direct IM injection of rat heart. Thus, constitutive viral regulatory sequences (vs. tissue-specific muscle promoter) may be optimal even for IM expression of exogenous genes due to their inherently higher activity. It is possible, however, that applying modifications cited above (15, 40) to the CMV vector used here might yield more robust gene expression.

The duration of gene expression in the current series of experiments was nevertheless sufficient to permit augmented collateral vessel development. This is consistent with the time course of collateral development reported previously in this animal model following administration of the recombinant protein, in which maximal endothelial cell proliferation is observed within 5 d following VEGF therapy (59). Provided that a satisfactory clinical benefit has been realized, early cessation of gene expression may represent a safety feature of the strategy proposed in this report, in that the recipient is not exposed indefinitely to increased levels of the transgene product.

Role of protein in determining the success of gene transfer

In summary, experience with intra-arterial and intra-muscular gene transfer of VEGF to date illustrates in prototypical fashion how features of the gene, protein, and target tissue may all contribute to phenotypic modulation of the host despite a low transfection efficiency.

First, rhVEGF contains at its amino terminus the signal sequence which permits it to be actively secreted by intact cells.

Second, heparin-avidity of the intermediate and longer VEGF isoforms, $VEGF_{165}$ and $VEGF_{189}$ respectively, promotes binding to cell surface and matrix heparan sulfates that may create a biological reservoir of the secreted protein, enhancing the temporal opportunity for bioactivity.

Third, while ECs were previously viewed solely as the target for VEGF, it is now clear that ECs under stress, in particular hypoxia, can synthesize VEGF as well (47). This autocrine feature of VEGF creates the opportunity for amplifying the effects of even a small amount of exogenous VEGF, as EC proliferation in the ischemic territory creates additional potential sites of VEGF synthesis and secretion.

Fourth, VEGF inhibits apoptosis (Losordo, D. W. unpublished data), apparently by upregulating EC expression of fibronectin and $\alpha v \beta 3$ and thus promoting the critical step of EC attachment to the extracellular matrix. Such reduction in EC apoptosis would be expected to complement the mitogenic effect of VEGF, resulting in a further net increase in EC viability.

Fifth, with regard to the target of gene therapy, it has been noted (33, 61, 62) that VEGF-induced angiogenesis is not indiscriminate or widespread, but is instead restricted to sites of ischemia. This appears to result from paracrine upregulation of the principal high-affinity VEGF receptor (Kdr) in response to factors released from hypoxic skeletal myocytes (10). Receptor upregulation on ECs within the region of lower limb or myocardial ischemia thus enables these cells to act as magnets for any VEGF secreted into the ischemic milieu.

These considerations underscore the notion that the success of gene therapy is not solely a function of vectors or transfection efficiency While it is clear that better vectors with which to augment transfection efficiency should remain a principal goal of gene therapy, features of the gene and target may independently increase or decrease the likelihood of a favorable outcome. Modifications in any of these respects, including the use alone or in combination of other angiogenic growth factors, will receive intensive scrutiny in the coming months to optimize angiogenesis as a useful treatment option for lower extremity and myocardial ischemia.

References

1. Acsadi G, Jani A, Massie B, Simoneau M, Holland P, Blaschuk K, Karpati G (1994) A differential efficiency of adenovirus-mediated in vivo gene transfer into skeletal muscle cells of different maturity. Human Molecular Genetics 3: 579–584
2. Asahara T, Bauters C, Pastore CJ, Kearney M, Rossow S, Bunting S, Ferrara N, Symes JF, Isner JM (1995) Local delivery of vascular endothelial growth factor accelerates reendothelialization and attenuates intimal hyperplasia in balloon-injured rat carotid artery. Circulation 91: 2793–2801
3. Asahara T, Bauters C, Zheng LP, Takeshita S, Bunting S, Ferrara N, Symes JF, Isner JM (1995) Synergistic effect of vascular endothelial growth factor and basic fibroblast growth factor on angiogenesis in vivo. Circulation 92: II-365–II-371
4. Asahara T, Chen D, Kearney M, Rossow S, Passeri J, Symes JF, Isner JM (1996) Accelerated re-endothelialization and reduced neointimal thickening following catheter transfer of phVEGF$_{165}$. J Am Coll Cardiol 27: 1A (Abstract)
5. Baffour R, Berman J, Garb JL, Rhee SW, Kaufman J, Friedmann P (1992) Enhanced angiogenesis and growth of collaterals by in vivo administration of recombinant basic fibroblast growth factor in a rabbit model of acute lower limb ischemia: Dose-response effect of basic fibroblast growth factor. J Vasc Surg 16: 181–191
6. Banai S, Jaklitsch MT, Shou M, Lazarous DF, Scheinowitz M, Biro S, Epstein SE, Unger EF (1994) Angiogenic-induced enhancement of collateral blood flow to ischemic myocardium by vascular endothelial growth factor in dogs. Circulation 89: 2183–2189
7. Banai S, Jaklitsch MT, Casscells W, Shou M, Shrivastav S, Correa R, Epstein SE, Unger EF (1991) Effects of acidic fibroblast growth factor on normal and ischemic myocardium. Circ Res 69: 76–85
8. Bauters C, Asahara T, Zheng LP, Takeshita S, Bunting S, Ferrara N, Symes JF, Isner JM (1994) Physiologic assessment of angiogenesis induced by vascular endothelial growth factor in a rabbit ischemic hindlimb model. Am J Physiol 36: H1263–H1271
9. Bauters C, Asahara T, Zheng LP, Takeshita S, Bunting S, Ferrara N, Symes JF, Isner JM {1995) Site-specific therapeutic angiogenesis following systemic administration of vascular endothelial growth factor. J Vasc Surg 21: 314–325
10. Brogi E, Schatteman G, Wu T, Kim EA, Varticovski L, Keyt B, Isner JM (1996) Hypoxia-induced paracrine regulation of VEGF receptor expression. J Clin Invest 97: 469–476
11. Brown LF, Yeo K-T, Berse B, Yeo T-K, Senger DR, Dvorak HF, Van De Water L (1992) Expression of vascular permeability factor (vascular endothelial growth factor) by epidermal keratinocytes during wound healing. J Exp Med 176: 1375–1379
12. Buttrick PM, Kass A, Kitsis RN, Kaplan ML, Leinwand LA (1992) Behavior of genes directly injected into the rat heart in vivo. Circ Res 70: 193–198
13. Chapman GD, Lim CS, Gammon RS, Culp SC, Desper JS, Bauman RP, Swain JL, Stack RS (1992) Gene transfer into coronary arteries of intact animals with a percutaneous balloon catheter. Circ Res 71: 27–33
14. Clowes AW, Reidy MA, Clowes MM (1983) Kinetics of cellular proliferation after arterial injury. I. Smooth muscle growth in the absence of endothelium. Lab Invest 49: 327–333
15. Coleman ME, DeMayo F, Yin KC, Lee HM, Geske R, Montgomery C, Schwartz RJ (1995) Myogenic vector expression of insulin-like growth factor I stimulates muscle cell differentiation adn myofiber hypertrophy in transgenic mice. J Biol Chem 270: 12109–12116
16. Connolly DT, Hewelman DM, Nelson R, Olander JV, Eppley BL, Delfino JJ, Siegel RN, Leimgruber RS, Feder J (1989) Tumor vascular permeability factor stimulates endothelial cell growth and angiogenesis. J Clin Invest 84: 1470–1478
17. Danko I, Fritz JD, Jiao S, Hogan K, Latendresse JS, Wolff JA (1994) Pharmacological enhancement of in vivo foreign gene expression in muscle. Gene Therapy 1: 114–121
18. Davis HL, Whalen RG, Demeneix BA (1993) Direct gene transfer into skeletal muscle in vivo: factors affecting efficiency of transfer and stability of expression. Human Gene Ther 4: 151–159
19. Detmar M, Brown LF, Claffey KP, Yeo K-T, Kocher O, Jackman RW, Berse B, Dvorak HF (1994) Overexpression of vascular permeability factor/vascular endothelial growth factor and its receptors in psoriasis. J Exp Med 180: 1141–1146
20. Donnelly JJ, Friedman A, Maretinez D, Montgomery DL, Shiver JW, Motzel SL, Ulmer JB, Liu MA (1995) Preclinical efficacy of a prototype DNA vaccine: Enhanced protection against antigenic drift in influenza virus. Nature Med 1: 583–587

21. Drake CJ, Little CD (1995) Exogenous vascular endothelial growth factor induces malformed and hyperfused vessels during embryonic neovascularization. Proc Natl Acad Sci USA 92: 7657–7661
22. Dvorak HF, Brown LF, Detmar M, Dvorak AM (1995) Vascular permeability factor/vascular endothelial growth factor, microvascular hyperpermeability, and angiogenesis. Am J Pathol 146: 1029–1039
23. European Working Group on Critical Leg Ischemia (1991) Second European consensus document on chronic critical leg ischemia. Circulation 84: IV-1–IV-26
24. Feldman LJ, Steg PG, Zheng LP, Chen D, Kearney M, McGarr SE, Barry JD, Dedieu JF, Perricaudet M, Isner JM (1995) Low-efficiency of percutaneous adenovirus-mediated arterial gene transfer in the atherosclerotic rabbit. J Clin Invest 95: 2662–2671
25. Ferrara N, Henzel WJ (1989) Pituitary follicular cells secrete a novel heparin-binding growth factor specific for vascular endothelial cells. Biochem Biophys Res Commun 161: 851–855
26. Fitzgerald PJ, Ports TA, Yock PG (1992) Contribution of localized calcium deposits to dissection after angioplasty. An observational study using intravascular ultrasound. Circulation 86: 64–70
27. Folkman J (1995) Clinical applications of research on angiogenesis. N Engl J Med 333: 1757–1763
28. Gitay-Goren H, Cohen T, Tessler S, Soker S, Gengrinovitch S, Rockwell P, Klagsbrun M, Levi B-Z, Neufeld G (1996) Selective binding of $VEGF_{121}$ to one of the three vascular endothelial growth factor receptors of vascular endothelial cells. J Biol Chem 271: 5519–5523
29. Hall-Craggs ECB (1980) Early ultrastructural changes in skeletal muscle exposed to the local anaesthetic bupivacaine (marcaine). Br J Exp Pathol 61: 139–149
30. Houck KA, Leung DW, Rowland AM, Winer J, Ferrara N (1992) Dual regulation of vascular endothelial growth factor bioavailability by genetic and proteolytic mechanisms. J Biol Chem 267: 26031–26037
31. Hsu C-H, Chua K-Y, Tao M-H, Lai Y-L, Wu H-D, Huang S-K, Hsieh K-H (1996) Immunoprophylaxis of allergen-8induced immunoglobulin E synthesis and airway hyperresponsiveness in vivo by genetic immunization. Nature Med 2: 540–544
32. Ingo F, von Reutern M, Drexler HCA, Syed-Ali S, Risau W (1995) Overexpression of vascular endothelial growth factor in the avian embryo induces hypervascularization and increased vascular permeability without alterations of embryonic pattern formation. Dev Biol 171: 399–414
33. Isner JM, Pieczek A, Schainfeld R, Blair R, Haley L, Asahara T, Rosenfield K, Razvi S, Walsh K, Symes J (1996) Early report: clinical evidence of angiogenesis following arterial gene transfer of $phVEGF_{165}$. Lancet 348: 370–374
34. Isner JM, Walsh K, Symes J, Pieczek A, Takeshita S, Lowry J, Rosenfield K, Weir L, Brogi E, Jurayj D (1996) Arterial gene transfer for therapeutic angiogenesis in patients with peripheral artery disease. Human Gene Ther 7: 959–988
35. Keck PJ, Hauser SD, Krivi G, Sanzo K, Warren T, Feder J, Connolly DT (1989) Vascular permeability factor, an endothelial cell mitogen related to PDGF. Science 246: 1309–1312
36. Keyt BA, Nguyen HV, Berleau LT, Durate CM, Park J, Chen H, Ferrara N (1996) Identification of vascular endothelial growth factor determinants for binding KDR and FLT-1 receptors. J Biol Chem 271: 5638–5646
37. Lachman AS, Spray TL, Kerwin DM, Shugoll GI, Roberts WC (1977) Medial calcinosis of Monckeberg. Am J Med 63: 615–622
38. Lemarchand P, Jones M, Yamada I, Crystal RG (1993) In vivo gene transfer and expression in normal uninjured blood vessels using replication-deficient recombinant adenovirus vectors. Circ Res 72: 1132–1138
39. Losordo DW, Pickering JG, Takeshita S, Leclerc G, Gal D, Weir L, Kearney M, Jekanowski J, Isner JM (1994) Use of the rabbit ear artery to serially assess foreign protein secretion after site specific arterial gene transfer in vivo: Evidence that anatomic identification of successful gene transfer may underestimate the potential magnitude of transgene expression. Circulation 89: 785–792
40. Manthorpe M, Cornefert-Jensen F, Hartikka J, Felgner J, Rundell A, Margalith M, Dwarki V (1993) Gene therapy by intramuscular injection of plasmid DNA: studies on firefly luciferase gene expression in mice. Human Gene Ther 4: 419-431
41. McDonnell WM, Askari FK (1996) DNA vaccines. N Engl J Med 334: 42–45
42. Miles AA, Miles EM (1952) Vascular reactions to histamine, histamine liberators or leukotoxins in the skin of the guinea pig. J Physiol 118: 228–257
43. Millauer B, Wizigmann-Voos S, Schnurch H, Martinez R, Moller NPH, Risau W, Ulrich A (1993) High affinity VEGF binding and developmental expression suggest Flk-1 as a major regulator of vasculogenesis and angiogenesis. Cell 72: 835–846
44. Minutes Recombinant DNA Advisory Committee (RAC) of National Institutes of Health, Sept 13, 1994. RAC #9409-088 approved in final form 11/15/94
45. Nabel G (1994) Proposed amendment to Appendix D of the NIH Guidelines Regarding a Human Gene Therapy Protocol Entitled Immunotherapy of Malignancy by In Vivo Gene Transfer into Tumors. Human Gene Ther 5: 236–240
46. Nabel EG, Gordon D, Yang Z-Y, Xu L, San H, Plautz GE, Wu B-Y, Gao X, Huang L, Nabel GJ (1992) Gene transfer in vivo with DNA-liposome complexes: lack of autoimmunity and gonadal localization. Human Gene Ther 3: 649–656

47. Namiki A, Brogi E, Kearney M, Wu T, Couffinhal T, Varticovski L, Isner JM (1995): Hypoxia induces vascular endothelial growth factor in cultured human endothelial cells. J Biol Chem 270: 31189–31195

48. Park JE, Keller G-A, Ferrara N (1993) The vascular endothelial growth factor (VEGF) isoforms: Differential deposition into the subepithelial ECM and bioactivity of ECM-bound VEGF. Mol Biol Cell 4: 1317–1326

49. Pearlman JD, Hibberd MG, Chuang ML, Harada K, Lopez JJ, Gladston SR, Friedman M, Sellke FW, Simons M (1995) Magnetic resonance mapping demonstrates benefits of VEGF-induced myocardial angiogenesis. Nature Med 1: 1085–108

50. Pepper MS, Montesano R (1990) Proteolytic balance and capillary morphogenesis. Cell Differ Devel 32: 319–328

51. Pickering JG, Weir L, Jekanowski J, Kearney MA, Isner JM (1993) Proliferative activity in peripheral and coronary atherosclerotic plaque among patients undergoing percutaneous revascularization. J Clin Invest 91: 1469–1480

52. Plate KH, Breier G, Weich HA, Mennel HD, Risau W (1994) Vascular endothelial growth factor and glioma angiogenesis: Coordinate induction of VEGF receptors. Distribution of VEGF protein and possible in vivo regulatory mechanisms. Int J Cancer 59: 520–529

53. Plouet J, Schilling J, Gospodarowicz D (1989) Isolation and characterization of a newly identified endothelial cell mitogen produced by AtT-20 cells. EMBO J 8: 3801–3806

54. Pu LQ, Jackson S, Lachapelle KJ, Arekat Z, Graham AM, Lisbona R, Brassard R, Carpenter S, Symes JF (1994) A persistent hindlimb ischemia model in the rabbit. J Invest Surg 7: 49–60

55. Pu LQ, Sniderman AD, Brassard R, Lachapelle KJ, Graham AM, Lisbona R, Symes JF (1993) Enhanced revascularization of the ischemic limb by means of angiogenic therapy. Circulation 88: 208–215

56. Riessen R, Rahimizadeh H, Blessing E, Takeshita S, Barry JJ, Isner JM (1993) Arterial gene transfer using pure DNA applied directly to a hydrogel-coated angioplasty balloon. Hum Gene Ther 4: 749–758

57. Ross R (1993) The pathogenesis of atherosclerosis: a perspective for the 1990s. Nature 362: 801–805

58. Takeshita S, Isshiki T, Sato T (1996) Increased expression of direct gene transfer into skeletal muscles observed after acute ischemic injury in rats. Lab Invest 74: 1061–1065

59. Takeshita S, Rossow ST, Kearney M, Zheng LP, Bauters C, Bunting S, Ferrara N, Symes JF, Isner JM (1995) Time course of increased cellular proliferation in collateral arteries following administration of vascular endothelial growth factor in a rabbit model of lower limb vascular insufficiency. Am J Pathol 147: 1649–1660

60. Takeshita S, Losordo DW, Kearney M, Isner JM (1994) Time course of recombinant protein secretion following liposome-mediated gene transfer in a rabbit arterial organ culture model. Lab Invest 71: 387–391

61. Takeshita S, Tsurumi Y, Couffinhal T, Asahara T, Bauters C, Symes JF, Ferrara N, Isner JM (1996) Gene transfer of naked DNA encoding for three isoforms of vascular endothelial growth factor stimulates collateral development in vivo. Lab Invest 75: 487–502

62. Takeshita S, Zheng LP, Asahara T, Pu L-Q, Ferrara N, Symes JF, Isner JM (1993) Therapeutic angiogenesis: A single intra-arterial bolus of vascular endothelial growth factor augments collateral vessel formation in a rabbit ischemic hindlimb. Circulation 88: I-370 (Abstract)

63. Takeshita S, Zheng LP, Brogi E, Kearney M, Pu LQ, Bunting S, Ferrara N, Symes JF, Isner JM (1994) Therapeutic angiogenesis: A single intra-arterial bolus of vascular endothelial growth factor augments revascularization in a rabbit ischemic hindlimb model. J Clin Invest 93: 662–670

64. Tang DJ, DeVit M, Johnston SA (1992) Genetic immunization is a simple method for eliciting an immune response. Nature 356: 152–154

65. Terman BI, Dougher-Vermazen M, Carrion ME, Dimitrov D, Armellino DC, Gospodarowicz D, Bohlen P (1992) Identification of the KDR tyrosine kinase as a receptor for vascular endothelial cell growth factor. Biochem Biophys Res Commun 187: 1579–1586

66. Tischer E, Mitchell R, Hartmann T, Silva M, Gospodarowicz D, Fiddes J, Abraham J (1991) The human gene for vascular endothelial growth factor: multiple protein forms are encoded through alternative exon splicing. J Biol Chem 266: 11947–11954

67. Tsurumi Y, Takeshita S, Chen D, Kearney M, Rossow ST, Passeri J, Horowitz JR, Symes JF (1996) Direct intramuscular gene transfer of naked DNA encoding vascular endothelial growth factor augments collateral development and tissue perfusion. Circulation 94: 3281–3290

68. Ulmer JB, Donnelly JJ, Parker SE, Rhodes GH, Felgner PL, Dwarki VJ, Gramkowski SH, Deck RR, DeWitt CM, Friedman A, Hawe LA, Leander KR, Martinez D, Perry HC, Shiver JW, Montgomery DL, Liu MA (1993) Heterologous protection against influenza by injection of DNA encoding a viral protein. Science 259: 1745–1749

69. van der Zee R, Murohara T, Luo Z, Zollmann F, Passeri J, Lekutat C, Isner JM (1997) Vascular endothelial growth factor (VEGF)/vascular permeability factor (VPF) augments nitric oxide release from quiescent rabbit and human vascular endothelium. Circulation 95: 1030–1037

70. Vincent CK, Gualberto A, Patel CV, Walsh K (1993) Different regulatory sequences control creatine-kinase-M gene expression in directly injected skeletal and cardiac muscle. Mol Cel Biol 13: 1264–1272

71. Vitadello M, Schiaffino M, Picard A, Scarpa M, Schiaffino S (1994) Gene transfer in regenerating muscle. Human Gene Ther 5: 11–18
72. Walder CE, Errett CJ, Ogez J, Heinshon H, Bunting S, Lindquist P, Ferrara N, Thomas GR (1996) Vascular endothelial growth factor (VEGF) improves blood flow and function in a chronic ischemic hind limb model. J Cardiovasc Pharmacol 27: 91–98
73. Waltenberger J, Claesson-Welsh L, Siegbahn A, Shibuya M, Heldin C-H (1994) Different signal transduction properties of KDR and Flt1, two receptors for vascular endothelial growth factor. J Biol Chem 269: 26988–26995
74. Wells DJ, Goldspink G (1992) Age and sex influence expression of plasmid DNA directly injected into mouse skeletal muscle. FEBS Lett 305: 203–205
75. Wolff JA, Ludtke JJ, Acsadi G, Williams P, Jani A (1992) Long-term persistence of plasmid DNA and foreign gene expression in mouse muscle. Human Molecular Genetics 1: 363–369
76. Wolff JA, Malone RW, Williams P, Chong W, Acsadi G, Jani A, Felgner PL (1990) Direct gene transfer into mouse muscle in vivo. Science 247: 1465–1468
77. Wolff JA, Williams P, Acsadi G, Jiao S, Jani A, Chong W (1991) Conditions affecting direct gene transfer into rodent muscle in vivo. Biotechniques 11: 474–485
78. Yang Y, Nunes FA, Berencsi K, Furth EE, Gonczol E, Wilson JM (1994) Cellular immunity to viral antigens limits E1-deleted adenoviruses for gene therapy. Proc Natl Acad Sci USA 91: 4407–4411
79. Yanagisawa-Miwa A, Uchida Y, Nakamura F, Tomaru T, Kido H, Kamijo T, Sugimoto T, Kaji K, Utsuyama M, Kurashima C, Ito H (1992) Salvage of infarcted myocardium by angiogenic action of basic fibroblast growth factor. Science 257: 1401–1403

Author's address:
Jeffrey M. Isner, M.D.
St. Elizabeth's Medical Center
736 Cambrige St.
Boston, MA 02135, USA
E-mail: VeJeff@aol.com

Genetic engineering for human bypass vein grafts

M. J. Mann

Brigham and Women's Hospital/Harvard Medical School, Boston, MA, USA

Abstract

Practical genetic therapies require both an adequate understanding of the molecular and genetic underpinnings of a disease process as well as an effective means to alter patterns of gene expression in a clinically significant manner in living tissues. One early avenue for the application of gene therapy techniques that meets these criteria is in the engineering of bypass vein grafts to resist neointimal disease, accelerated atherosclerosis and failure. Vein graft disease leads to such failures in up to 50 % of such grafts placed in the coronary and lower limb circulations, and a biologic manipulation that alters this process is, therefore, likely to significantly impact the treatment of occlusive arterial disease. The following discussion will review the fundamentals of genetic manipulation involving gene blockade, the molecular basis for vein graft failures, and a strategy for vein graft engineering now being tested in human clinical trials that is based on the blockade of cell cycle gene expression via intra-operative transfection of vein grafts with E2F decoy oligonucleotides.

An increasing understanding of the molecular biology of cardiovascular disease has made possible the design of initial approaches to treat these disorders through the manipulation of the genetic machinery that controls all cellular biology and physiology. Gene therapy can be broadly defined as any such manipulation of genes that play a role in normal or abnormal cellular function. Target genes the protein products of which play a critical role in disease onset and progression can potentially be silenced, whereas the genes for proteins that might ameliorate a disease process, if expressed at the appropriate levels in cells of the appropriate tissues, could be delivered and regulated by the gene-based clinician. Although the tools currently available for the manipulation of genetic function in intact tissues in vivo are limited by issues of safety and efficiency, a number of novel strategies have evolved that may overcome these limitations and provide early evidence of the feasibility of genetic therapy in a human clinical setting.

One such approach involves the genetic engineering of bypass vein grafts to resist occlusive failure. Bypass grafting remains a mainstay of therapy for approximately 1 million patients with ischemic disease of the heart and limbs annually. Nevertheless, failures continue to occur in up to 50 % of grafts (8), leading to recurrent morbidity and mortality and a growing number of repeat procedures. Vein graft failures have been linked to the development of neointimal hyperplasia as a part of vein graft adaptation and a subsequent aggressive form of atherosclerosis. This vein graft disease has been prevented in an experimental model via an intra-operative treatment that blocks the activation of specific genes, and a human clinical trial of this vein graft gene therapy has recently been initiated.

Gene blockade

The transfection of cells with oligonucleotides represents the most common approach for specific inhibition of target gene expression. These short chained nucleic acids can be utilized in a number of different ways to block target genes in a sequence-specific manner. Specific gene targeting may allow more precise therapeutic intervention than can be achieved with traditional drugs, as side effects relating to the common non-specific interactions of pharmacologic agents with non-target proteins can be minimized or avoided. The first oligonucleotides to be widely used for gene blockade are known as antisense oligodeoxynucleotides (ODN). These single stranded DNA molecules are generally 15–20 bases in length and bear a sequence that is complimentary in a Watson-Crick base-pairing sense to a segment of the target gene. Antisense ODN are beleived to inhibit gene expression via binding to mRNA transcripts from which translation into protein is subsequently blocked. Although a number of mechnisms have been proposed, DNA-RNA hybrid destruction by RNAse H is likely to be a primary mechanism of antisense action. Ribozymes are somewhat larger RNA molecules the sequences of which contain both a catalytic region that can cleave other RNA segments in a sequence-specific manner, and an adjacent sequence that confers the specificity of the target. A variety of ribozymes have been described that differ primarily in their three dimensional structures. Because the sequence recognition portion of ribozymes is generally limited to approximately 6 bases, these gene

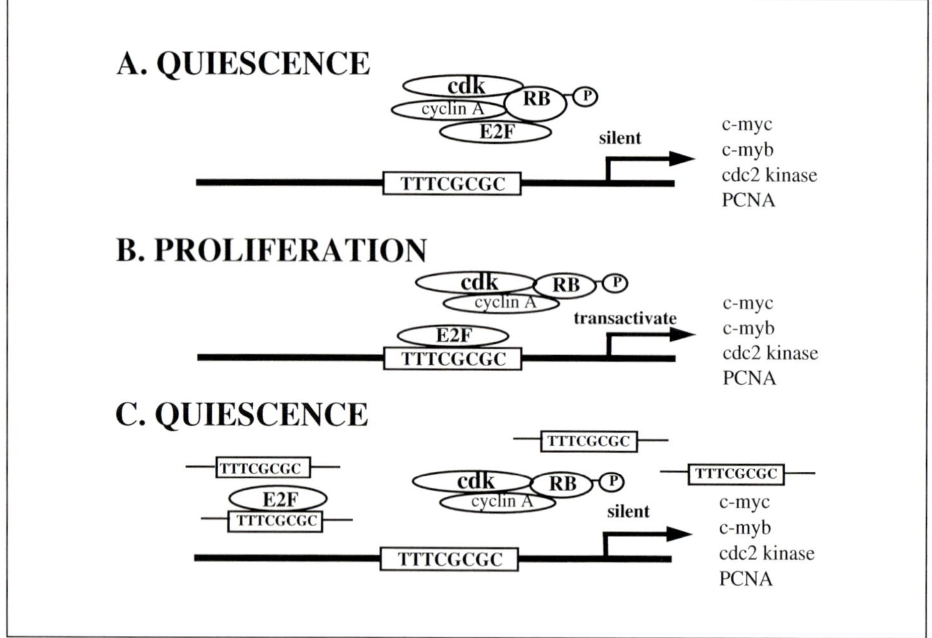

Fig. 1. The transcription factor "decoy" approach. The trascription factor E2F is bound to a regulatory complex and is inactive in quiescent cells (A). Upon activation, E2F is released and is free to interact with the consensus binding site in promoters of target genes (B). "Decoy" ODN bearing the consensus binding site compete for transcription factor binding and prevent gene transactivation (C).

inhibitory agents are generally more susceptible to non-specific interactions than their antisense counterparts.

More recently, a third oligonucleotide gene blockade strategy has emerged for use as an in vivo or ex vivo gene therapy (20). Transcription factor decoys are genrally double stranded ODN that bear a consensus binding site for a target transcription factor. When delivered to the nucleus of a target cell, the decoy oligonucleotide can bind to free transcription factor protein, and block that factor's interaction with the promoter region of the target genes under its transcriptional regulation (Fig. 1). Alternatively, decoy oligonucleotides against a negative transcription factor may act to enhance expression of an otherwise supressed gene. Decoy oligonucleotides have been used successfully in vitro and, more importantly, in cells in vivo in intact tissues to modulate gene expression in animal models. They have been used in a variety of forms, ranging from short, 10–20 base pair ODN to plasmid DNA containing multiple repeats of the consensus sequence (29). To enhance the efficacy and duration of activity of these oligonucleotides, phosphorothioate ODN that are resistant to nuclease activity have often been used.

The biology of vascular proliferative disease

Vascular proliferative disorders, including atherosclerosis, post-angioplasty restenosis, and bypass vein graft disease, are among the most common causes of morbidity and mortality in developed countries. They are characterized by an abnormal proliferation of vascular cells, particularly vascular smooth muscle cells (VSMC), which results in the formation of a lesion that can progressively encroach upon the vessel lumen, limiting and possibly threatening the conduit's capacity to carry blood flow to downstream tissues. Given the normal quiescent nature of these vascular cells in healthy vessels, the regulation of entry into and progression through the cell cycle represents a critical pathway for the pathogenesis of vascular proliferative disease. Elucidation of the elaborate molecular events involved in cell cycle regulation has revealed a pattern of upregulated expression of genes that encod cell cycle regulatory proteins at various criticial points during the cycle of DNA replication and cell division. These findings have in turn made possible therapeutic strategies of gene blockade designed to halt the activation of vascular cells and inhibit the development of proliferative lesions.

Neointimal hyperplasia refers to the growth of a new inner lining of the blood vessel, one that is comprised largely of cells that have migrated from the middle muscular layer and have undergone rapid proliferation. Vein graft occlusions have been linked to neointimal hyperplasia within the first 12–24 months after operation, and this abnormal neointimal layer is believed to provide the pathologic environment in which accelerated atherosclerosis later develops and results in graft failures after post-operative year two (2). Researchers have, therefore, looked toward the inhibition of vein graft neointimal hyperplasia as a means to significantly improve the long-term success of surgical revascularization. Aspirin and other anti-platelet therapies have succeeded in reducing the incidence of acute thrombosis in bypass grafts (9), but the vast majority of graft failures are due to fibrointimal hyperplasia and subsequent graft atherosclerosis (3). To date no pharmacologic approach has successfully influenced the development of graft neointimal hyperplasia (2). Advances in our understanding of the cellular and molecular bases of vein graft disease have, therefore, prompted the consideration of novel, gene-based approaches to prolonging graft function.

Although the molecular and cellular biology of neointimal hyperplasia have been best characterized in animal models of arterial injury such as balloon angioplasty, studies have verified a similar pattern of vascular cell biology during the adaptive remodeling of autologous vein grafts after surgery. Neointimal hyperplasia begins with the activation of medial VSMC, and their subsequent proliferation and migration across the internal elastic lamina. Numerous factors have been found to stimulate VSMC proliferation in vitro, including basic fibroblast growth factor (bFGF) and platelet derived growth factor (PDGF) (6), and these factors have been identified in the vessel wall in vivo in arterial and venous models of neointimal hyperplasia, as well (10). Increased platelet adherence and degranulation and release from injured vascular cells were initially thought to be the primary sources of PDGF and bFGF, respectively, although it is now recognized that vascular cells themselves initiate the autocrine and paracrine production of these factors after arterial injury and vein grafting (27).

Proliferation of medial VSMC proliferation peaks within the first 1–2 weeks after balloon arterial injury (23). Cell division subsequently slows, while further increases in neointimal thickness result primarily from continued extracellular matrix production. In addition to PDGF and bFGF, other factors, such as transforming growth factor β (TGFβ), angiotensin II and insulin-like growth factor-1 (IGF-1), are also expressed in the arterial wall after injury (13). An increase in VSMC DNA synthesis has also been documented during the first week after operation in experimental vein grafts (30). Zwolack and colleagues found that in rabbit jugular to carotid interposition grafts, proliferation returned to a low rate by post-operative weeks 2–4, by which time a thick, highly cellular neointimal layer had been formed. Neointimal thickening proceeded over the subsequent 4–8 weeks primarily via increased extracellular matrix production and the neointima remained stable up to 12 months, establishing a pattern of cellular kinetics parallel to those observed after rat carotid balloon injury. Francis et al. (7) succeeded in demonstrating the release of PDGF in porcine vein grafts at 1 and 4 weeks after surgery, while Hoch et al. (11) established the time course of both TGF-β1 and PDGF-A expression by rat vein graft cells and the relationship of this growth factor expression to the development of graft neointimal hyperplasia. Further studies have since documented the elaboration of cytokines such as interleukin 1-β (IL 1β), tumor necrosis factor (TNF), and monocyte chemoattractant protein 1 (MCP-1) in the vein graft wall during the first 1–4 weeks after operation; these proteins may play roles in the further "activation" of vascular cells, and may enhance the infiltration of the vessel wall by pro-inflammatory cells.

The molecular control of cellular growth and proliferation involves an elaborate system of checkpoints and regulatory events (Fig. 2). Although a number of details have been found to vary slightly in different cell types and in different species, a remarkably conserved pattern of gene upregulation and enzymatic activity has been observed during the movement of cells through the various stages of new DNA synthesis and cellular division. In this context, several classes of molecules have been described as playing well-defined roles in the management of cell cycle progression, and studies have confirmed many of these roles in VSMC in vitro.

One of the first responses of cells to stimulation by growth factors or other mitogens is the upregulated expression of a series of proto-oncogenes, also known as immediate early genes. Among these genes, *c-fos* and *c-myc* are known to be important not only for entry of cells into the cell cycle, but for successful progression through all four stages as well. The protein products of these genes act as transcription factors that increase the expression of other molecules (in particular the cyclin-depedent kinases described below) whose

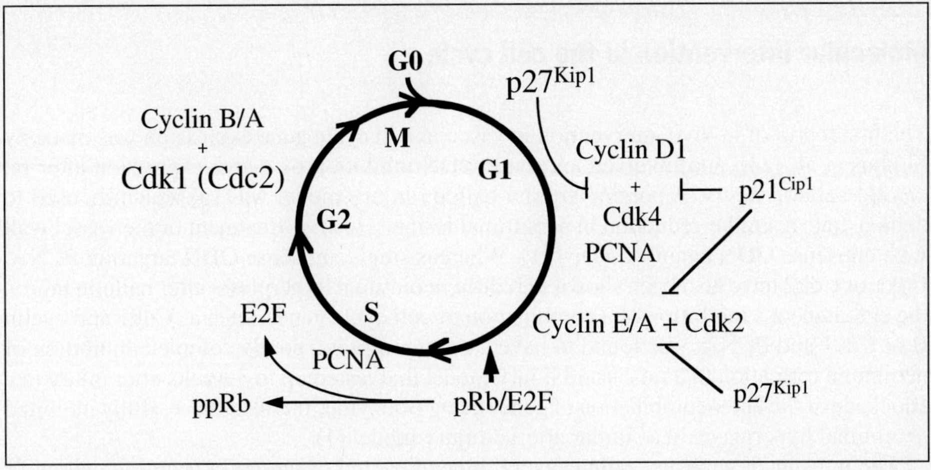

Fig. 2. The cell cycle. The upregulated expression and coordinated activation of cyclin-dependent kinases (Cdk's) is required at various points during cell cycle progression. These enzymes are regulated by inhibitory proteins such as p27 and p21. At the R point, the hypophosphorylated retinoblastoma gene product (pRb) is hyperphosphorylated by G1 Cdk's, releasing the transcription factor E2F, which in turn transactivates up to a dozen genes that encode proteins required for completion of the cell cycle.

activities are required to trigger cell cycle switches. The product of another proto-oncogene, *c-myb*, acts similarly to upregulate cell cycle proteins, whereas the *ras* gene encodes a membrane-bound, guanine nucleotide binding protein that couples signals from surface tyrosine kinase growth factor receptors to cytoplasmic secondary messenger systems (22).

The cyclin-dependent kinases (Cdk's) form another class of molecules that directly regulate the progression of cells through the cell cycle. Other proteins, termed cyclins, act as co-factors for the Cdk's, and the binding of specific cyclins to specific Cdk's leads to formation of active holoenzymes. Both cyclins and Cdk's are expressed only at low levels in quiescent cells, and are upregulated at various intervals after stimulation of the cell into cell cycle progression. Once upregulated, Cdk expression remains high as long as the cell continues to progress through rounds of the cell cycle, whereas cyclin protein levels fluctuate at different points through cell cycle progression. Early in the G1-phase, cyclin D and Cdk4 are upregulated and form a complex together with another cell cycle regulatory protein, proliferating cell nuclear antigen (PCNA). Cdk4 further requires phosphorylation by a Cdk activating kinase (CAK) to complete its activation. Cdk2, which forms a holoenzyme with cyclin E, is the other primary G1-phase Cdk, and it is responsible, along with cyclin D/Cdk4, for hyperphosphorylation of the retinoblastoma gene product Rb (19).

In quiescent cells, Rb exists in its hypophosphorylated form, pRb, and resides in a complex with cyclin A, Cdk2 and the transcription factor E2F. Hyperphosphorylation to the ppRb state results in a release of E2F-1 from this complex (28). E2F-1 then transactivates a number of other genes whose products are essential for progression through the S-, G2-, and M-phases of the cell cycle (4). These genes include proto-oncogenes such as *c-myc*, genes encoding enzymes such as dihydrofolate reductase, and those for cell cycle regulatory proteins such as Cdk2 and cyclin E. Hyperphosphorylation of Rb and activation of E2F comprises the restriction point R in the cell cycle, beyond which the cell is committed to DNA synthesis and after which the cell cycle can be completed without further stimulation from external growth factors (25).

Molecular intervention in the cell cycle

The first report of in vivo intervention in vascular cell cycle gene expression was made by Simons et al. (24), and involved antisense ODN inhibition of *c-myb* expression after rat carotid balloon injury. A porcine arterial balloon injury model was subsequently used to demonstrate a similar reduction in neointimal lesion size after treatment of the vessel wall with antisense ODN against *c-myc* (21). Whereas single antisense ODN targeting PCNA, Cdk1 or Cdk2 have also been shown to reduce neointimal hyperplasia after balloon injury, the simultaneous inhibition of a combination of cell cycle genes, such as Cdk1 and cyclin B or Cdk1 and PCNA, was found to have a more profound, nearly complete inhibition of neointima formation in a rat carotid injury model that lasted up to 8 weeks after injury (5). Blockade of the latter combination of genes using ribozymes has also successfully inhibited neointimal hyperplasia in a similar arterial injury model (1).

The transfer of genes encoding several bioengineered or naturally occuring cell cycle inhibitory proteins has also succeeded in reducing neointimal hyperplasia after arterial balloon injury. For example, neointima formation has similarly been reduced via transduction of porcine femoral arteries with a non-phosphorylatable mutant of Rb and of rat carotid arteries with a dominant negative mutant of Ras (12, 15). Cell cycle interruption via gene transfer, however, is likely to require a very high transduction efficiency to achieve a clinically significant effect on VSMC proliferation and neointimal growth, since cell cycle progression will be blocked only in transduced cells. The studies described all utilized replication-deficient, recombinant adenoviral vectors to achieve transgene delivery to the target vessels. Although these recombinant adenoviruses are the most widely studied and efficient vectors yet described in vascular tissue, transgene expression is generally limited to approximately 30–50 % of cells in an arterial wall, and only after some form of vessel wall injury. Furthermore, infection with these vectors is associated with a prominant inflammatory reaction, transient gene expression, and the hazard of possible viral mutation. Non-viral means of manipulating cell cycle gene expression may, therefore, provide a more practical opportunity at the present time for influencing vascular proliferative disease in both human arteries and vein grafts.

The synergy observed with inhibition of multiple cell cycle regulatory genes led to studies of in vivo inhibition of the transcription factor E2F using decoy ODN transfection after carotid injury (21). Fusigenic liposomes comprised of coat proteins from inactivated hemagglutinating virus of Japan (HVJ) particles and neutral lipids were used to enhance delivery of the decoy ODN. Free E2F is responsible for the transactivation of up to a dozen cell cycle regulatory proteins, including C-myc, Cdk1, and PCNA, and its blockade with the single decoy ODN proved as effective as combinations of antisense ODN directed against multiple cell cycle gene targets.

Vein graft genetic engineering

The role of neointimal hyperplasia in the pathogenesis of autologous vein graft failure is related not only to the direct encroachment of the neointima upon the vessel lumen, but also

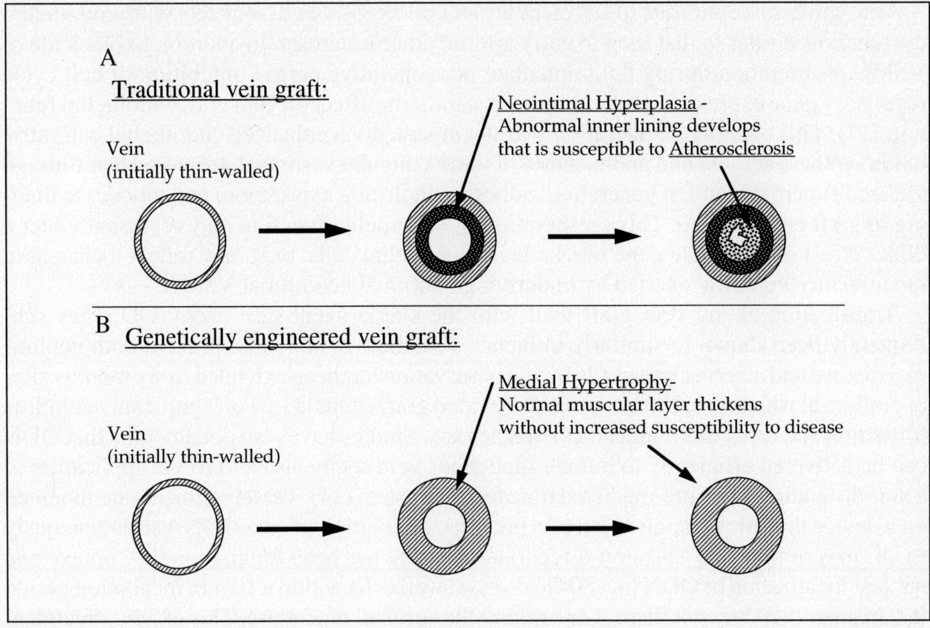

Fig. 3. A) Vein grafts remodeling involves significant neointimal hyperplasia, and subsequent wall thickening results in a return of wall stress to normal arterial levels. The neointima, however, provides a substrate for accelerated atherosclerosis that leads to graft failure. B) Inhibition of the genetic machinery necessary for VSMC proliferation prevents neointimal hyperplasia, but allows the graft to respond to the arterial circulation via medial hypertrophy.

to its role as a substrate for accelerated graft atherosclerosis. Neointima formation is a well-characerized response to multiple forms of vascular injury, ranging from gentle denudation to dessication to balloon distension. The ischemic, mechanical, and inflammatory injuries associated with vein graft harvest and implantation are, therefore, likely to provide a strong stimulus for neointima formation. It has been hypothesized that blockade of gene expression necessary for cell cycle progression can prevent the initiation of neointimal hyperplasia as a response to these multiple factors and stimuli. Furthermore, once graft healing has progressed and the stimulation from these injuries has subsided, the graft can respond to the hemodynamic impetus for wall thickening via vascular hypertrophy and medial thickening. Stabilization of vascular cell phenotype and function during the post-operative period of graft healing may, therefore, allow vein graft adaptation to the hemodynamic stresses of the arterial circulation without incurring increased susceptibility to graft disease and failure associated with neointimal hyperplasia (Fig. 3).

This hypothesis was first tested in a series of experiments utilizing the delivery of ODN to cells of rabbit jugular veins at the time of grafting into the carotid artery. A combination of antisense ODN against both Cdk1 and PCNA inhibited neointimal hyperplasia by 90 %, and this inhibition persisted for up to 10 weeks after grafting (16). By week 6, however, adaptive graft wall thickening approached levels seen in untreated grafts largely through hypertrophy of the medial layer. This thickening translated into an effective reduction in tangential wall stress. Most importantly, in the absence of significant neointimal hyperplasia, these genetically engineered grafts resisted the accelerated, diet-induced deposition of foam cells and generation of atherosclerotic plaque observed in control grafts.

Vein graft susceptibility to accelerated atherosclerosis is associated with endothelial dysfunction similar to that seen in early arterial atherosclerosis. In addition to blockade of VSMC proliferation during the immediate post-operative period, inhibition of cell cycle regulatory gene expression had a long-term stabilizing effect on vein graft endothelial function (17). This phenotypic alteration was documented via enhanced endothelial cell nitric oxide synthase activity and maintenance of normal jugular vasoreactivity, as well as through reduced superoxide anion generation, adhesion molecule expression, and monocyte binding to graft endothelium. This preservation of endothelial function may represent either a direct effect of cell cycle gene blockade in endothelial cells, or it may reflect a change in the influence normally exerted by underlying abnormal neointimal VSMC.

Transfection of the vein graft wall with the single agent E2F decoy ODN has subsequently been shown to similarly influence vein graft biology and prevent both neointimal disease and atherosclerosis (26). This observation has been extended to six months after operation, at which time E2Fdecoy ODN-treated grafts remain free of significant neointima formation and resist diet-induced atherosclerosis. Studies have also documented that ODN can be delivered efficiently to human saphenous vein segments ex vivo via application of a non-distending, pressure-mediated transfection system (14). Vessel segments are mounted on a device that allows application of a pressurized solution of naked DNA simultaneously to all sides of the vein. This non-directional pressure has been found to induce uptake and nuclear localization of ODN in > 80 % of vessel wall cells within a 10 min incubation period in a manner that does not disrupt or prolong the surgical procedure. This ex vivo treatment spares the patient systemic exposure to a significant quantity of the active DNA agent, and yields the safe and efficient DNA delivery that is anticipated to be necessary for successful application of an in vivo gene blockade strategy.

In an organ culture system both antisense and decoy ODN have inhibited target gene function in a sequence specific manner in human saphenous vein. These findings have served as the basis for initiation of a human clinical trial to test the efficacy of intra-operative vein graft engineering via E2F decoy ODN transfection in preventing infrainguinal bypass graft failures. This study represents the first attempt at integrating a gene therapy strategy into a routine cardiovascular surgical procedure, and the first definitive testing of our ability to influence cell cycle biology and its role in human vascular pathogenesis. This study is a prospective, randomized double-blind analysis of the efficacy of E2F decoy ODN transfection at preventing vein graft failure, and preliminary results from a small group of patients treated in an open label manner indicate that intra-operative treatment of vein grafts with E2F decoy ODN can, in fact, reduce levels of cell cycle regulatory gene expression in vascular cells (18).

In vivo genetic manipulation promises to greatly broaden the scope of therapeutic tools available to clinicians, particularly in their fight against disorders such as vascular proliferative disease that have remained recalcitrant to traditional pharmacologic and interventional approaches. A number of factors have made the treament of bypass vein grafts with E2f decoy ODN a unique opportunity to test an early application of this type of gene therapy strategy. The harvest of the vein allows the surgeon direct access to the target tissue in an ex vivo manner, enabling highly efficient ODN transfection in a safe and completely localized manner. Furthermore, grafting represents a precise point in time after which a well-characterized sequence of events initiates the disease process in tissue that had been relatively healthy. Such early clinical experiences should provide researchers with new insights into our ability to apply molecular science to the complex situation of human pathology and may, therefore, lay the groundwork for new inroads into the amelioration of disease in the cardiovascular system, and the body as a whole.

References

1. Chang MW, Barr E, Seltzer J, Jiang YQ, Nabel GJ, Nabel EG, Parmacek MS, Leiden JM (1995) Cytostatic gene therapy for vascular proliferative disorders with a constitutively active form of the retinoblastoma gene product. Science 267: 518–522
2. Clowes AW, Reidy MA (1991) Prevention of stenosis after vascular reconstruction: Pharmocologic control of intimal hyperplasia – A review. J Vasc Surg 13: 885–891
3. Cox JL, Chaisson DA, Gotleib AI (1991) Stranger in a strange land: The pathogenesis of saphenous vein graft stenosis. Prog Cardiovasc Dis 34: 45–68
4. Degregori J, Kowalik T, Nevins Jr (1995) Cellular targets for activation by the E2f1 transcription factor include DNA synthesis- and G1/S-regulatory genes. Mol Cell Biol 15: 4215–4224
5. Dev V, Parikh A, Ren M, Goldenberg T, Fishbein MC, Eigler N, Rossi J, Litvack F (1995) Ribozymes to cell division cycle (Cdc-2) kinase and proliferating cell nuclear antigen (Pcna) prevent intimal hyperplasia in rat carotide artery (abstract). Circ (Suppl I) 92: I-634
6. Faries PL, Marin ML, Veith FJ, Ramirez JA, Suggs WD, Parsons RE, Sanchez LA, Lyon RT (1996) Immunolocalization and temporal distribution of cytokine expression during the development of vein graft intimal hyperplasia in an experimental model. J Vasc Surg 24: 463–471
7. Francis SE, Hunter S, Holt CM, Gadsdon PA, Rogers S, Duff GW, Newby AC, Angelini GD (1994) Release of platelet-drived growth factor activity from pig venous arterial grafts. J Thor Cardiovasc Surg 108: 540–548
8. Grondin CM, Campeau L, Thornton JC, Engle JC, Cross FS, Schreiber H (1989) Coronary artery bypass grafting with saphenous vein. Circ 79: I-24–I-29
9. Goldman S, Copelan J, Moritz T, Henderson W, Zadina K, Ovitt T et al. (1989) Saphenous vein graft patency 1 year after coronary artery bypass surgery and of antiplatelet therapy. Circ 80: 1190–1197
10. Hamdan AD, Misare B, Contreras M, Logerfo FW, Quist WC (1996) Evaluation of anastomotic hyperplasia progression using the cyclin specific antibody Mib-1. Am J Surg 172: 168–170
11. Hoch Jr, Stark VK, Turnipseed W (1995) The temporal relationship between the development of vein graft intimal hyperplasia and growth factor gene expression. J Vasc Surg 22: 51–58
12. Indolfi C, Avvedimento Ev, Rapacciuolo A, Di Lorenzo E, Esposito G, Stabile E, Feliciello A, Mele E, Giuliano P, Condorelli G (1995) Inhibition of cellular Ras prevents smooth muscle cell proliferation after vascular injury in vivo. Nat Med 1: 541–545
13. Majeski MW, Lindner V, Twardzik DR, Reidy MA (1991) Production of transforming growth factor beta-1 during repair of arterial injury. J Clin Invest 88: 904–910
14. Mann MJ, Dzau VJ (1997) Gene therapy of cardiovascular disease (Excerpta Medica, Amsterdam)
15. Mann MJ, Gibbons GH, Kernoff RS, Diet FP, Tsao P, Cooke JP, Kaneda Y, Dzau VJ (1995) Genetic engineering of vein grafts resistant to atherosclerosis. Proc Natl Acad Sci USA 92: 4502–4506
16. Mann MJ, Gibbons GH, Tsao PS, Von Der Leyen HE, Buitrago R, Kernoff R, Cooke JP, Dzau VJ (1997) Cell cycle inhibition preserves endothelial function in genetically engineered vein grafts. J Clin Invest 99: 1295–1301
17. Mann MJ, Kernoff R, Dzau VJ (1997) Intra-operative transfection with E2f decoy oligonucleotide yields long term resistance to vein graft atherosclerosis. J Investigative Med 45: 224a
18. Mann MJ, Whittemore AD, Donaldson MC, Belkin MA, Orav EJ, Polak J, Dzau VJ (1997) Preliminary clinical experience with genetic engineering of human vein grafts: Evidence for target gene inhibition. Circ 96: I4
19. Morgan DO (1995) Principles of Cdk regulation. Nature 374: 131–134
20. Morishita R, Gibbons GH, Horiuchi M (1995) A novel molecular strategy using cis element "decoy" of E2f binding site inhibits smooth muscle proliferation in vivo. Proc Natl Acad Sci USA 92: 5855–5859
21. Morishita R, Gibbons GH, Kaneda Y, Dzau VJ (1994) Pharmacokinetics of antisense oligodeoxynucleotides (cyclin B1 and Cdc2 kinase) in the vessel wall in vivo: Enhanced therapeutic utility for restenosis by Hvj-liposome delivery. Gene 149: 13–19
22. Pardee AB (1989) G1 events and regulation of cell proliferation. Science 246: 603–608
23. Reidy MA, Fingerle J, Lindner V (1992) Factors controlling the development of arterial lesions after injury. Circ 86: Iii43–46
24. Simons M, Edelman ER, Dekeyser JL, Langer R, Rosenberg RD (1992) Antisense C-Myb oligonucleotides inhibit intimal arterial smooth muscle cell accumulation in vivo. Nature 359: 67–70
25. Shi Y, Fard A, Galeo A, Hutchinson HG, Vermani P, Dodge GR, Hall DJ, Shaheen F, Zalewski A (1994) Trans-catheter delivery of C-Myc antisense oligomers reduce neointimal formation in a porcine model of coronary artery balloon injury. Circ 90: 944–951
26. Von Der Leyen HE, Mann MJ, Braun-Dullaeus RC, Zhang L, Dzau VJ (1998) A pressure-mediated, non-viral method for efficient in vivo arterial transfection. Keystone Symposia on the Molecular and Cellular Biology of Gene Therapy: 67

27. Walker LN, Bowen-Pope DF, Ross R, Reidy MA (1986) Production of platelet-derived growth factor-like molecules by cultured arterial smooth muscle cells accompanies proliferation after arterial injury. Proc Natl Acad Sci USA 83: 7311–7315
28. Weinberg RA (1995) The retinoblastoma protein and cell cycle control. Cell 81: 323–330
29. Weintraub SJ, Prater C, Dean DC (1992) Retinoblastoma protein switches the E2f site from positive to negative element. Nature 358: 259–261
30. Zwolak RM, Adams MC, Clowes AW (1987) Kinetics of vein graft hyperplasia: Association with tangential stress. J Vasc Surg 5: 126–136

Author's address:
Michael J. Mann, M.D.
Brigham & Women's Hospital
Harvard Medical School
Div. of Cardiology Med.
75 Francis Street
Boston, MA 02115, USA

Molecular cardiology and the physician

S. H. Taylor

University of Leeds, England

In recent years, and particularly during the last decade, knowledge of the molecular basis of health and disease, not least that of the cardiovascular system, has undergone a quantum leap and opened up avenues of information previously unimagined. The cardiological physician is now in an era of knowledge totally different from that of his training which threatens of overwhelm his understanding and by so doing prevent him from appreciating its ultimate value to his discipline. He is left only with the forlorn hope that the deluge of information will be eventually distilled into a format that can be applied to the detection, diagnosis, and treatment of his patients' diseases. The kaleidoscope of information now available is difficult for the practising physician to comprehend. The mysterious vistas of the molecule that occasionally appear in cardiological publications reinforce his intellectual apprehension of this new and exciting field. There are a number of reasons for this default, not least of which is the failure of basic scientists to appreciate the physician's lack of understanding of the new molecular biology. The gap developing between the knowledge available and its practical application to the sick patient are compounded not only by the clinicians lack of training in this new discipline but also by the totally new language that has developed. Swynghedauw in his outstanding monograph on the subject cites 94 new words introduced in this field, the majority of which are totally foreign to the practising cardiologist (4). It takes little prescience to realise that these tribulations in understanding the new molecular biology and the related genetic controlling influences will eventually afford the cardiological physician many outstanding contributions to the care of his cardiological patients. Few advances will benefit medicine in general and cardiology in particular as will those of molecular biology. In fact it is now clear that knowledge of their molecular basis is vital for more successful prevention of cardiovascular disease syndromes and their better treatment.

The new biology encompassing the chemical basis of heredity is based on knowledge of the structure of the deoxyribonucleic acids (DNA) and the ribonucleic (RNA) molecules, their organisation, synthesis and degradation within the cell and their control of the intracellular synthesis of proteins from amino acids. The structure and function of cells are determined entirely by their chemical structure in terms of proteins. In turn, proteins comprise innumerable amino acids, all with different molecular structures. The amino acid composition of the different proteins is transmitted as a genetic code provided by the molecules of DNA present the nucleus of all cells. The DNA molecule residing in the cell nucleus consists of a series of nucleotides joined together in a linear arrangement in right handed coil (Fig. 1). Each nucleotide of the DNA molecule contains a pentose sugar, a phosphate group and a nitrogenous base of either adenine, cytosine, thymine or guanine. The sequence whereby the nitrogenous bases are joined together provides the genetic code. The DNA molecule contains specific segments in which all genetic information is stored. The genotype is translated by various changes into the phenotype specific to the vast variety

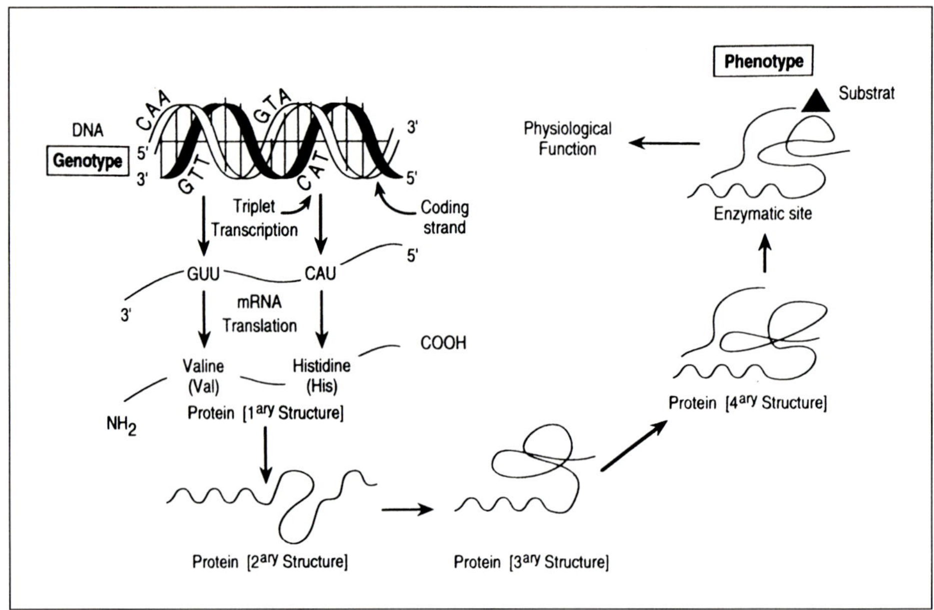

Fig. 1. Diagrammatic illustration of the translation of the DNA genotype to the tissue-specific protein of the phenotype (4).

of different cells in the different tissues (Fig. 1). For example, the genotype of a cardiac myocyte and a leukocyte are identical in the same individual but the phenotype depends on the tissue of which the cell is attached. Between the DNA genotype and its phenotype tissue expression the vital messenger RNA (mRNA) allows the cell to translate the code into the specific tissue protein (Fig. 2). Genes account for less than 10 % of the whole DNA molecule but each has the required nucleotide encoded for the synthesis of a specific protein responsible for all the functions of that particular cell. The synthesis of the proteins on which cell function depends is a complex process initiated with the transcription of double-stranded DNA to single-stranded RNA. The RNA leaves the cell nucleus to enter the cytoplasm where it facilitates the synthesis of protein from amino acids joined together in a sequence specified by the mRNA template. The joining together of specific amino acids is controlled by 3 nucleotides (a "condon"). Should even one of the nucleotides be defective, the condon will become ineffective and the synthesis of normal protein molecules from the encoded amino acids may be radically changed, constituting a mutation that may induce disease. The cell or tissue location of the mutation will determine whether disease develops and a change in just one of the 3 billion nucleotides present in the body may induce disease. If the mutation affects the germinal cells, the disease will be transmitted to the next generation and become familiar.

Knowledge of the molecular basis for the health and disease of the cardiovascular system continues to accrue at ever increasing pace. The genetic codes for proteins in the cardiovascular system have now nearly all been described and their amino acid composition and arrangement defined. However fascinating such academic knowledge, the cardiological physician is likely to be far more interested in the impact of disease on the various aspects of molecular transformation. The molecular basis of contractility of the myocardium

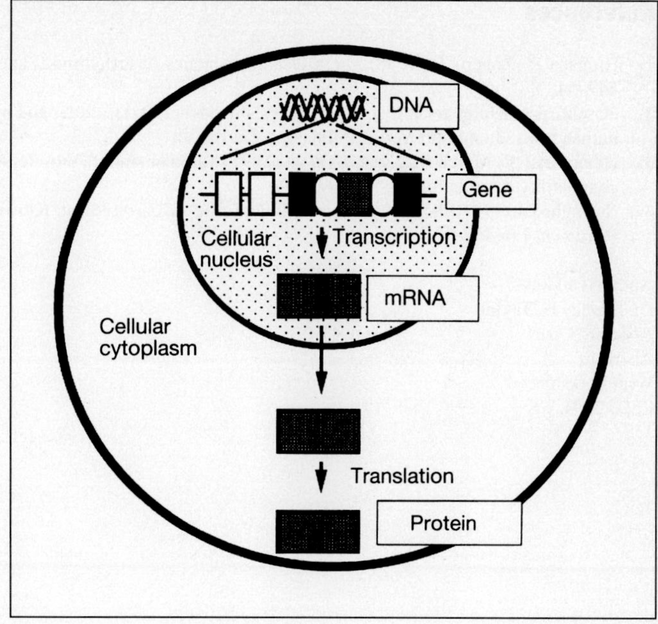

Fig. 2. The DNA molecule is distributed in 23 pairs of chromosomes. The gene is the inheritance unit and possesses all the material required for the synthesis of RNA. When relocated in the cytoplasm the RNA amino acid sequence is used as a pattern for the synthesis of the cell protein (1).

and vascular smooth muscle (3) and the molecular biology of the failing myocardium (2) are understandably of substantially more practical interest to him. Unfortunately as yet, many of the new findings in this field remain to be translated into methods the cardiologist can apply to improve his diagnostic abilities and enhance his therapeutic understanding. Whilst it is now possible to provide a molecular explanation for most cardiovascular disease syndromes, their prevention and treatment have yet to be benefited by such knowledge.

The changes in genetic expression that occur as a result of cardiovascular disease contrast starkly with abnormalities resulting from primary gene defects. Genetic diseases arise from changes in the gene structure of the parents that are transmitted to the offspring. Their detection in the former awaits further clarification and it is only when this hiatus is bridged that earlier detection, diagnosis and treatment will be available.

How far have these many new exciting developments achieved an improvement in cardiovascular therapeutics? Undoubtedly the new molecular biology has opened up the vista if not yet the practice of many new therapeutic avenues. It allows consideration of how new drugs may de developed to alter beneficially the molecular adaptations that are the biochemical hallmarks of disease. It will probably be some considerable time before gene therapy is available to the cardiologist. Fortunately this offers him the intellectual "breathing space" during which he may familiarise himself with the fundamental features of this vital new science and ready himself to assimilate the advances in the detection, diagnosis and therapy of cardiovascular diseases that are certainly on the horizon.

References

1. Brugada R, Roberts R (1998) The molecular genetics of arrhythmias and sudden death. Clin Cardiol 21: 547–54
2. Hasenfuss G, Holubarsch C, Just H, Alpert NR (eds) (1992) Cellular and molecular alterations in the failing human heart. Steinkopff Verlag Publishers; Darmstadt
3. Hathaway DR, March KL, Lash JA et al. (1991) Vascular smooth muscle. A review of the molecular basis of contractility. Circulation 83: 382–97
4. Swynghedauw B (1995) Molecular cardiology for the cardiologist. Kluwer Academic Publishers; Boston/ Dordrecht/London

Author's address:
Dr. Stanley H. Taylor
Aberford Court
Aberford
West Yorkshire
LS25 3AH, UK